The Natural History of Alcoholism Revisited

The Natural History of Alcoholism Revisited

∼ George E. Vaillant

HARVARD UNIVERSITY PRESS

Cambridge, Massachusetts
London, England
1995

LIBRARY OF CONGRESS CATALOGING-IN-PUBLICATION DATA

Vaillant, George E., 1934–
    The natural history of alcoholism revisited / George E. Vaillant.
        p.   cm.
    Contains entire text of the 1983 publication, The natural history of alcoholism, plus new
sections updating the research.
    Includes bibliographical references and index.
    ISBN 0-674-60377-X (cloth : alk. paper). — ISBN 0-674-60378-8 (pbk. : alk. paper)
    1. Alcoholism.   2. Alcoholism—Longitudinal studies.
I. Vaillant, George E., 1934–   . II. Title.
    [DNLM: 1. Alcoholism.   2. Longitudinal Studies.   WM 274 V131n 1995]
RC565.V332   1995
616.86′1—dc20
DNLM/DLC
for Library of Congress   94-41749

For Emery, John, Henry, Anne, and Joanna
with much love

Acknowledgments

The title page of this book is misleading, for it suggests a single authorship. In truth, this book represents a vast collaborative effort that has continued for 45 years. The effort began in the late 1930s as two separate studies: a study of juvenile delinquency by Sheldon and Eleanor Glueck at Harvard Law School, and the Grant Study by Clark Heath and Arlie Bock at the Harvard University Health Services. In 1972 the two studies were brought together under the auspices of the Harvard Medical School as the Study of Adult Development. I have written this book as one member of a very large team, and I have played for the team for only a third of its 45 years. Many others can also claim authorship.

Clearly, I am most deeply indebted to the several hundred erstwhile college sophomores and Boston schoolboys who are the study's subjects. Since 1940, they have generously shared their time, their lives, and their experiences. This work is also indebted to the two independent teams of researchers who conceived, sustained, funded, and guided this longitudinal research for the first 30 years of its existence. The mere listing of names grossly understates the enormous devotion and painstaking hard work required to follow more than 600 individuals for 40 years.

Sheldon Glueck and Eleanor Glueck were responsible for the creation of the Core City sample, as a control group for their classic text, *Unravelling Juvenile Delinquency.* In their work many helped them—especially Mildred

Cunningham, Mary Moran, Ernest Schachtel, John Burke, Sheila Murphrey, and George McGrath.

With philanthropic help and imaginative interest from William T. Grant, Arlie Bock and Clark Heath were responsible for the creation of the Grant Study of Adult Development (the College sample). Among the many who helped them were Frederic Wells, Carl Selzer, and especially Lewise Gregory Davies, who is the only still-active staff member who was there at the birth. Charles McArthur, the director of the Grant Study from 1954 to 1972, played a crucial role in the continuity of the study and in facilitating my own involvement.

In the 10 years since the Grant and the Glueck studies were consolidated into the Study of Adult Development, many individuals have played critical roles. For nine years Eva Milofsky has been the keystone to the Study's staff and has taken a major part in every facet of the Study's execution. Phyllis Remolador was invaluable at the beginning. Caroline Vaillant manifested an uncanny knack for finding "lost" subjects, and Robert Richards showed equal skill in tactfully interviewing them once they were found. Nancy Mogielnicki, Gregory Clark, Catherine Cyrus, Daniel Hobbing, Jeffrey Kopp, and Victoria Wulsin were also valued colleagues and interviewers.

I owe special thanks to my teachers, who must bear responsibility for what in this book is true. Hilma Unterberger, a gifted leader and teacher, created the Cambridge and Somerville Program for Alcoholism Rehabilitation (CASPAR) and thereby provided the educational arena in which many individuals, including Harvard Medical School faculty members like me, could correct previous miseducation about alcoholism. William Clark, the first director of CASPAR and the creator of this book's Clinic sample, has been a wonderful colleague. Over the years he has stimulated and guided my efforts to understand the disease. For 15 years, Griffith Edwards has patiently and modestly provided me with a role model for balanced scholarship in the field of addictions. Last but not least, many members of Alcholics Anonymous—especially John B. and Bunny—have taught me invaluable truths about alcholism. Over the last 10 years, I have attended about 50 AA meetings; I would recommend the same to any serious student of the disease. Perhaps no one understands alcoholism treatment as well as those who have overcome the illness in themselves.

Not only has this work had many collaborators, it has enjoyed many patrons. The first explanation that I received for the name of the Grant Study was: "Well, it took an awful lot of grants to support the study for 30 years."

If wrong in fact, the explanation was right in spirit. Among the financial benefactors who helped found the two studies on which this book is based were the William T. Grant, the Nathan Hofheimer, the Field, and the Ford Foundations; generous help was also received from the Commonwealth Fund and the National Institute of Mental Health. Since 1967 I have received funding from the William T. Grant and the Spencer Foundations, the Milton Fund, Grant AA-01372 from the National Institute of Alcohol Abuse and Alcoholism, and Grants MH–38798, MH–32885, and KO5–MHO364 from the National Institute of Mental Health. Over the years, four broad-minded department chairmen—Paul Myerson, John Mack, Lee Macht, and Miles Shore—have helped to ensure that I had time for this study. As director of the Harvard University Health Services, Warren Wacker has been my host and adviser throughout.

Writing this book would have been impossible without the stimulation and sanctuary provided by a sabbatical year in 1978–79 at the Center for Advanced Study in the Behavioral Sciences in Stanford, California. While I was the, Carol Trainor and Lynn Gale earned special thanks by making the computer a friend and not a foe.

Finally, anyone who has ever written an academic text knows that it is editors, research assistants, medical artists, and typists smarter than oneself who make such books possible and the reader's task bearable. Credit for authorship belongs to them as well as to the initial scribbler. In this regard, I render special thanks to Eric Wanner, Linda Son, and Camille Smith. Nancy Knysh, Kate Hughes, John Oberbeck-Friedlich, Liv Bjornard, and Lianne Carlin also played valuable roles.

I hope that the many others who have helped me to create this book but whose names do not appear will understand that the limiting factor is space and not gratitude.

G.E.V.
1983

～ Acknowledgments Revisited

Almost 15 years have passed since the above acknowledgments were written and *The Natural History Of Alcoholism Revisited,* like its predecessor, has benefited from the help of many people. The most important contributors to the book, of course, have been the more than 600 surviving men of the College and the Core City samples who have collaborated with the Study of

Adult Development for more than 55 years. Special gratitude is owed those men who, despite being afflicted with alcoholism, have continued to share their lives with the Study so that others might benefit.

Besides those already acknowledged in 1983, many others collaborated on this updated version of the book. Over the years, Sara Koury, Tara Mitchell, Sally Allen, Darsie Riccio, and Mimi Shields helped to keep the files current, telephoned men who did not complete questionnaires, and organized and rated the many waves of data. Leigh McCullough, Maria Naples, David Adler, Julie Goldman, and Kimberly Lee interviewed study members who had been lost for years. Charlene Drake, William Beardslee, and Stephanie Meyer served as independent raters and greatly enriched the data base. Henry Vaillant, Ilan Kutz, William Branch, and especially Paul Gerber provided independent evaluations of the men's physical health. Jo Steele, Carolyn Sherman, Paula Schnurr, and John Baron, each in a different way, helped to turn raw data into understandable science. Ludilla Biñas and Robin Western typed and shaped the text to make it fit for the printers. Many of these persons helped with more than one of the identified tasks.

Over the past fifteen years the Study of Adult Development and I have continued to receive generous support. From 1983 to 1992, Dartmouth Medical School provided me with the security of the Raymond Sobel professorship, and the National Institutes of Mental Health, of Aging, and of Alcohol Abuse and Alcoholism supported my research. As Director of the Harvard University Health Services, David Rosenthal continued to give the Study a secure institutional home. Gary Tucker and Peter Silberfarb at Dartmouth Medical School and, more recently, Jonathan Borus at Brigham and Women's Hospital supplied me with a rich and protected environment in which to work. In addition, in 1992 Charles O'Brien, director of the University of Pennsylvania Treatment Center, offered me a stimulating refuge in which to spend a sabbatical. During this time the past fifteen years of the lives of the alcohol-abusing men of the Study of Adult Development were collated and reanalyzed.

Finally, Angela von der Lippe and Camille Smith, editors at Harvard University Press, deserve my thanks for their creative guidance and help in transforming my typescript into a finished book.

G.E.V.
1995

Contents

II. Patterns of Recovery

III. Methodology

IV. Lessons for Treatment

The Natural History of
Alcoholism Revisited

$\backsim$ *The Problem*

Alcoholism is a disorder of great destructive power. Depending on how one defines alcoholism, it will afflict, at some time in their lives, between 3 and 10 percent of all Americans. In the United States alcoholism is involved in a quarter of all admissions to general hospitals, and it plays a major role in the four most common causes of death in males aged 20 to 40: suicide, accidents, homicide, and cirrhosis of the liver. The damage it causes falls not only on alcoholics themselves but on their families and friends as well—and this damage touches one American family out of three.

Such a serious and widespread problem demands to be studied, yet our lack of knowledge about alcoholism is astonishing. If to the casual bystander the disorder is obvious, some experts who have studied alcohol abuse for years doubt that any such entity as alcoholism exists. The reason is that alcoholism has an unstable, chameleon-like quality that makes it difficult to pin down at any given time.

Thus, the professional literature on alcohol abounds in controversy; and controversy, if unresolved, may add to uncertainty and actually detract from knowledge. For example, is alcoholism caused by heredity or by environment? Is it a cause or a result of mental illness? Is it a sin or a sickness? Some experts contend that calling alcoholism a disease is merely a semantic trick to counter the lingering belief that it is a vice. Others view alcoholism as an insidious disease that makes itself known with the first drink. Until we know the answers to such questions, we will be unable to devise rational ways to treat individuals with alcoholism.

But obtaining the answers is not easy. To be trusted, information should come from meticulously conducted long-term prospective studies—studies in which individuals are selected for study *before* they develop problems with

1

alcohol and then followed for many years. Hundreds of retrospective papers have been written about the genesis of alcoholism, but there are almost no prospective studies of its development in a normal population. Most of the existing studies have a cross-sectional design—a design that captures the characteristics of alcoholics at a certain point in their lives but reveals little about how they got to that point or what will happen to them thereafter. Alcoholism often lasts a lifetime, and it is hard to believe that virtually no studies have followed alcoholics for more than five years.

In the search for answers about alcoholism, longitudinal study offers many advantages. For one thing, since alcoholism is a chronic affliction, both its victims and the nature of their disability change over time. Thus, a cross-sectional view of an alcoholic's life will never adequately capture the nature of the disorder. Second, alcoholism is a malady about which there are no black and white answers, and longitudinal study is far better suited than cross-sectional study to elucidate clinical "grays." Third, unlike most habits and conditions, alcoholism has direct, as well as indirect, effects upon the central nervous system. Alcoholism affects personality and perceptions about the past so markedly that the true facts of an alcoholic's life can often be discovered only by prospective study.

The insights about alcoholism that I present in this book come from such a prospective study, the Harvard Medical School's Study of Adult Development. This project has followed 660 men from 1940 to 1980, from adolescence into late middle life. Information has been collected about many aspects of their lives, including their use of alcohol. The 660 subjects fall into two groups: 204 in the upper-middle-class College sample, chosen for study when they were sophomores at an elite college; and 456 in the less privileged Core City sample, chosen when they were inner-city boys of junior high school age. The data about these men's lives are supplemented by information from a third, very different group of subjects, the Clinic sample: 100 alcohol-dependent men and women followed for eight years after being admitted to a clinic for detoxification. Taken together, these three diverse samples yield a fund of information about alcohol use and abuse that no other published study can match.

∾ The Problem Revisited

Fifteen years have passed since the above was written and the data were collected for the earlier version of this book; 12 years have passed since the literature was reviewed to provide comment on, challenge to, and confirmation of its data. Much has changed; much has stayed the same. Rather than alter the original text, I have chosen to add data collected and literature reviewed since 1980 in new sections, under headings marked with the symbol 〜 and the word *Revisited*. (Additional brief new passages appear in occasional footnotes.) One purpose of using separate sections for new material is to underscore the relativity that time imposes upon "truth." A second purpose is to highlight the power of further long-term follow-up to add to our understanding of complex social problems.

The Seven Questions

There are at least seven controversial questions that longitudinal study of alcoholism might help to resolve: (1) Is alcoholism a symptom or a disease? (2) Does alcoholism usually get progressively worse? (3) Are alcoholics, *before* they begin to abuse alcohol, different from nonalcoholics? (4) Is abstinence a necessary goal of treatment, or can insisting on abstinence sometimes be counterproductive? (5) Is returning to safe social drinking possible for some alcoholics? (6) Does treatment alter the natural history of alcoholism? (7) How helpful is Alcoholics Anonymous in the treatment of alcoholism?

Let me pose these seven questions in greater detail. First, is alcoholism a symptom, a social problem, or a disease? As long ago as 1804 Thomas Trotter wrote unambiguously: "In medical language, I consider drunkenness, strictly speaking, to be a disease produced by a remote cause in giving birth to actions and movements in a living body that disorder the functions of health" (p. 2). Yet in 1882, in a pamphlet entitled "Drunkenness a Vice, Not a Disease," J. E. Todd wrote: "Every human soul is worth saving; but what I mean is, that if a choice is to be made, drunkards are about the last class to be taken hold of." And a century and a half after Trotter, McGoldrick (1954) could still write: "Alcoholism is no more a disease than thieving or lynching. Like these, it is the product of a distortion of outlook, a way of life bred of ignorance and frustration." Perhaps it was more from charity than conviction that the World Health Organization in 1951 decreed that "Alcoholism (or rather certain forms of it) is a disease process."

Since the WHO report, writers like Robinson (1972) have suggested that the term "alcoholism" is too vague to have meaning. Others (Roman and Trice 1968) have reviewed the multiple dangers of the medical model and the labeling of alcoholics. Some writers have even suggested that the disease label can provide alcohol abusers with a means of avoiding responsibility.

Gitlow has argued from authority: "The American Medical Association,

American Psychiatric Association, American Public Health Association, American Hospital Association, American Psychological Association, National Association of Social Workers, World Health Organization, and the American College of Physicians have now each and all officially pronounced alcoholism as a disease. The rest of us can do no less" (1973, p. 8).

Others, however, identify this kind of statement for what it is, a sociopolitical generalization (Pattison et al. 1977; Blane 1978). They remind us that in delineating the disease concept of alcoholism, Jellinek (1960) was far more cautious, and they suggest that there is no single entity which can be defined as alcoholism. Their point is that alcoholism cannot be reified but reflects a collection of various symptoms and episodic behaviors that collectively make up perhaps as many alcoholisms as there are alcohol abusers.

The debate goes on not only between individuals, but also within individuals. For example, a few years ago Hodgson and his colleagues wrote: "Whenever alcoholics are said to be characterized by a particular attribute then we can be sure some are and some are not" (1978, p. 339). The next year the same authors suggested: "the syndrome of alcohol dependence is given expression and in various ways . . . but remains nevertheless, a unitary syndrome" (1979, p. 9). In other words, alcoholism is and is not a disease.

But the debate over whether alcoholism is a disease is far more than just a semantic argument. Is alcohol abuse the cart or the horse? Is it the underlying cause or the sometime result of the patient's disordered personality, culture, or lifestyle? Our answer to this question will define our approach to treatment.

The most compelling empirical evidence against the existence of a sharp distinction between alcohol use and the disorder, alcoholism, has been Cahalan's (1970) study of a national panel of alcohol users, which suggests that drinkers cannot be divided into social drinkers and alcoholics, but that the categories of alcohol users and alcohol abusers merge with each other depending upon one's definition of abuse. Alcohol abuse is not black and white; it is gray. One of my purposes in this book, therefore, in following 600 men for four decades, is to watch individual lives unfold and to examine the different shades of gray expressed through their drinking behavior. I shall apply several different definitions of alcoholism and try to determine the circumstances under which the disease model seems legitimate.

In this context a paradox must be acknowledged. For purposes of conceptualization, I shall examine alcoholism within the medical model. But I must concede at the outset that however dexterously alcoholism may be shoehorned into a medical model, both its etiology and its treatment are largely social. Indeed, in modern medicine there may be no other instance of sociology's contributing so much to our understanding of a so-called disease. Thus, a major focus of this book will be to contrast social and medical models of alcoholism to see if they are congruent.

Related to whether alcoholism is a disease is the second unanswered question: Is alcoholism inevitably progressive? Once a regular pattern of alcohol abuse is established, once dependence, whether psychological or physiological, seems clear, does the disorder take on a life of its own? Does alcoholism, like Huntington's chorea, multiple sclerosis, and diabetes, manifest the statistical tendency to get worse without treatment? One side of the debate is set forth in Jellinek's model of phases in the drinking history of alcoholics (1952); this model represents alcoholism as an insidious, progressive disease that if not arrested ends eventually in death. This model is also a basic tenet of Alcoholics Anonymous. The other side of the debate is set forth in a paper by Drew (1968) who found that after age 50 there was a progressive decline in the number of alcoholics presenting themselves for treatment. By minimizing the contribution of death to this decline, Drew suggests that spontaneous return to normal drinking and spontaneous abstinence account for the improvement.

Because we lack longitudinal studies of both treated and untreated alcoholics, the current student of alcoholism can go no further than to agree with Cahalan (1970), who pointed out that with passage of time some alcoholics will die, some will become abstinent, some will return to social drinking, and some will be unchanged. The proportion of alcoholics following any single route is unknown. Positions taken on the progressive nature of alcoholism often depend more upon the treatment orientation of the observers than upon the adequacy of their data. Whether or not alcoholism is inevitably progressive can only be determined by following large numbers of alcoholics for long periods of time without significant attrition and without the bias that results from selecting a clinic population.

The third question about which there is sustained controversy is whether alcoholics are premorbidly different from nonalcoholics. Is their biochemistry different? Is their heredity different? Is their childhood environment different? Is their premorbid personality different? Recent years have seen most of the hypothesized biochemical differences between alcoholics and nonalcoholics put to rest (Jellinek 1960; Pattison et al. 1977; Mello and Mendelson 1978). There is no good evidence that alcoholism is caused by hypoglycemia, vitamin deficiency, disordered metabolic pathways, or "allergy" to alcohol in other than the most metaphorical sense. But the other etiological questions are not as easily answered.

In 1938 Karl Menninger could make the bold statement: "the older psychiatrists . . . considered alcoholism to be an hereditary trait. Of course, scarcely any scientist believes so today, although it's still a popular theory. Alcoholism cannot possibly be an hereditary trait, but for a father to be an alcoholic is an easy way for a son to learn *how* to effect the retaliation he later feels compelled to inflict" (p. 177). Modern evidence unseats Menninger's certainty. While it is unlikely that alcoholism represents a genetic disorder caused by a single aberrant allele, there is increasing evidence that genetic factors play a significant role (Goodwin 1976; Wolff 1972). Studies of adopted children (Goodwin 1976) suggest that alcohol abuse by the adoptee's *biological* parents plays a greater role in alcohol abuse in the adoptee than does alcohol abuse in his *environment.*

But if in recent years it has become increasingly clear that environmental patterns of alcohol abuse are relatively unimportant as a cause of alcoholism, cultural patterns of alcohol *use* are very important. The attitudes toward drinking and the socially sanctioned drinking practices surrounded by which a child learns to drink play an important role in the development of subsequent alcoholism (Jellinek 1960; Pittman and Snyder 1962; Heath 1975). Economic factors and patterns of legislation appear to be equally important (Bruun et al. 1975).

If genes and society both play a role in alcoholism, what is the effect of childhood environment? Retrospective studies (Blum 1966) speculate that childhood factors are critical to the genesis of alcoholism. The much better designed prospective studies by the Gluecks (1968), the McCords (1960), and Robins (1966) certainly suggest that childhood environment contributes to antisocial behavior; and in delinquent populations *premorbid* antisocial behavior is associated with *subsequent* alcohol abuse. However, in the past there have been no prospective studies of middle-class or nondelinquent blue-collar families that have produced enough alcoholics to answer the question: do most alcoholics or only premorbidly sociopathic alcoholics have disturbed childhoods? In the present follow-up of 600 nondelinquent adolescents with well-characterized childhoods, it should be possible to answer this question.

An equally important area of disagreement in the alcohol literature is whether the alcoholic is premorbidly mentally ill or at least premorbidly manifests a specific personality style. Jellinek wrote: "In a large proportion of alcoholics—the predominant species of alcoholism on the North American continent—prealcoholic, high psychological vulnerability is essential" (1960, p. 153). Wallerstein expressed the view that "alcoholism is a *symptomatic* expression of a deep-seated emotional difficulty" (1956, p. 228); and in a retrospective study of 161 alcoholics, Sherfey (1955) maintained that in every one of them, drinking was secondary to an abnormal psychiatric condition. Finally, as recently as 1973, in his widely used textbook on clinical psychiatry, Kolb wrote: "In spite of the conviction of most alcoholics that they would be quite normal if they ceased drinking, psychologically well-adapted personalities are seldom found during periods of sobriety" (1973, p. 205).

But opponents of this view are equally emphatic. In an often quoted review, Syme wrote: "it is rather clear that, on the basis of the evidence (all available relevant literature published from 1936 to 1956), there is no warrant for concluding that persons of one type are more likely to become alcoholics than persons of another type" (1957, p. 301). Syme did quote one MMPI (Minnesota Multiphasic Personality Inventory) study where the author wrote that the more maladjusted the individual the more need he seemed to have for alcohol as a crutch. However, in a prospective study of the MMPI, Kammeier and colleagues (1973) demonstrated that after the development of alcoholism previously normal MMPI's are distorted into the very patterns thought typical of alcoholism. In an undocumented editorial on alcoholism for the *Annals of Internal Medicine,* Enoch Gordis wrote: "Changes in personality or mood are now recognized to be largely the consequence of alcoholism, not its cause" (1976, p. 823). Obviously, if these different viewpoints are to be reconciled, prospective studies of premorbidly well-defined populations are needed.

Jellinek warns us: "the idea that presents itself to an omnivorous reader of the alcohol literature is usually that alcoholism is either an economic, a psychological, a physiological or a sociological problem to the exclusion of other aspects" (1960, p. 13). What is needed is not an argument that one or another factor is the most important cause of the development of alcoholism, but rather an effort to understand the relative etiological contributions of each variable to the total clinical picture. Only a longitudinal design allows both an individual's alcoholism and the relevant premorbid variables to be conceptualized as independent continua.

But which premorbid variables are relevant? An important strength of the long-term prospective nature of the Study of Adult Development is that it enables us to distinguish premorbid variables (such as ethnicity, strengths or weaknesses of childhood environment, boyhood competence, and parents' social class) and to determine which of them predict various adult outcomes. Both the childhood variables and the adult outcome variables other than alcoholism (such as global mental health, sociopathy, marital stability, and social class) are presented in detail, and their interrelationships are traced, in Chapter 7.

The question of which childhood variables predict alcoholism is addressed in Chapter 2. To help to resolve controversies regarding the etiology of alcoholism, in my discussion of these men from the upper middle class and from the inner city I shall attempt to match up their hereditary *and* their ethnic *and* their psychological *and* their childhood environmental backgrounds with their subsequent patterns of social drinking or alcohol abuse. In such a task prospective study is invaluable.

The fourth unanswered question in the alcoholism literature is whether abstinence should be a primary goal of treatment. If Keller is right that "if an alcoholic takes a drink, he can never be sure he will be able to stop before he loses control and starts on a bout" (1972, p. 160), then sustained remission is likely to be achieved only through abstinence. This is the view taken by the National Council on Alcoholism and by Alcoholics Anonymous.

This position, however, has been seriously challenged on the basis of a variety of evidence. First, there is a common, if undocumented, fear that by setting lifelong abstinence as a goal for treatment, alcohol clinics may drive away potential patients. Second, under monitored laboratory conditions, alcoholics are able to drink in a quite controlled fashion (Cohen et al. 1973; Merry 1966). Third, there is increasingly impressive evidence that some alcoholics can return to social drinking (Armor et al. 1978). Fourth, according to a follow-up study by Gerard and colleagues (1962), abstinent alcoholics do not necessarily function better than actively drinking alcoholics. The above evidence has led Pattison and colleagues to suggest that "abstinence may be neither a necessary nor a desirable goal in terms of drinking outcome" (1977, p. 200). Each piece of evidence against abstinence as a goal of treatment can, in turn, be criticized. Thus, without long-term, multivariate studies, we are left with no real solution to the debate. In the present investigation special attention will be paid to the effects of long-term abstinence.

The fifth question is whether it is possible for "real" alcoholics to return to social drinking. There are many researchers who see the dictum "once an alcoholic always an alcoholic" as no more than a slogan. They can point to a large number of short-term studies of alcoholics that identify a significant percentage who return to social drinking (Pattison et al. 1977). Cahalan and Room (1974) even suggest that returning to social drinking is more the rule than the exception. In contrast to researchers, the clinicians most actively involved in treating alcoholics continue to believe that "real" alcoholics can virtually never return to social drinking. As Fox put it: "'Cure' in terms of being able to get back to moderate social drinking is considered impossible by most doctors working with alcoholics, although there may be an occasional patient who can do so. Among my own approximately 3,000 patients not one has been able to achieve this, although almost every one of them has tried to" (1963, p. 117). After 20 years, Davies's (1962) study of seven alcoholics who did return to asymptomatic drinking is still quoted as a major datum to support the return-to-social-drinking hypothesis. Confronted by thousands of clients who are unable to control their drinking, clinicians are understandably unimpressed.

But, of course, once an alcoholic patient returns to social drinking, the clinician loses track. Unlike researchers, clinicians maintain contact only with problem drinkers. Understandably, Fox acknowledges that her work as a practitioner has prevented her from conducting adequate follow-up studies. Whom are we to believe, clinician or researcher? Only a long-term follow-up of a large sample of alcoholics, of clinic attenders *and* nonattenders, can convincingly demonstrate whether or not alcoholics can return to sustained social drinking. If return to social drinking is possible, then only a prospective follow-up can decide for which patients a return to social drinking can be advised.

The sixth unanswered question is, do our current modes of treatment really alter the natural history of alcoholism? And if so, what kinds of treatment are most effective? The evidence is contradictory. There is no question that in the first half of this century every new enthusiastically administered treatment of alcoholism produced promising results, but proper control groups were always lacking.

More recently, treatment effectiveness may have been exaggerated not so much by novel and pioneering spirits, but in an effort to justify to Congress and to health insurance companies their enormous expenditures in the treatment of alcoholism. According to the National Institute of Alcoholism and Alcohol Abuse, "56% of the patients who have gone through the alcoholism programs at D.C.'s St. Elizabeth Hospital have stayed sober from one to five years according to a recent survey there. The program is one of the few in the country keyed to long-term rehabilitation involving in-patient treatment averaging 6 to 8 months with some stays up to 2 years" (1972, p. 4). The Rand Report suggests that 67 percent of patients attending federally funded alcohol clinics were significantly improved at the end of 18 months (Armor et al. 1978).

Such hopeful statistics, however, are flatly contradicted by other reports. An editorial in the *Annals of Internal Medicine* announces: "The treatment of alcoholism has not improved in any important way in 25 years . . . only a minority of patients who enter treatment are helped to long-term recovery" (Gordis 1976, p. 821). The most careful, controlled treatment study done to date (Orford and Edwards 1977) is in close agreement with this editorial. Orford and Edwards suggest that commonsense advice plus the natural history of the disorder may be just as effective as adding hospitalization, family therapy, referral to AA, and Antabuse to the treatment regimen.

But Orford and Edwards's careful two-year follow-up also points out why we have such difficulty in assessing whether treatment is worthwhile. We have a very poor understanding of the natural history of alcoholism. In their fine-grained analysis of posttreatment drinking behavior, Orford and Edwards noted that, over the course of a year, even their poorest outcomes spent an average of 21 weeks abstinent and only 15 weeks drinking the equivalent of five quarts of beer or more a day. Even the wives of poor-outcome alcoholics saw their husbands' drinking as unacceptable for only 21 weeks out of 52. Such an outcome will be viewed differently by optimists and pessimists. Do we label a tumbler of water half empty or half full? Once again answers to the riddles posed by alcoholism appear relative and not absolute.

To understand a picture made up of grays, not blacks and whites, we need to stand back from the canvas. Obviously, a longitudinal study of many years' duration will clarify some of the ambiguities of the outcome of treatment for alcoholism. Indeed, the conclusion at which Orford and Edwards arrive expresses a central point of this book: "Alcoholism treatment research should increasingly embrace the closer study of natural forces which can be captured and exploited by planned therapeutic intervention" (1977, p. 3).

This brings us to the seventh unanswered question: How helpful is Alcoholics Anonymous in the treatment of alcoholism? One point of view is summarized by an old chestnut: A wise physician, asked to explain how Alcoholics Anonymous works, replies, "Alcoholics Anonymous works very well, thank you." A contrasting view is maintained by investigators who suggest that AA is useful to only a small minority (Orford and Edwards 1977; Pattison et al. 1977; Armor et al. 1978). One difficulty is that investigations of clinic populations tend to focus upon the AA failures, while AA members tend to see only the successes. Whom should we believe? Clearly a complete community sample is critical. In a naturalistically derived population of problem drinkers, what proportion of alcoholics will find help through AA and what proportion will find help through clinic treatment programs? Are there differences in the two populations? This is the final question that I try to answer in this book.

My purpose in the subsequent chapters will be to respond to the challenge that Shadwell presented to alcohol research 80 years ago: "Surely, some general lessons can be drawn from all this mass of material which would raise the question a little out of the chaotic confusion surrounding it and keep it from being so often the sport of theory, assumption, sentiment, passion, prejudice and self interest" (1902, p. 176).

In many ways in this book, by focusing on more than 600 men prospectively followed for almost 40 years, I will be treading new ground. But this type of research is well suited to answering these questions about alcoholism. As Rohan suggested: "If there is a return to studying drinking behavior itself, as it occurs, and if the way people actually drink is accurately observed, it would be possible to cut through the ideological barriers, discard unnecessary assumptions and perceive and describe the objective components of the problem. With the help of further research the factors which lead to increases or decreases in alcohol consumption may be identified and controlled. The criteria would be of value in identifying characteristic consequences of problematical drinking, and in establishing a continuum of negative consequences, rather than as serving to diagnose the explanatory fiction of 'alcoholism'" (1978, p. 217). In this book I will try to meet this challenge and identify alcoholism as a "continuum of negative consequences"—but, as we shall see in the next chapter, one end of this continuum may be best viewed as a disease.

〜 The Questions Revisited

The power of the earlier version of this book to address unanswered questions in the field of alcoholism came from its longitudinal design and the fact that it followed community samples of adolescents for 35 years. The power of this new version comes from the fact that almost all the alcohol abusers identified in the first edition have been followed for an additional 15 years, a total of

50 years in all. The new information presented here comes from continued follow-up of the men in both samples with questionnaires every two years and with physical exams every five years. Those who did not return questionnaires were interviewed by telephone every five years. During any given five-year period no more than 2–3 percent of the subjects were lost; and only 1 percent of the sample appear permanently lost. National and state death registers have been searched to identify mortality among men who either withdrew from the study or could not be located.

In this updated version, to simplify the diagnosis of alcoholism and to obtain greater statistical power in the follow-up studies, the two samples in this book have been slightly enlarged. The number of identified alcohol abusers among the 443 men in the Core City sample on whom we have adequate data was increased from 120 to 150 by the following two steps. First, I used the less stringent DSM III definition of Alcohol Abuse instead of four problems on the Problem Drinking Scale (PDS) as described in Chapter 1. This step increased the number of individuals labeled alcohol abusers from 120 to 142. Second, since the Core City men were last interviewed more than 15 years ago, 8 additional men have developed alcohol abuse, increasing the total to 150.

The number of alcohol abusers among the College sample was expanded from 26 to 52 by the following three steps. First, changing the diagnostic criteria of alcohol abuse from those of the PDS to those of DSM III increased the number of identified alcohol abusers from 26 to 35. Next, including 64 College men from the classes of 1939–1941, who had been studied identically to the 204 from the classes of 1942–1944 already included in the sample, further increased the number of alcohol abusers to 51. Third, an additional College man first met the criteria for alcohol abuse at age 65; this addition raised the total to 52.

Fifteen years later, at least three additional unanswered questions regarding alcoholism remain "the sport of theory, assumption, sentiment, passion, prejudice and self-interest"; these questions can be answered only by follow-up longer than that reported in the earlier book. First, why does the prevalence of alcohol abuse decline sharply after age 50? Is the explanation for this decline stable abstinence, return to asymptomatic drinking, high mortality, or poor case finding among the elderly?

Second, how long must abstinence or return to controlled drinking persist before an individual's recovery can be considered secure? In cancer, remission must often last five years before relapse is considered unlikely. In treatment studies, however, investigators often speak of recovery after the alcohol abuser has been symptom-free for six months or one year; two years of abstinence is considered an adequate criterion for candidacy for liver transplant. Is that long enough?

Third, why do smoking, depression, and alcohol abuse so often occur together? Each of these three conditions is associated with high mortality. Only by studying individuals for a lifetime is it possible to unravel the relative dangers and the etiological importance of each of these variables.

Continuing to follow the Core City men until age 62 and the College men until age 70 has addressed these three new questions and has also cast additional light on some of the original seven questions. For example, Chapter 3 adds to the data with which to assess the question of whether alcoholism is progressive and also addresses the question of why the prevalence of alcohol abuse declines after age 50. Over the last 15 years the number of studies following alcoholics for 10–30 years has doubled, and the number of alcohol abusers in the College and Core City samples who have died has trebled. These additions to Chapter 3 underscore that premature death and stable abstinence are the chief reasons for the "disappearance" of alcohol abuse with age.

Continued follow-up of the expanded College sample has also allowed examination of the relative roles of heavy smoking and alcohol abuse in this increased morbidity. Although modest alcohol use is good for the heart, alcohol abuse is bad for the heart. Of the 176 College and Core City alcohol abusers on whom we had recent follow-up information, 61 had died by 1992—19 from heart disease.

Chapter 4 provides a straightforward answer to the question of how many years an alcoholic must remain abstinent until recovery can be deemed secure. The chapter also reviews the last 12 years of research by others to provide further information pertaining to question 7: how helpful is Alcoholics Anonymous? Chapter 5 provides additional data with which to answer question 5: Is return to social drinking possible for some alcoholics? Another type of addition appears in Chapter 2, which takes advantage of research by others during the last 12 years to examine the relevance of the findings of this book to women.

I ～ What Is Alcoholism?

1 ～ Is Alcoholism a Unitary Disorder?

Scientists and clinicians do not always agree about the best model for conceptualizing alcohol abuse. No other habit or culturally determined behavior pattern creates more medical problems than does alcohol abuse; no other social "deviance" leads to more somatic pathology. But at the same time, there is no other so-called disease in which both etiology and cure are more profoundly dependent upon social, economic, and cultural variables.

Doctors—and clinicians generally—tend to diagnose people as being either blind or sighted, feeble-minded or of normal intelligence, alcoholic or non-alcoholic. Social scientists generally prefer to see sight, intelligence, and drinking behavior as continua. Whether a person is blind, feeble-minded, or alcoholic depends upon a host of independent cultural, motivational, interpersonal, and economic factors. Yet these are complexities for which an engrossed clinician may have little patience. Besides, when a patient comes to a clinic for help, there is often a certain crispness of definition as to what the real problem is. After all, the patient has already decided to go to expense and inconvenience to seek help for a self-acknowledged dis-ease. In contrast, when an epidemiologist or anthropologist happens upon the same individual in the community, patienthood and diagnosis are not so easily determined.

An illuminating study by Campbell and colleagues (1979) reveals that doctors share real uncertainty regarding what conditions should be called diseases. About 85 percent of general practitioners agree that alcoholism is a disease—the same proportion that regard coronary thrombosis, hypertension, and epilepsy as diseases. In contrast, only 50 percent of medical academicians would consider any of these four disorders diseases. More would view malaria and diabetes as diseases; fewer would regard gallstones and piles as diseases.

So, what is a disease? I shall use coronary artery disease and hypertension as examples to throw light on the advantages and limitations of regarding alcoholism as a medical disorder—a disease. Twenty years ago, coronary heart *disease* was regarded by most clinicians as a unitary diagnosis with a relatively clear etiology: atherosclerosis. Since then, compelling research on Type A and B personalities, on smoking and exercise habits, on life stress, on cross-cultural variables, and on interpersonal variables have all pointed in one direction. The etiology of coronary heart disease is best conceived as a result of psychosocial instability and of bad habits engendered by modern Western society. Atherosclerosis is no more the "cause" of coronary heart disease than cirrhosis of the liver is the cause of alcoholism. As Marmot and Syme explain it:

> Among men of Japanese ancestry, there is a gradient in the occurrence of coronary heart disease (CHD). It is lowest in Japan, intermediate in Hawaii, and highest in California. This gradient appears *not* to be completely explained by differences in dietary intake, serum cholesterol, blood pressure or smoking. To test the hypothesis that social and cultural differences may account for the CHD differences between Japan and the United States, 3809 Japanese-Americans in California were classified according to the degree to which they retained a traditional Japanese culture. The most traditional group of Japanese-Americans had a CHD prevalence as low as that observed in Japan. The group that was most acculturated to Western culture had a three- to five-fold excess in CHD prevalence. This difference in CHD rate between most and least acculturated groups could not be accounted for by differences in the major coronary risk factors. (1976, p. 225)

Simultaneously, modern doctors have learned to confess greater uncertainty about the diagnosis of coronary heart disease. Thus "typical angina" in a young person with modest ST segment depression (that is, pathology) in his electrocardiogram reveals only a 50 percent likelihood of coronary artery disease. Reviewing these findings, Diamond and Forrester write: "the diagnosis of coronary artery disease has become increasingly complex. Many different results, obtained from tests with substantial imperfections, must be integrated into a diagnostic conclusion about the probability of disease in a given patient" (1979, p. 1350). How much that sounds like recent reviews of the disease concept of alcoholism.

Effective treatment of early coronary heart "disease" probably depends far more upon changing bad habits than upon receiving medical treatment

(Farquhar 1978). Thus, in our conceptualization of the treatment and pre-vention of coronary heart disease, the medical model deserves no more than a modest place. But although other models are also helpful, the medical model does add to, rather subtract from, our overall understanding of coronary heart disease. I believe the same holds true for the medical model of alcoholism.

The manifold dangers of a medical model for alcoholism have been sum-marized by Armor and colleagues (1978). First, alcohol abuse is a habit under considerable volitional control and conforms to no Koch's postulates. Second, although there is compelling evidence that variations in alcohol consumption are distributed along a relatively smooth continuum (de Lint and Schmidt 1968), the medical model suggests that in any individual alcoholism is either present or absent. Third, to treat alcoholism as a disease is to allow it to be used both by the individual and by society to explain away or to obscure major underlying problems—poverty, mental deficiency, crime, and the like. Without attention to the latter factors, efforts at prevention, treatment, and understanding may be for naught. Fourth, to diagnose someone as alcoholic is to label that someone in a way that can cause damage both to self-esteem and to public acceptance. Fifth, if alcoholism is merely a symptom of under-lying personality disorder, it should not be considered a disease. Is not alcoholism just a bad habit?

Let me try to refute these objections to the medical model. First, it may be true that alcoholism conforms to no Koch's postulates and there is no known underlying biological defect. Rather, alcohol abuse reflects a multi-determined continuum of drinking behaviors whose determinants are differ-ently weighted for different people and include culture, habits, social mores, and genes. But the same can be said of hypertension.

The point of using the term *disease* is simply to underscore that once an individual has lost the capacity consistently to control how much and how often he drinks, then continued use of alcohol can be both a necessary and a sufficient cause of the syndrome that we label alcoholism. Like an automo-bile driver who chooses to drive rapidly down a busy highway in a car with defective brakes and ends up spending two years in an orthopedic rehabili-tation clinic, the alcoholic may consciously have made some early decisions related to his eventual disorder. But such conscious choice becomes less and less important with the passage of time.

Like essential hypertension, alcoholism has no known specific etiology, but both conditions are a cause of resulting somatic pathology. Hypertension lies on a physiological continuum which defies precise definition and which varies according to procedures for measurement and according to psychological circumstances. Hypertension, like alcoholism, is powerfully affected by social factors and has become epidemic among young urban black males. In other words, there are multiple factors that lead to alcohol dependence, as to hypertension. The point at which one chooses to intervene in the chain of a disease sequence is often the one that governs how we label the disorder.

The second objection to using the medical model to conceptualize alcoholism is that there is no clear line that separates the alcoholic from the heavy drinker. One supposedly either has a disease or does not have it; diagnosis should depend upon signs and symptoms, not upon value judgment. But again, consider the example of hypertension. We regard it as a medical disease, albeit one of diverse and often poorly understood etiologies. There is no fixed point where we can decide that normal variation in blood pressure has evolved into an abnormal elevation. Rather, in the early stages, the diagnosis of hypertension is relative; and its clinical assessment is often inaccurate (Spence et al. 1978). The more numerous and severe the signs the more certain the diagnosis, but value judgment is always involved. So it is with alcoholism. Normal drinking merges imperceptibly with pathological drinking. Culture and idiosyncratic viewpoint will always determine where the line is drawn. Ultimately, the diagnosis of both hypertension and alcoholism depends upon a longitudinal perspective. In the opinion of Room (1977), who studied many borderline problem drinkers diagnosed by rather inclusive criteria (Cahalan 1970), problem drinking is a very unstable diagnosis. In the opinion of most alcohol clinicians, who usually see only advanced cases, alcoholism is a diagnosis stable for a lifetime.

A third objection to the medical model is that alcoholism is often affected by so many situational and psychological factors that the disorder must often be viewed as reactive (Sugarman et al. 1965). Some people drink uncontrollably only after a serious loss or when they are in a specific situation. Again, some alcoholics, by an act of will, return to normal drinking. But these observations are equally true of hypertension, which often has an extremely important reactive component. Avoiding specific living situations and exerting willpower over salt and caloric intake are sometimes enough to cause the "disease" of hypertension to disappear. The less advanced along the hypertensive continuum the patient happens to be, the more significant will be the components of willpower and emotional crisis, and the less stable will be the diagnosis.

The fourth objection to calling alcoholism a disease is that such a decision involves both labeling and a disparagement of free will. In alcoholism, I believe neither of these processes is antitherapeutic. Some people believe that the label "alcoholic" transforms a person into an outcast akin to a leper. But, if leprosy is a disease, should a doctor who has proof that a person has leprosy keep that fact a secret lest he label the person a leper? Is not the real challenge for the doctor to continue making the diagnosis and to change society's views toward leprosy?

Some people believe that if alcoholics are taught to regard alcoholism as a disease they will use this label as an excuse to drink or as a reason why they should not be held responsible for their own recovery. But the facts are that once patients understand that they have a "disease" they become more, not less, responsible for self-care. This is why the self-help group Alcoholics Anonymous places such single-minded emphasis on the idea that alcoholism is a disease. This is also why physicians are learning the value of *early* diagnosis of hypertension. Being told that one probably has hypertension is rarely a desired occurrence, but it can provide a rational explanation for hitherto "neurotic" or irrational headaches. At the same time, the diagnosis of hypertension can show a patient *how* to assume responsibility for his or her own care. For years, alcoholics have labeled themselves wicked, weak, and reprehensible; being offered a medical explanation for their behavior does not lead to irresponsibility—just to hope and improved morale. There is an enormous difference between diagnosis and name-calling.

The fifth argument against calling alcoholism a disease is the most compelling. Uncontrolled, maladaptive ingestion of alcohol is not a disease in the sense of biological disorder; rather, alcoholism is a disorder of behavior. Thomas Szasz drives this point home with a sledgehammer: "Excessive drinking is a habit. If we choose to call bad habits 'diseases,' there is no limit to what we may define as a disease" (1972, p. 84). The argument may be legitimately made that there is no more reason to subsume alcohol abuse under the medical model than to include compulsive fingernail biting, gambling, or child molesting in textbooks of medicine.

Alcoholism does reflect deviant behavior that can be often better classified by sociologists than by physiologists; alcoholism is often better treated by psychologists skilled in behavior therapy than by physicians with all their medical armamentarium. But unlike giving up gambling or fingernail biting, giving up alcohol abuse often requires skilled medical attention during the period of acute withdrawal. Unlike gamblers and fingernail biters, most alcoholics as a result of their disorder develop secondary symptoms that do require medical care. Unlike gamblers and fingernail biters, alcoholics have a mortality rate two to four times as high as that of the average person. In order to receive the medical treatment they require, alcoholics need a label that will allow them unprejudiced admission to emergency rooms, access to medical insurance coverage, detoxification, and paid sick leave—all of which are denied to (and rarely required by) compulsive gamblers, child molesters, and nail biters.

The final argument for making a disease out of a behavior disorder is that, unlike gambling and fingernail biting, the behavior disorder known as alcoholism leads to marked mistreatment of the alcoholic's loved ones, and hence to profound guilt. Outside of residence in a concentration camp, there are very few sustained human experiences that make one the recipient of as much sadism as does being a close family member of an alcoholic. As a result, the behavior disorder model (which conveys a concept of misbehavior) generates far more denial in the guilt-ridden alcoholic than does the disease model, which implies behavior that lies outside of voluntary control.

In other words, calling alcoholism a disease, rather than a behavior disorder, is a useful device both to persuade the alcoholic to admit his alcoholism and to provide a ticket for admission into the health care system. I willingly concede, however, that alcohol dependence lies on a continuum and that in scientific terms *behavior disorder* will often be a happier semantic choice than *disease*.

In short, in our attempts to *understand* and to *study* alcoholism, it behooves us to employ the models of the social scientist and of the learning theorist. But in order to *treat* alcoholics effectively we need to invoke the model of the medical practitioner. As Jellinek warned in 1960: "The usefulness of the idea that alcoholism is a medical and public health problem depends, to a large extent, upon the recognition of social and economic factors in the etiology of all species of alcoholism" (p. 158). Sixteen years later, Mark Keller, as editor of the *Journal of Alcohol Studies,* wrote that he was comfortable that the concept of "disbehaviorism" perhaps described alcoholism better than "disease," and that quite possibly alcoholism "comes into being as an interactive effect of sufficient alcohol with constitutional, personality, psychological and social co-factors." Nevertheless, he closed his article by trumpeting: "So I shall not settle for less than—alcoholism is a disease" (1976, p. 1714).

Let me offer a more personal anecdote which underscores the same paradox. My research associate had been reviewing the lives of 100 patients who had been hospitalized eight years previous for detoxification from alcohol.

She wrote to me of her mistrust of the diagnosis, alcoholism. To illustrate her mistrust, she described one man who had been detoxified for alcohol abuse and who continued heavy drinking for six years. Neither he nor his wife acknowledged his drinking as a problem. However, in the minds of the hypercritical staff of the alcohol clinic his heavy drinking had been labeled alcoholic. Finally, in the seventh year of follow-up study, the man required a second detoxification, and the clinic staff could claim that their value system was right. "How can you call such behavior a disease," my associate wrote, "when you cannot decide if it represents a social problem or alcohol-dependent drinking?" But, then, oblivious of the contradiction, she shifted her attention from that single tree to the whole forest of the other 99 tortured lives she had been reviewing. She concluded her letter: "I don't think I ever fully realized before I did this follow-up what an absolutely devastating disease alcoholism is."

Empirical Evidence

Having argued for retaining the medical model as one means of conceptualizing alcoholism, I shall now use data from the Core City longitudinal study to define alcoholism.* Studied in cross-section, alcoholism reveals itself in so many guises and in so many stages of development that definition seems impossible. Longitudinal study simplifies but does not solve the problem of definition. For alcoholism is a continuum—and an individual's position on the continuum depends on many different factors.

The most obvious dimension is that of quantity and frequency of consumption. However, alcohol consumption per se is of little help in making the diagnosis. A yearly intake of absolute alcohol that would have represented social drinking for the vigorous, 100-kilogram Winston Churchill with his abundant stores of fat would spell medical and social disaster for a skinny epileptic woman or a 60-kilogram airline pilot with an ulcer. Individual differences mean everything. Besides, although social drinkers can often give reliable histories of how much they drink, problem drinkers are extremely

---

*The Core City sample manifested a higher rate of alcoholism than the College sample: 110 of the 456 Core City men abused alcohol at some time in their lives, as contrasted with only 26 of the 204 College men. Therefore, in this book I shall focus my analysis on the Core City sample—with reference where appropriate to the College sample. The Clinic sample will come into the discussion in Chapter 3. (The Core City and College samples and the measures used to evaluate them are described in detail in Part III, Methodology.)

inaccurate. At present the relation of alcohol intake to problem drinking is unknown beyond the rule of thumb that multiple alcohol-related problems usually do not begin until after blood alcohol levels exceed 100 mg per 100 cc of blood and/or daily intake exceeds five drinks a day.

More important, it is not how much a person drinks that matters, but what symptoms result. But if we try to measure symptoms, which symptoms should we trust? Not only is there no single symptom that defines alcoholism, but often it is not who is drinking but who is watching that defines a symptom. A drinker may worry that he has an alcohol problem because of his impotence. His wife may drag him to an alcohol clinic because he slapped her during a blackout. Once he is at the clinic, the doctor calls him an alcoholic because of his abnormal liver-function tests. Later society labels him a drunk because of a second episode of driving while intoxicated. A Bordeaux vintner who drinks a liter and a half of wine a day can seem quite normal to his French wife, but a drunkard to his Israeli son-in-law. On a Saturday evening, the members of a motorcycle gang may see their use of beer as recreational, socially acceptable, and under total voluntary control, while the residents of the town they terrorize may judge their episodic consumption as the most heinous abuse.

Indeed, the diagnosis of alcoholism depends so much upon definition that some individuals believe that all dimensions are meaningless and suggest there are as many alcoholisms as there are drinkers. One person drinks a pint of whiskey a day for a month after a broken engagement and needlessly fears irreversible alcoholism. Another person drinks two liters of wine (a greater amount of absolute alcohol than the pint of whiskey) a day for 20 years and no one worries until he is admitted to the hospital for terminal hepatic failure. A third is a housewife who on half a bottle of compulsively drunk sherry a night drives her family to distraction, but who spends her mornings and afternoons quite sober. A fourth is a college sophomore who spends Friday and Saturday nights blind drunk and is proud to vomit on the courthouse steps and spend Sunday night in jail. To address this problem of different alcoholisms Jellinek (1960) devised his system of types of alcohol abuse: alpha (symptoms and psychological but not physical dependence), beta (medical symptoms but no physical dependence), gamma (symptoms *and* physical dependence), delta (physical dependence but few or no symptoms), epsilon (binge drinking). While serving as a useful cross-sectional classification, Jellinek's scheme breaks down if studied longitudinally. Over time, patterns of alcohol abuse do not remain constant. The "epsilon" disappointed fiancé

TABLE 1.1. Different definitions of the frequency of alcohol abuse in the Core City sample (total n = 400).

Criterion	Subjects meeting criterion	
	n	%
1+ alcohol-related problems ever (Cahalan)	240	60
Alcohol abuse ever (DSM III)	131	33
Alcohol abuse ever (PDS)	110	28
Admits problem with control ever	91	23
Alcohol dependent ever (DSM III)	71	18
Alcohol abuse ever (Cahalan)	70	18
Ever diagnosed alcoholic by a clinician	44	11
Alcohol abuse at present (PDS)	43	11

may return to social drinking, the "alpha" housewife may progress to become a skid-row "gamma" alcoholic, and the unclassified college student may develop the ulcer of a "beta" alcoholic. Thus, any definition of alcoholism must include the dimensions of how much loss of control, how much physical dependence, and how irritating the drinking and to whom.

Finally, it helps to keep criteria for alcoholism simple. There have been many efforts to develop complex, well-constructed instruments to measure alcoholism. In his review monograph Jacobsen (1976) described 13. None have met with widespread acceptance.

The diagnosis of alcoholism seems terribly vague to a professor of sociology or a WHO epidemiologist (Room 1977), and estimates of the number of alcoholics in both the United States and England vary over a tenfold range from 0.8 percent to 8 percent of the adult population (Mulford and Miller 1960; Orford and Edwards 1977). Nevertheless, the diagnosis of alcoholism is frighteningly clear to a Salvation Army worker, to a victim of a score of drunken beatings, or to a thankful member of Alcoholics Anonymous.

For the present I shall adopt the solution suggested by Room (1977, p. 78) and attributed to Bruun: "One way to avoid the negative effects of the black/white thinking easily introduced by the dichotomy of alcoholics/non-alcoholics is to try to use not only one but two or three measures thereby indicating the vagueness of our definitions . . . this will force the user to discuss what is behind these measures." Table 1.1 introduces our efforts to follow this advice and to employ multiple measures. The rest of this chapter examines "what is behind these measures." Alcohol abuse is diagnosed by the variety and not by the specificity of alcohol-related problems; and different diagnostic schemes are assessed to see if the use of one definition rather than another affects the conclusions. As Table 1.1 illustrates, the frequency with which alcohol abuse was diagnosed depends upon the definition of alcoholism, the data source, and the time frame. Depending on the definition, the frequency of alcohol abuse in the Core City sample varied from 11 percent to 60 percent.

The rates of alcohol abuse among the Core City men are higher than the rates reported in most published studies; and this increased rate may be attributed to three causes. First, the sample was at high risk to develop alcohol abuse (Cahalan 1970); the sample was of lower social status, urban, male, aged 45–49, without college degrees, and either Catholic or Protestant "of no specific denomination." Second, in general, the rates reflect lifetime incidence (until age 47) rather than cross-sectional prevalence. Third, drinking behavior was assessed from different observational vantage points, a tactic that permitted fewer problem drinkers to slip through the cracks. Edwards (1973) has offered evidence that in a given year the number of "problem drinkers" in a community will be perhaps nine times greater than the number known to any agency. Thus, in only one of the definitions in Table 1.1 was it essential that the subject have come to clinic attention; that definition, of course, produced the lowest rate of problem drinking.

Table 1.1 includes the three scales used to identify alcohol abuse among the Core City men—the PDS (Vaillant 1980a), the Cahalan scale (Cahalan 1970) and the DSM III (American Psychiatric Association 1980). Throughout this book the Problem Drinking Scale (PDS) is used to define *alcohol abuse* and the DSM III scale is used to define *alcohol dependence*. The criteria for the PDS are outlined in Table 1.2. The PDS was devised to combine the emphasis on physiological dependence derived from the medical model of alcoholism and the concept of social deviance derived from the sociological model of problem drinking. Although I shall examine the validity of such a definition, the focus of this book is to study paths into and out of problem drinking, not to determine the exact prevalence of alcoholism. Thus, the cutting point on the PDS used to define alcohol abuse—four or more problems—was deliberately set low to include a relatively large proportion of problem drinkers.

Of all the 456 men in the Gluecks' original sample, 400 could be rated with confidence on all the individual items in the PDS. Core City men with no

TABLE 1.2. The problem drinking scale (PDS) compared with other scales for diagnosing alcoholism.

Problem (all items weighted equally)	Frequency in Core City sample (n = 397±3)	Presence of items on other scales[a]			
		Cahalan	MAST	Orford and Edwards	DSM III
Employer complains	11%	x	x		x
Multiple job losses	8				
Family/friends complain	34	x	x		x
Marital problems	21	x	x		x
Medical problem	19	x	x		x
Multiple medical problems	5		x		
Diagnosis by clinician	11				
Alcohol-related arrest	28	x	x		
3 + alcohol-related arrests	14				x
Single hospital, clinic, or AA visit	14		x[b]		
3+ visits to clinics	7		x		
2 + blackouts	23		x	x	x
Going on wagon	25				x
Morning tremulousness/drinking	20		x	x[b]	x[b]
Tardiness or sick leave	13		x	x	x
Admits problem with control	23	x	x		x

a. The following items were not included in the PDS but were included in other scales:
(1) Cahalan: frequent intoxication, psychological dependence, financial problems, belligerence, binge drinking.
(2) MAST: belligerence, family sought help, binge drinking.
(3) Orford and Edwards: morning nausea, hallucinations, financial problems, secret drinking.
(4) DSM III: tolerance, belligerence, binges, nonbeverage alcohol.
b. Indicates heavy weighting.

more than one problem on this scale were by definition classified as asymptomatic drinkers (n = 256). Men with four or more problems were defined as alcohol abusers (n = 110). Of the 400 men most clearly studied, the remaining 34, those with two or three problems, represented an intermediate group.

Of the 456 men in the original sample, 56 were less completely studied. Of these, there were 42 whose data sets were sufficiently complete to rate them as probable asymptomatic drinkers (n = 32) or probable alcohol abusers (n = 10). Of the remaining 14 men whose pattern of alcohol use was totally unknown, 10 had died before the age of 40, 2 had dropped out of the study, and 2 were known to be alive but could not be located.

Table 1.2 contrasts the items on the PDS with other scales defining alcoholism. The PDS ignores some of the social problems emphasized by the Cahalan scale, and it focuses less upon physiological dependence than does the Orford and Edwards trouble score (1977). In many ways, the PDS is similar to the Michigan alcohol screening test (MAST; Selzer 1971); the most important difference is that the MAST gives higher weights to theoretically more important problems. Capitalizing on a longitudinal design, the PDS was constructed to give double weighting to problems that occurred frequently.

Table 1.3 compares the frequency of the PDS items among alcohol abusers in the Core City and the College samples. The purpose of this comparison was to determine to what extent items on the PDS were class-dependent. Would the items be equally common, or uncommon, in a group of men with much greater education and with alcoholism of later onset? The Core City men were more likely to experience alcohol-related arrests, blackouts, morning drinking, and missed time from work because of alcohol. The men in the College sample were more likely to acknowledge that they had a problem controlling their alcohol use and that their wives regarded their drinking as a problem.

There were profound differences both in the social class of the two samples of men and in the methodology of identifying them as alcohol abusers (Vaillant 1980a). However, many of the most important items occurred with equal frequency in both samples. Such items included having ever received a diagnosis of alcoholism by a clinician, multiple clinic visits, and medical complications. It should be noted, however, that the lifetime incidence of alcohol abuse, as defined by four or more PDS problems, was 28 percent in the Core City sample and only 13 percent in the College sample.

The fifth definition of alcoholism listed in Table 1.1 is alcohol dependence. This is a more stringent definition of alcoholism and is defined by the American Psychiatric Association (see Appendix) in its Diagnostic and Statistical Manual (1980)—more commonly referred to as the DSM III. The term "alcohol dependence" may be considered roughly synonymous with "alcoholic addiction," "physiological dependence," and Jellinek's "gamma" alcoholic. By age 47, 18 percent of the Core City men met the DSM III criteria for alcohol dependence, and by age 55 only 5 percent of the College sample had met the same criteria. To be assigned a diagnosis of "alcohol abuse" by the DSM III an individual must show evidence of pathological alcohol use

TABLE 1.3. Percentage of alcohol abusers in the Core City and College samples exhibiting each PDS item.

PDS item	Core City sample (n = 110)	College sample (n = 26)
Employer complains	38%	31%
Multiple job losses	28	8
Family/friends complain	87	100
Marital problems	66	88
Medical problem	55	54
Multiple medical problems	19	19
Diagnosis by clinician	40	42
Alcohol-related arrest	73	19
3+ alcohol-related arrests	47	8
Single hospital, clinic, or AA visit	46	31
3+ visits to clinics	24	23
2 + blackouts	69	42
Going on the wagon	70	58
Morning tremulousness/drinking	65	42
Tardiness or sick leave	43	12
Admits problem with control	72	92

and impairment of social or occupational functioning *and* duration of a month or more. In order to receive the DSM III diagnosis of "alcohol dependence," in addition to the criteria for alcohol abuse the person must show evidence either of physical tolerance or of physiological withdrawal. It was possible to rate 399 of the Core City men by the DSM III criteria. Of these, 71 (18 percent) met the criteria for alcohol *dependence* and an additional 60 (15 percent) met the definition for alcohol *abuse*. As Table 1.1 illustrates, the DSM III definition of alcohol abuse (which encompassed 131 men) was more inclusive than the definition I use in this book—four or more symptoms on the PDS.

The sixth definition listed in Table 1.1, the Cahalan scale, constructed by sociologists, depends heavily on drinking problems identified by others: 7 of the 11 items on this scale reflect belligerence, frequent intoxication, or job, marital, social, legal, or financial problems; whereas only one item reflects alcohol dependence and only one item reflects medical problems. (The other two items are binge drinking and psychological dependence.) At first glance, this emphasis appears to exaggerate the alcohol-related difficulties experienced by younger alcohol abusers, and the scale might be expected to be

TABLE 1.4. Intercorrelation of the scales used to estimate alcohol abuse in the Core City sample.

Scale	PDS	Cahalan	DSM III	% of adult life abusing alcohol
PDS (n = 400)	—			
Cahalan (n = 399)	.91	—		
DSM III (n = 399)	.90	.87	—	
% of adult life abusing alcohol (n = 398)	.82	.77	.77	—
Alcoholism in heredity (n = 400)	.23	.28	.26	.19*

*r > .15, significant at p < .001 (Pearson product-moment correlation coefficient).

insensitive to alcohol abuse in the Core City sample men who are now over the age of 47.

Table 1.4, however, suggests such a concern to be groundless. There were 398 men in the Core City sample who received ratings on all three scales for problem drinking. Table 1.4 contrasts the intercorrelation of duration of alcohol abuse and a crude assessment of familial alcoholism in these men with the three alternative scales for quantifying alcohol abuse that have already been described. The Cahalan scale was as highly correlated with all other indices of alcohol abuse as were the PDS and the DSM III scales. Viewed from a longitudinal perspective, there may not be as many different alcoholisms as some investigators fear.

Table 1.5 compares the frequency of the alcohol-related problems that make up the Cahalan scale in the Core City sample and the frequency of these problems in Cahalan's national sample of adult American males. In comparing the two groups it must be remembered that the period of observation for Cahalan's men was three years and for the Core City men it was 35 years. Only 159 (40 percent) of the entire Core City sample had experienced no problems at all on the Cahalan scale; 70 (17 percent) of the men had experienced seven problems or more. (We used 7 symptoms out of 11 on the Cahalan scale as the arbitrary cutting point to diagnose "problem drinking.") In their own work Cahalan and co-workers also labeled men problem drinkers who had fewer than seven symptoms if the symptoms were severe (Cahalan 1970). Thus, on the basis of an average of three to four different symptoms, 15 percent of Cahalan's sample were labeled problem drinkers. Within their longer period of observation, 35 percent of the Core City men met such a definition of alcohol abuse.

TABLE 1.5. Frequency of alcohol-related problems in a national panel of adult males and in the Core City men.

Problem	Cahalan[a] (n = 751)	Core City sample[b] (n = 399)
Frequent intoxication	17%	54%
Binge drinking	3	21
Symptomatic drinking	16	30
Psychological dependence	39	39
Problems with spouse or relatives	16	39
Problems with friends or neighbors	7	11
Job problems	6	16
Problems with police or accidents	1	28
Health problems	12	21
Financial problems	9	12
Belligerence associated with drinking	12	19
Identified as a problem drinker	15[c]	17[d]
Problem score of 0	57	40
Mean number of symptoms identified in a "problem drinker"	3–4	9

a. Moderate or serious problems in previous 3 years.
b. Moderate or serious problems at any time during adult life.
c. 7+ of a maximum weighted problem score of 58.
d. 7+ of a maximum unweighted problem score of 11.

Defined by physicians, the DSM III criteria lean more heavily upon symptomatic drinking and medical complications. Thus, where the Cahalan scale described drinking largely in terms of problems to society, the DSM III perceives alcoholism largely in terms of problems to the individual. As a result, only three-quarters of the men identified by the DSM III as alcohol-dependent would be problem drinkers on the Cahalan scale (Table 1.6), and only three-quarters of the men called problem drinkers by Cahalan and two-thirds of those called alcohol abusers by the PDS would also be called alcohol-dependent by the DSM III. However, 99 percent of the men called problem drinkers by the Cahalan criteria and 96 percent called alcohol-dependent met the criteria of the PDS for alcohol abuse. Like Table 1.1, Table 1.6 illustrates that, depending on scale employed to measure abuse, different (if overlapping) groups of men become identified as alcohol abusers.

For the rest of this book, the arbitrary categories of alcohol use in Table 1.6 will be adhered to. *Asymptomatic drinking* will refer to those 240 (256 when drops and dead are included) men with one or fewer problems on the

TABLE 1.6. Agreement between categories of alcohol use and scales of alcohol abuse.

Category of alcohol use	Scales of alcohol abuse		
	PDS (4+ symptoms) (n = 110)	Cahalan (7+ symptoms) (n = 70)	DSM III (Alcohol-dependent) (n = 71)
Asymptomatic drinking (n = 240)[a]	0%	0%	0%
Alcohol abuse (n = 110)[a]	100 (110)	99 (69)	96 (68)
Alcohol dependence (n = 71)	65 (71)	76 (53)	100 (71)

a. Because 50 men (12 percent) had too many problems on the PDS to be called asymptomatic drinkers but too few to meet the criteria for alcohol abuse, the number of asymptomatic drinkers plus alcohol abusers does not add up to 400.

PDS and for whom an adequate history exists. As will be elaborated in Chapter 3, this item includes 80 virtual teetotalers. The term *alcohol abuse* will refer to the 110 (120 when drops and dead are included) men who received a score of four or more on the PDS. The term *alcohol dependence* will refer to those men who met the criteria of the DSM III. It must be stressed, however, that the diagnosis of alcoholism is relative. As these men grow older, additional men will meet the diagnosis of alcoholism. At the same time, lest the forest of consistency in the diagnosis of alcoholism be lost among the trees of inconsistency, the very high correlations among the various scales used for diagnosis (Table 1.4) must be emphasized.

Another way of measuring alcoholism was the percentage of his adult life during which a man had a drinking problem. Operationally, alcohol abuse was defined as beginning at that point in a man's life when he received his fourth point on the PDS, and to end when he had spent a full year without evidence of any problems due to alcohol use. Thus, once the criteria for alcohol abuse were met, a man was considered to be an alcohol abuser if he had continued to evidence just one or two problems a year. Obviously, this estimate is crude; but over a 30-year period even if such an estimate was off by two years it still would alter a man's percentage of lifetime problem drinking by only 7 percent.

Before analyzing the nature of alcohol abuse further, it seems germane to describe in some detail how the men's alcohol-related symptoms were identified. On the basis of the interview, each man's interviewer made tentative ratings on the PDS and the Cahalan scales and provided written documentation for each item. (The interview schedule is described in the Appendix.) To these items a second rater added additional symptoms of alcohol abuse, revealed in medical records and the men's prison and mental health records. To these also were added symptoms of alcohol abuse found in the interviews conducted when the men were 25 and 31. If there were ambiguities, a third rater read all current data. The final alcohol symptomatology scores on the Cahalan scale, the DSM III, and the PDS were by consensus. In all cases, ratings of alcohol symptomatology were made by individuals who had not seen the men's childhood records.

Although alcohol abusers cannot always tell the truth about their alcohol intake, they are more accurate regarding symptoms. The very high rates of alcohol abuse identified in this study attest to the fact that the methodology was adequate to identify at least a large percentage of symptomatic alcohol abusers. Other researchers have found that alcoholics describe their own excessive drinking practices more accurately than their relatives describe them (Guze et al. 1963; Haberman 1966). Sobell and Sobell (1975) have also documented that the symptomatic diagnosis of alcoholism can in fact be reliably made from the patient if certain rules are followed. Subjects should be without a clouded sensorium and relatively sober at the time of interview. They should be questioned by a sophisticated interviewer who asks the "right" questions, who is not in a position to threaten the alcoholic's right to drink, who obtains reasonable rapport, and who has time to conduct an adequate interview. The methodology of the present study observed these rules.

Certainly, in interviews of chronic emergency room patients, in the courtroom, and in many medically hospitalized alcoholics the criteria set forth by the Sobells are missing. It is largely for this reason that physicians perceive alcoholics as poor informants and as exhibiting so much denial. Also, there is little doubt that in the end stages of alcohol dependence, especially when there is a cognitive deficit, patterns of denial may become relatively fixed. Thus, individuals who are most symptomatic and thus most frequently seen in medical clinics may also manifest the most flagrant denial. Such individuals made up perhaps 5 percent of the Core City alcohol abusers.

However, for many Core City men who initially presented themselves as social drinkers, it became clear as the interview progressed that they had lost control over their use of alcohol. Conversely, other men appeared to be extremely heavy drinkers and yet extensive interview and longitudinal follow-up established that they were in fact asymptomatic. Two case examples are illustrative and reveal how the questions used in the structured interview served to distinguish alcohol abuse from asymptomatic drinking.

One man had said he now drank "very little" and had especially cut down his drinking during the last two months (from the perspective of this study, two months was an inconsequential period of time). Since the subject had "cut down," he reported, he now had only "a couple dozen" beers at a party and drank only five beers during the week. Before two months earlier, his pattern had been not to drink for a few days and then to consume 20 or 30 beers two or three times a week. He said he had never been on a binge, which by his definition was "drinking for five days without sleeping," but during weeks when he drank heavily, he would "have a few drinks in the morning to straighten my stomach out." He protested "It's been quite a while since this happened"—seven months before the interview. (By the criteria of the Rand Report—Armor et al. 1978—this man had returned to social drinking.)

As the interviewer systematically took the subject's history, the following pattern emerged. Both the subject's mother and his wife complained about his drinking, and therefore he tried to stay away from relatives when he drank. He used to take time off work to drink; and after drinking heavily the night before, he would come to work late. During the 1950s he had attended several AA meetings; the last of his multiple blackouts had been seven months earlier, when he had smashed up his car without being able to remember what happened. He rationalized that "except when I wake up in the morning," he never thought he had a drinking problem; he boasted that he was able to "control" his morning shakes. Thus, in spite of his initial assertion that he now was drinking "very little," he met the criteria for alcohol abuse on the PDS, the Cahalan, and the DSM III scales.

In contrast, a second man boasted that his weekly intake was "at least 60" drinks and sometimes was as high as "80." Further questioning revealed that this 200-pound man possessed great tolerance for alcohol and that he had been maintaining this pattern of drinking for 20 years. Careful questioning revealed that he consumed closer to 40 drinks a week: he would have a couple of drinks after work and a couple during bowling, and would drink Saturday evenings from eight o'clock until closing time. Review of all his records revealed no alcohol-related problems with the law, with his job, or with friends. In 1980, five years after his age 47 interview, he was observed to have a palpable liver. He had continued his previous pattern of drinking five to eight drinks daily. Thus, in 1980, he could be assigned one point on the PDS, two on the Cahalan, and by the criteria of DSM III, he was still asymptomatic.

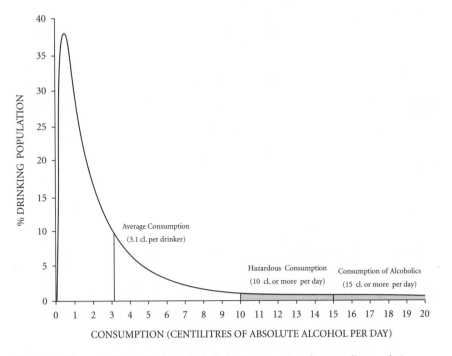

Figure 1.1 Theoretical distribution of adults in Ontario, Canada, according to their consumption of alcoholic beverages (reproduced with the permission of W. Schmidt).

What do the data reveal regarding whether alcoholism is a discrete medical problem or merely one end of a continuum of alcohol use? Our evidence suggests that both views are correct.

If alcoholism were a discrete disease with a fully independent life of its own (analogous, for example, to multiple sclerosis rather than hypertension) one might expect that individual alcohol consumption would be bimodal. Unable to control how much they drank, alcoholics should cluster at the right-hand side of a distribution curve of alcohol consumption, and they should uniformly drink more than asymptomatic social drinkers. Instead, the curve of individual alcohol consumption appears to be smooth (de Lint and Schmidt 1968). This suggests that the alcohol consumption of alcoholics blends imperceptibly with that of nonalcoholics. Figure 1.1 illustrates the so-called Ledermann curve of the distribution of alcohol consumption in the general population (Ledermann 1956). The only generalization possible is that people who are labeled alcoholic will be clustered at the right-hand side of the curve.

TABLE 1.7. Frequency of alcohol-related problems among the total sample and among those men with commonsense evidence of alcoholism.

Number of problems (Cahalan and PDS scales combined)	n^a	Admits problem with control (n = 91)	DSM III alcohol-dependent (n = 71)	Diagnosis of alcoholism (n = 43)
0	157	0%	0%	0%
1-4	83	1	0	0
5–8	48	28	4	0
9–12	38	58	34	11
13–16	28	64	57	25
17–20	21	76	91	67
21–24	12	92	100	75
25–27	9	100	100	100

a. As in previous tables, the total n is less than 400 because of slightly incomplete data sets.

However, those who believe that alcoholism is a discrete disease can reply that alcohol consumption is an unreliable gauge of alcohol abuse. Many severe alcoholics drink only episodically; many are often hospitalized or on the wagon. Thus, the alcoholic's total consumption over a year may average out to be no more than that of a heavy asymptomatic drinker. Accepting this argument, if alcoholism were really distinct from social drinking, advocates of the disease concept might still expect a bimodal curve for alcohol problems. The social drinker should have virtually no problems, and once control of alcohol is lost the number of symptoms should increase, especially over time. Thus, if the conceptual model of alcoholism as a progressive disease were correct, in a sample like the Core City sample—where all the men were older than 45—one might expect to find that men had either no problems or many problems. As Table 1.7 illustrates, this assumption proved incorrect. When the number of symptoms on the Cahalan scale and the PDS were summed, 157 men manifested no problems at all and 9 men manifested the maximum of 25–27 problems. The data in Table 1.7, however, suggest a smooth asymptotic curve—not a bimodal one. From such a perspective alcoholism truly reflects a continuum.

Table 1.7 also suggests what will become a major conclusion of this chapter, namely that the concept "alcoholism" defines a unitary syndrome and that each of the commonly accepted symptoms of alcohol abuse in Table 1.2 may be of roughly equal diagnostic import. By this I mean that it is the number and frequency of alcohol-related problems, not just their specificity, that define the clinical phenomenon known as alcoholism. On the one hand, efforts to fit all individuals who appear to be problem drinkers—to themselves or to society or to clinicians—into a single rigid definition will prove procrustean. On the other hand, available evidence suggests that alcoholism may be conceptualized as a unitary syndrome. But to be believed, such assertions must be examined in detail.

Table 1.7 illustrates that commonsense definitions of alcohol abuse—"diagnosis of alcoholism by a clinician" or "admits problem with control"—were highly correlated with the number of alcohol problems an individual manifested. Perceived loss of control of alcohol consumption appeared to be a more inclusive definition, but its occurrence practically guaranteed that an individual would display six or more *other* alcohol-related problems; physical dependence was somewhat less inclusive; and actually having been labeled an alcoholic by a clinician encompassed a group of individuals who manifested an average of 17 other alcohol-related problems.

In other words, labels can be meaningful and yet not be black or white. Intelligence lies along a continuum but we reserve the diagnosis "genius" for individuals with I.Q.'s of 140 or more. In similar fashion, men do not appear to be called alcoholic until they clearly lie at the extreme of the distribution curve for alcohol-related problems. The twin fears that the diagnosis "alcoholism" is so bound up with individual variation as to be meaningless or so bound up with societal value judgment as to be dangerous appear to be groundless. In Table 1.7 the 43 men ever labeled alcoholic by a clinician shared a common characteristic: they all exhibited at least eight (an average of 17) other alcohol-related problems.

Seeley (1959), Room (1977), and many others have questioned the legitimacy of using social disabilities to indicate a "disease" state. Their concern is that problem drinking can be viewed as possessing two dimensions: socially deviant drinking and alcohol addiction. Perhaps each dimension defines different populations. What is interesting here is that for the Core City men studied over a long period of time, these two dimensions did not actually define two different alcoholisms. As Table 1.4 suggests, the medical model of alcoholism is not more highly correlated with familial alcoholism than is the sociological model.

Because it is easier to measure alcohol-related misbehavior than it is to measure the ephemeral concepts of "loss of control" or "addiction," it becomes important to examine how well social disabilities correlate with dependence. Table 1.8 suggests that the correlation is very high. Along the left-hand side of the table are listed the six items that best define alcoholism from

TABLE 1.8. Intercorrelations of evidence of individual discomfort caused by alcohol abuse with evidence of causing discomfort to others.[a]

	Frequent intoxication	Alcohol-related arrests	Problems with job	Family or friends complain
Morning tremulousness/drinking	.46	.46	.49	.55
Problems with health	.46	.44	.53	.55
Going on the wagon	.50	.42	.47	.52
Diagnosis of alcoholism by clinician	.33	.44	.55	.54
Symptomatic drinking	.58	.54	.54	.41
Admits problem with control	.52	.45	.51	.60
DSM 111 scale	.60	.63	.68	.70

	Marital problems	Belligerence associated with alcohol	Total number of problems on Cahalan scale
Morning tremulousness/drinking	.54	.49	.70
Problems with health	.54	.48	.73
Going on the wagon	.47	.40	.66
Diagnosis of alcoholism by clinician	.53	.38	.62
Symptomatic drinking	.55	.47	.81
Admits problem with control	.54	.41	.70
DSM III scale	.69	.57	.87

a. All correlations significant at $p < .001$ (Spearman Pearson correlation coefficient). Correlations between symptoms are minimized by the fact that symptoms were coded as dichotomous variables.

the point of view of the medical model; these are individually highly correlated with the items along the top of the table, which do not specify alcohol addiction but only reflect social deviance. The net effect of these high individual intercorrelations is that the 3-point rating scale produced by the DSM III definition of physiological dependence correlates with the 11-point Cahalan scale of socially deviant drinking with an r of .87. In other words, despite their theoretical differences, physicians and sociologists are really talking about the same syndrome—each group simply focuses on individual symptoms that the other tends to ignore.

In summary, when a longitudinal view of alcoholism is substituted for the cross-sectional view, there do not appear to be many different alcoholisms. The clinicians' "disease" and the sociologists' "continuum" appear quite congruent. Certainly, the possibility must be entertained that the correlations in Table 1.8 are relevant only to American male alcoholics. Only empirical study will determine whether these same high correlations will be observed in countries like Portugal and France where many individuals physiologically dependent upon alcohol are alleged to be otherwise asymptomatic.

It probably makes sense to talk about different alcoholisms only when each is caused by different yet necessary and sufficient etiological factors. For example, there are many different pneumonias. Pneumonia secondary to cardiac failure is different from pneumococcal infection. However, the only necessary and sufficient agent in alcoholism is unwanted alcohol consumption. For treatment purposes, we may wish to accent the differences between a young male sociopath who binge drinks in New York City and an elderly matriarch who daily drinks two liters of wine in Lisbon. If these two individuals both had diabetes, we would also want to treat them differently. But as Tables 1.7 and 1.8 illustrate, the more that alcohol consumption develops a life of its own, the more it results in a common syndrome.

Statistical analysis confirms that it is the number and not the specificity of symptoms that defines alcoholism. Each of the 27 items that make up the Cahalan and the PDS inventories was evaluated for its ability to distinguish the 110 men labeled alcohol abusers from the 256 asymptotic drinkers (Table 1.9). The 34 men with intermediate scores on the PDS were excluded. In Table 1.9, the 14 items (out of a total of 27) that had the greatest discriminating power in distinguishing alcohol abusers from social drinkers are arrayed.

Among the variables not included in Table 1.9 because they did not discriminate between alcohol users and alcohol abusers was the Cahalan variable "psychological dependence." People who really drink for a reason often remain in control of their alcohol use. In other words, many moderate social drinkers reported psychological dependence, while many alcohol abusers did not. Consistent with the concept of progression, the number of years that an individual abused alcohol correlated highly with his receiving the diagnosis of alcoholism, but it did not correlate well with psychological dependence.

Four statistical techniques were employed to try to select items in Table 1.9 that would yield the fewest false positives and the fewest false negatives. The first technique was to examine percentages of asymptomatic drinkers,

TABLE 1.9. The symptoms of problem drinking that most effectively define alcoholism.

	% in diagnostic categories manifesting symptom			Rank order by different criteria		
Symptom^a	Alcohol abuse (PDS) (n = 110)	Alcohol-dependent (DSM III) (n = 68)^b	Asymptomatic drinker^c (n = 240)^b	Correlation with all 4 definitions	Stepwise discriminant analysis	Fewest errors in prediction
Symptomatic drinking^d(C)	85%	96%	4%	1	*	—
Admits problem with control (V)	72	90	1	2	6	8
Family/friends complain (V)	87	93	8	3	4	—
Morning drinking (V)	65	76	1	4	2	2
Problems with health (C)	62	78	1	5	*	6
Problems with job (C)	55	67	0	6	1	1
Blackouts (V)	69	80	3	7	—	—
Going on the wagon (V)	70	79	5	8	7	3
Diagnosis by clinician (V)	40	56	0	9	*	3
Marital problems (V)	66	71	2	10	3	10
3+ alcohol-related arrests (V)	47	61	0	—	5	4
Single hospital, clinic, or AA visit (V)	46	59	0	—	—	7
Financial problems (C)	39	49	0	—	*	5
Employer complains (V)	38	50	0	—	—	8

a. V = PDS item; C = Cahalan item.
b. Because not all 400 men had complete data sets for all 3 scales of alcohol abuse, these figures are slightly smaller than the ones in the text.
c. This group showed no more than 1 symptom on the PDS.
d. Synonymous with physical dependence.
*In top 5 in importance on one of the stepwise discriminant analyses of the split samples.

alcohol abusers, and alcohol-dependent individuals who manifested each item. Such analysis again underscores the necessity for viewing alcoholism as a continuum. When 400 inner-city men were successfully followed and studied for three decades at least a third had family or friends who believed that they misused alcohol, but only 11 percent of the men were ever diagnosed alcoholic by a clinician. Defining alcohol abuse by the complaints of family or friends captured most of the alcohol abusers at the expense of including 20 drinkers who otherwise were problem-free; defining it by having been ever diagnosed alcoholic included no false positives but missed 44 percent of those who were physiologically dependent on alcohol.

The second technique in delineating alcoholism was to rank each symptom according to the strength of its correlations with each of the four definitions of alcohol abuse in Table 1.4. This ranking appears in column 4 of Table 1.9. It is significant that symptoms that reflect the medical model and physical dependence are evenly interspersed with symptoms that reflect deviance and the social model of alcoholism.

The third technique was the use of stepwise discriminant analysis to rank the 16 PDS and the 11 Cahalan items that best separated 75 "alcoholic" men who met the criteria for problem drinking in two or more of the three scales (that is, 4+ symptoms on the PDS, 7+ symptoms on the Cahalan scale, or the criteria for alcohol dependence on the DSM III) from the 312 "non-alcoholic" men who did not. (Out of the total of 400 data sets, 13 were excluded because they contained one or more missing values.)

The problem addressed was to find the smallest subset of dichotomous variables that captured the information necessary to distinguish "alcoholic" from "nonalcoholic" subjects. We employed a stepwise discriminant analysis which enters variables one at a time into a discriminant function according to a predetermined criterion for best separating the subjects into the two groups. The criterion used was minimization of an estimate of the proportion of variance in the group (dummy) variable *not* explained by the discriminating variables under consideration (Nie et al. 1975). In the case of only two groups, this is equivalent to the procedure of maximizing the Mahalanobis distance between the groups. Once a suitable subset of variables has been chosen, the standardized discriminant function coefficients indicate the relative contributions of their associated variables. Realizing the almost certain lack of normality and difference in covariance structure of the two populations, we avoided interpretation of F values and significance levels and simply judged the value of our discriminant functioning by using it to classify our data at hand.

We carried out this analysis on 75 "alcoholics" and 312 "nonalcoholics." The first seven variables chosen are rank ordered (in decreasing order of their standardized coefficients) in column 5 of Table 1.9. The resulting classification scheme incorporates the discriminant function and also prior probabilities for group membership based on the relative group sizes.

Since we would expect a discriminant function to perform well on the subjects from which it was derived, we sought cross-validation. We split the subjects into two separate samples, and used the first sample's discriminant function to classify the second sample's subjects and vice versa. The two variable lists generated in this way shared only one variable. In other words, different subsets of variables probably define "alcoholism" equally well, and the selection of a given "best" subset is sensitive to particular interactions among variables in any given sample.

The fourth statistical technique for identifying the most powerful discriminating variables was to use the computer to select from the 27 symptoms those from which a combination of five variables could be chosen that would allow the sharpest discrimination between 75 men classified as "alcoholic" and all others. Merely selecting the five items with the highest individual correlations with the Cahalan, the DSM III, and the PDS was inadequate; many of these five variables measured the same dimension and there were interactions between variables. In practice, each of several clusters of variables that were most accurate in dichotomizing the men (96 percent correct classification) included symptoms from both the medical and the social models. For example, presence of three or more of the following five-symptom cluster: symptomatic drinking (C), problems with job (C), marital problems (V), 3+ alcohol-related arrests (V), and going on the wagon (V) allowed correct placement of 96 percent of the men. But so did two or more items from the following quite different cluster: problems with job (C), morning drinking (V), problems with health (C), financial problems (C), diagnosis of alcoholism (V). (The notations C and V indicate whether an item was taken from the Cahalan scale or the PDS respectively.)

The last column in Table 1.9 ranks individual items that alone correctly identified roughly 9 out of 10 men classified "nonalcoholic" or "alcoholic" by two or more of the scales. Once again a different rank ordering is produced.

Table 1.9 includes only 14 of the 27 symptoms on the PDS and the Cahalan scale. Certain symptoms were found by all methods of statistical assessment to be relatively poor discriminators. Psychological dependence (C) has already been mentioned as resulting in many false positives and negatives. On the

PDS, the least helpful items—multiple clinic visits, multiple problems at work, and multiple problems with health—tended to produce too many false negatives. As is well known, dependence upon the clinical features of the skid-row alcoholic will blind clinicians to many severe alcoholics. As a sociologist might predict, "frequent intoxication" (C) occurred among almost a third of the men who were otherwise asymptomatic drinkers and was a very poor discriminator. As the "disease" model might predict, the item "admits problem controlling alcohol use" (V) proved a reliable criterion (Table 1.7). In other words, multiple alcohol-related problems result not from ingesting large amounts of alcohol but from being unable consistently to control when, where, and how much alcohol is consumed. Alcoholism is a unitary syndrome but one defined by the number, not by the specificity, of alcohol-related problems.

In his critique of the National Council on Alcoholism criteria for the diagnosis of alcoholism, Rohan writes that "alcoholism exists in our language and in our minds but not in the objective world around us" (1978, p. 211); he supports this by a *Lancet* editorial (1977) which suggests that "the bulk of alcohol induced damage is in fact being experienced by non-dependent drinkers whose troubles do not resemble the medical stereotype of alcoholism" (p. 1087). The empirical data in Table 1.7 suggest otherwise. Conservatively, the average man in this study who by PDS was called an "alcohol abuser" experienced 15 to 30 times as many alcohol-related problems as the average man among the 290 men who did not abuse alcohol. The pity is still that we diagnose alcoholism too late, not too early.

Longitudinal study of a community cohort such as the Core City sample teaches an important lesson: alcoholism is a unitary syndrome best defined by the redundancy and variety of individual symptoms. It is the variety of alcohol-related problems, not any unique criterion, that captures what clinicians really mean when they label a person alcoholic, when they believe, but can never prove, that the person's use of alcohol has a "life of its own." Perhaps, as Table 1.7 suggests, the subject's own perception of loss of control and his finally receiving a clinical diagnosis of alcoholism may in fact serve as the most accurate indices of early and of late alcoholism. But even the individual's concern over control of his use of alcohol, as Clark (1976) has pointed out, is but one of many indicators of alcoholism. The failure of Table 1.9 and discriminant function analysis to improve on the simple clarity of Table 1.7 adds support to the disappointing observation that newer and more complex scales and high-powered statistical techniques have never been our allies in defining alcoholism. Jacobson (1976) reviewed four statistically sophisticated analyses of the symptoms of alcoholics, and the results are confusing. Using factor analysis, Wanberg and Horn (1970) found 11 first-order and three second-order factors; Pokorny and colleagues (1971) found one large factor and ten smaller factors; Park and Whitehead (1973) found four factors; and Hyman (1971), using latent cluster analysis, found three clusters. Since different data matrices, different populations, and somewhat different statistical techniques were used, it is not surprising that different dimensions of alcoholism were identified. But neither are such results encouraging.

Around the world, when kindergarten children play on a seesaw it is the number of children, not any special kind of children, that will be most discriminating in predicting which end will tip. So in the present study, it was the number of alcohol-related problems, not any particular cluster, that best predicted alcoholism. Likewise, it was the number of symptoms, not any particular symptoms, that best predicted two other indices suggestive of a unitary disorder: a familial history positive for alcoholism (Table 1.4) and the inability to resume asymptomatic drinking (Figure 5.1).

Medicine and sociology have much to teach each other. The etiology of many "diseases" lies outside of the simplicities and reductionism of the medical model. Good health will often be more dependent upon altering habits than upon visiting doctors. Indeed, the disease paradigm has probably slowed advances in management of diabetes, hypertension, and coronary heart disease. Had these disorders, like alcoholism, been reclassified as disorders of human behavior, greater emphasis would have been placed sooner on paramount issues of appropriate health-care delivery mechanisms, compliance monitoring, alteration of lifestyles, and the patient's motivation. Effective treatment will always gain much from undoing the simplistic thinking of the medical model.

At the same time, many of the criticisms of the medical model of alcoholism are based on naive conceptions about the specificity of the term "disease" in medicine. For one thing, in medicine the line between health and disease is always gray. In the treatment of peptic ulcer, in one individual the ulcer crater may be healed and yet the subjective symptoms remain severe; in another individual ulcer symptoms vanish but the ulcer crater will not be healed or even decreased in size (Peterson et al. 1977). Which individual shall we say has the disease?

Second, social factors are always important. For six months after the death of a spouse, mortality among widowers, especially cardiac mortality, is sharply increased (Young et al. 1963), yet we cannot regard a fatal heart attack as just a symptom of disturbed social networks.

Thus, as we shall see in the next three chapters, the etiology of alcoholism is multifactorial; morbidity is relative; and abstinence from alcohol and social recovery do not always coincide. But the fact that alcoholism is intricately woven into the individual's social fabric does not mean that alcoholism cannot also be regarded as a disease. Alcoholism becomes a disease when loss of voluntary control over alcohol consumption becomes a necessary and sufficient cause for much of an individual's social, psychological, and physical morbidity. Perhaps the best one-sentence definition of alcoholism available to us is the one provided by the National Council on Alcoholism (1976, p. 764): "The person with alcoholism cannot consistently predict on any drinking occasion the duration of the episode or the quantity that will be consumed."

As with coronary heart disease, we must learn to regard alcoholism as both disease and behavior disorder. To include any behavior disorder within the medical framework and to codify it with a unitary medical diagnosis, four criteria should be met: First, the diagnosis should imply causative factors that are independent of the presence or absence of social deviance. Alcohol addiction is often a necessary and sufficient cause for such social deviance as is observed, and alcohol dependence is significantly more likely when biologic relatives have also been alcoholic (Goodwin 1979). Second, the diagnosis should convey shorthand information about symptoms and course. As Table 1.7 illustrates, the diagnosis of alcoholism predicts that a whole constellation of symptoms are present. As Chapter 3 will illustrate, the diagnosis of alcoholism implies a disorder that lasts for several years. Third, the diagnosis should be valid cross-culturally and not dependent on mores or fashion. Certainly, alcoholism is no respecter of class, ethnicity, or historical epoch. Finally, the diagnosis should suggest appropriate medical response for treatment. Alcoholism, to the extent that it involves physical dependence, often requires detoxification in a medical setting, and, as Chapters 4 and 5 will document, specific treatment is often required in order to maintain sustained abstinence from alcohol.

2 ~ The Etiology of Alcoholism

One major intent in this chapter will be to try to determine which of the many factors to which alcoholism is attributed are of primary importance. Second, this chapter will focus attention on the fact that severe alcohol abuse may reflect a relatively unitary disorder that results from the coming together of multiple etiological risk factors. In other words, alcoholism is much more like coronary atherosclerosis—a single disorder with many interacting etiological factors—than like pneumonia—a term that encompasses multiple disorders, each of which has a fairly discrete etiology.

There is little question that unhappy children and depressed adults are at increased risk for all kinds of disease—and presumably this generalization includes alcoholism. But for the present I believe that we should relegate the same kind of role to psychological distress in the etiology of alcoholism that we relegate to bereavement or chronic depression in the etiology of atherosclerosis. Such factors exacerbate the condition and interfere with self-care, but they probably do not usually serve as primary causative agents.

Trying to specify the etiology of alcoholism is analogous to shooting a fish in the water. Because of the bending of light by the water, the fish is never where it appears to be. We can only discover where the fish really is in the water by requiring the fish to remain stationary while we experiment.

The etiology of alcoholism is equally difficult to pinpoint. The results of this chapter may defy the common sense of some readers. The experimental method reveals that the obvious etiologies of alcoholism, so patently clear to any observer, turn out to be illusory. For example, everybody knows that alcohol is used to reduce tension; thus, alcoholism must be a symptom of underlying anxiety. Clearly, alcoholism is either a self-destructive or a self-indulgent habit; hence, alcoholism should be the consequence of either a too traumatic or a too permissive childhood. Clearly, alcohol is physiologically addictive; thus, cure of alcoholism should result from a properly conducted withdrawal. Alcoholics, even when not addicted, often exhibit a desperate craving for alcohol; thus, perhaps alcoholism is a biochemical disorder, a disease like diabetes; perhaps an individual's inborn discrete metabolic defect leads to an insatiable desire for alcohol.

In the past decade, however, research workers have made important strides in demonstrating that the etiology of alcoholism resides in none of these four obvious locations. Work by Mello and Mendelson (1978) and others has demonstrated that alcohol is a poor tranquilizer. Cross-fostering studies by Goodwin (1979) and Schuckit and colleagues (1972), and prospective studies by McCord and McCord (1960) and Kammeier and colleagues (1973) have demonstrated that alcoholism is more often a cause than a result of personality disorder. The theoretical formulations of Bandura (1969) and the experimental work by investigators like Nathan and his co-workers (1970), Mello (1972), and Ludwig and Wikler (1974) have helped to demonstrate that compulsive alcoholism, like compulsive fingernail biting or gambling, is more rooted in learning theory than in pharmacological dependence per se. Finally, in the past 20 years, much of the best biochemically focused research on alcoholism has been to disprove poorly conceived prior metabolic theories, rather than to provide fresh evidence for metabolic causation of alcoholism.

In order to locate the etiology of alcoholism in the sea of speculation, we must look in less obvious places. In so doing I shall, admittedly, be holding the metaphorical fish stationary while I experiment. In other words, I shall be trying to draw conclusions from two parochial cohorts of men studied in only one historical era. Science, at best, is only an approximation of reality.

Prospective studies and critical literature reviews suggest that there are many scientifically better grounded, if less obvious, etiologies of alcoholism than the four mentioned above. In this chapter, because of the nature of the Core City sample, the importance of culture, genes, antisocial personality, and learning will be emphasized. Other factors will also be mentioned in passing, and the point most emphasized will be that the etiology of alcoholism must always be viewed as multifactorial.

Old theories die hard. Knight wrote: "Alcohol addiction is a symptom rather than a disease . . . There is always an underlying personality disorder evidenced by obvious maladjustment, neurotic character traits, emotional immaturity or infantilism" (1937, p. 234). Two decades later, Jellinek wrote:

"In spite of a great diversity in personality structure among alcoholics, there appears in a large proportion of them a low tolerance for tension coupled with an inability to cope with psychological stresses" (1960, p. 153). Two decades later still, Selzer discusses the etiology of alcoholism in the latest textbook of psychiatry: "Alcoholic populations do display significantly more depression, paranoid thinking trends, aggressive feelings and acts, and significantly lower self-esteem, responsibility and self-control than non-alcoholic populations. Despite occasional disclaimers, alcoholics do not resemble a randomly chosen population" (1980, p. 1629).

But just as light passing through water confounds our perceptions, the illness of alcoholism profoundly distorts the individual's personality, his social stability, and his own recollection of relevant childhood variables. Unfortunately, as the above quotes suggest, most etiological studies of alcoholism have ignored this distorting effect and not recognized the importance of prospective design.

Table 2.1 summarizes six previous prospective etiological studies of alcoholism. The first study cited is the most important. In 1956, the McCords undertook a very imaginative follow-up of the 325 boys in the Cambridge-Somerville study (Powers and Witmer 1959). Originally conceived as an experiment to prevent delinquency, this study was started in 1935 by a most innovative Massachusetts General Hospital physician, Richard Cabot—the same man who ten years earlier had stimulated the Gluecks' interest in delinquency. The Cambridge-Somerville study examined in a controlled fashion the effect of a five-year counseling program on antisocial grammar-school boys. The study's design had been to counsel both a control treatment group and a predelinquent treatment group. Each of the 325 youths in the treatment groups was seen at least weekly by a counselor who kept extensive progress notes. These notes and the original family investigation (undertaken to assess delinquency risk) allowed the McCords to make extensive judgments about the premorbid characteristics of these boys and their families. Fifteen years later, raters (blind to earlier judgments) obtained evidence for alcoholism from public records, clinics, probation officers, and social agencies. The "boys" were then between 30 and 35. The McCords defined an alcoholic as "one whose drinking has become a source of community or family difficulties or one who has recognized that excessive drinking is a primary problem to him" (p. 98). Operationally, this meant two or more arrests for alcoholism *or* being referred by a clinic or hospital for treatment *or* attending Alcoholics Anonymous. The McCords did not reinterview their subjects, and a disproportionate number of their alcoholics came from the predelinquent group.

TABLE 2.1. Prospective studies of the development of alcoholism.

Study	Age at follow-up	Original sample	Lost to follow-up	Alcohol abusers	Not also clearly antisocial	Proportion of alcohol abusers also dependent[a]	Recent interview	Multiple contacts over time
McCord and McCord 1960	30–35	325	70	29	11	2/3	No	No
Robins et al. 1962	c.43	367	81	78[b]	29	1/3	Yes	No
Jones 1968	36–38	106	40	6	6	?	Yes	Yes
Jones 1971	36–38	106	61	3[d]	3	?	Yes	Yes
Loper, Kammeier, and Hoffmann 1973	30–35	[c]	[c]	38	38	All	No	No
Vaillant 1980a	55	204	2	26	25	1/3	Yes	Yes
Core City sample	47	456	56	110	90	2/3	Yes	Yes

a. These proportions are our rough estimates of the severity of the alcohol abuse in the reviewed studies based on the authors' criteria for inclusion.

b. This figure includes the men who because they met Robins's diagnostic criteria for schizophrenia and sociopathy were excluded from her later report (Robins 1966). The figure excludes women and controls who abused alcohol.

c. This was a follow-back study.

d. In a more recent report (Jones 1981) this has been increased to 8.

Nevertheless, in their landmark study the McCords refuted several hypotheses regarding the etiology of alcoholism—refutations that have been upheld in subsequent prospective studies. They observed that, contrary to the findings of retrospective studies, men with nutritional disorders, glandular disorders, "strong inferiority feelings," phobias, and "more feminine feelings" were *not* more likely to develop alcoholism. More important, the men with "strong encouragement of dependency" from their mothers and manifest "oral tendencies" (thumb sucking, playing with their mouths, early heavy smoking, and compulsive eating) were actually *less* likely to develop alcoholism. Contrary to popular belief, prealcoholics were outwardly more self-confident, less disturbed by normal fears, more aggressive, hyperactive, and more heterosexual. In one stroke, the McCords brought into question many of the leading traits of the hypothetical prealcoholic personality.

The second important prospective study listed in Table 2.1 is that by Robins and her colleagues, who in the late 1950s followed up 524 children including 382 males admitted to a child guidance clinic 30 years previously at age $13\pm$ 2 years (Robins 1966; Robins et al. 1962). Robins was able to obtain reliable information for 286 of the 382 men. Although her original child guidance data were less rich than those of the McCords or the present Core City data obtained by the Gluecks, the follow-up was painstakingly thorough and included both interviews and search of public records. Unfortunately, half of her subjects were referred from juvenile courts and three-quarters were referred because of antisocial behavior. Thus, in her data evidence of emotional distress was often less available than evidence of misbehavior. Ethnicity was uncertain for many of her subjects, and information on mental illness in relatives other than parents was not available.

At some point in their lives 26 of her male subjects could be classified as "chronic alcoholics" and 52 as "probable" alcoholics. Robins's definition of alcoholism was "well established addiction to alcohol without recognizable underlying disorder." Empirically, this usually meant that two or more of the following were present: bender drinking, individual concern about ability to control drinking, family complaints, or social or medical problems related to abuse of alcohol. Only 12 of Robins's sample were ever hospitalized for alcoholism, but 20 had lost a job because of alcohol abuse. Perhaps one-third to one-half of Robins's sample would have met this book's definition for alcohol dependence. Premorbidly, the alcoholics in Robins's study differed from nonalcoholics in that they were more given to truancy, theft, inattention, and daydreaming; but they were not more likely than nonalcoholics to be regarded as impulsive, depressed, or unhappy. Inattention and daydreaming were the two traits that distinguished Robins's alcoholics from her sociopaths. In comparing the family life of future sociopaths and future alcoholics, Robins found virtually no significant differences. The exception was one also confirmed by the McCords' study: as children, alcoholics tended to have more consistent parental discipline than sociopaths.

At the Institute of Human Development at Berkeley, Jones (1968, 1971), studying a very small but repeatedly interviewed sample of middle-class youths, made similar observations. She used the Oakland Growth Study sample to compare heavy problem drinkers with moderate and light drinkers. All had been extensively studied in junior high school and high school and again in early and middle adulthood. Using personality traits defined by the Q-sort (Block 1961), Jones compared the high school evaluations of the 6 men who became problem drinkers with those of the 17 men who remained moderate drinkers. In high school, the heavy drinkers were characterized as "out of control, rebellious, pushing limits, self-indulgent and assertive" (Jones 1968). Among the girls, the heavy drinkers were more likely in high school to be "expressive, attractive, poised and buoyant" (Jones 1971). Jones's findings, and in fact all the above studies, conform to the hypothesis that in childhood, future alcohol abusers who progress to dependence have much in common with hyperactive children (Tarter et al. 1977).

In the fifth study reviewed in Table 2.1, Loper and colleagues (1973) compared the MMPI's (Minnesota Multiphasic Personality Inventories) of 38 college students who later developed alcoholism with the MMPI's of 148 matched male classmates. They observed that the prealcoholics were more compulsive, nonconforming, and gregarious and were more likely to answer "true" to items like: "In school, I sometimes was sent to the principal for cutting up," and "I like dramatics." Such observations are in keeping with those of other investigators who have observed that extroverted adolescents tend to engage in smoking, drug experimentation, and sexual behavior earlier than their peers.

In the same prospective study of MMPI's the authors noted that in college the original composite MMPI profile of their 38 alcoholic men had been within normal limits. However, when the men were hospitalized for alcoholism, their MMPI's were significantly elevated on the depression, psychopathic deviancy, and paranoia scales—to pathological levels. Once alcoholic, the men's composite profile revealed "the neurotic patterns consistent with self-centered, immature, dependent, resentful, irresponsible people who are unable to face reality." Once they had developed alcoholism, men were far more likely ($p < .01$) to answer "false" to "I am happy almost all the time" and "true" to "I shrink from facing a crisis," "I am high-strung," and "I am certainly lacking in self-confidence." In other words, they developed alcoholism first and *then* conformed to the hypothetical alcoholic personality (Kammeier et al. 1973; Hoffmann et al. 1974).

The sixth study (Vaillant 1980a) reports a prospective investigation of the mental health and alcohol use of the 184 men first studied during their college years—the College sample described in Chapter 6. When the men were 50 years old, a rater blind to childhood data and to other adult ratings classified the subject's adult alcohol use as little (n = 48), social (n = 110), or abuse (n = 26). The warmth of the men's childhood environments and their personality stability in college were assessed by other raters blind to data on their lives after college. Vignettes identifying "oral" adult behavior (pessimism, self-doubt, passivity, and dependence) were collected for each man by a rater blind to the subject's alcohol rating and to his childhood rating. Bleak childhood environments, personality instability in college, and adult evidence of premorbid personality disorder were all highly correlated with oral-dependent behavior but *not* with alcohol abuse. Furthermore, in the College sample, unhappy childhood led in adult life to mental illness, lack of friends, and low self-esteem (Vaillant 1974), but not to alcoholism. Many of the 26 problem drinkers seem to have become depressed and unable to cope *as a consequence* of their inability to control their alcohol consumption.

In other words, the earlier views on the etiology of alcoholism cited in the introduction were derived from data distorted by retrospection. Such views fail to consider the biological and psychological toll of alcoholism upon the personality (Bean and Zinburg 1981). In relatively healthy populations, alcohol abuse may be more analogous to any intractable habit (such as smoking or fingernail biting) than to mental illness. Such habits may develop independently of preexisting psychological vulnerability.

Unfortunately, there are methodological problems with all of the studies in Table 2.1. In summarizing their findings, the McCords suggest that parental conflict, the boy's conflict over dependency, and family role confusion lead to alcoholism. But in examining these conclusions, the reader is left wondering whether these allegedly etiological factors could not be secondary to alcoholism in the subject's parents and to the subject's own antisocial characteristics. First, alcoholism was much more common in the parents of the McCords' subjects who became alcoholic than in the parents of the nonalcoholics. The McCords, however, never factored out the effect of parental alcoholism as a source of role confusion, parental conflict, and the subject's unmet dependency needs. Second, the McCords' sample contained a disproportionate number of predelinquent youths. In their monograph, the McCords did not adequately emphasize the fact that the original sample was selected by matching the potentially most predelinquent youths in Cambridge and Somerville with an equal number of boys not at risk for delinquency. Of their 29 alcoholics, a disproportionate number were youths already diagnosed as predelinquent; and as adults, only 11 could not also be classified as "criminals." Third, the McCords' subjects were only 30 to 35 years old when they were followed up; identification of alcoholism depended not upon personal interview but upon arrest records or upon the subject's otherwise coming to public attention. Such criteria increase the chance of misidentifying as alcoholic those antisocial men who became drunk and disorderly but who never became physiologically dependent upon alcohol. The criteria also may have excluded law-abiding men, like those in the College sample, who rarely came to public attention or who did not lose control of their alcohol consumption until after age 40.

Finally, in many of their premorbid comparisons between alcoholics and nonalcoholics, the McCords excluded the 68 nonalcoholic criminals and their parents. Since many alcoholics were also criminals, the omission of nonalcoholic criminals from the statistical analyses exaggerated the importance of parental deviance in the genesis of alcoholism. That is, the parents of criminals were selectively included in the comparison only if their son was also an alcoholic.

Oversampling of antisocial children also prevented Robins and her colleagues from adequately identifying those antecedents of alcoholism which were clearly distinct from those of sociopathy. For example, if 75 percent of Robins's allegedly nonsociopathic alcoholics were frequently truant, only 10 percent of the 110 alcohol abusers in the Core City sample were premorbidly truant. Only 29 of Robins's 78 male alcohol abusers could not also be diagnosed sociopathic. Of these 29 nonsociopathic alcoholics, 83 percent had been originally referred for antisocial behavior; and half subsequently committed serious criminal offenses. Conversely, 76 percent of her 94 adult sociopaths would probably meet the DSM III criteria for alcohol abuse. Separating out sociopathy from alcoholism is not easy.

Table 2.1 illustrates the advantages of using the Core City sample to unravel important etiological factors in alcoholism. In this sample a large number of nonantisocial youths studied originally both for ethnicity and for family history of alcoholism were followed well into middle life by interview in a study that was deliberately prospective in design. The sample had little attrition and included both alcoholics who had and who had not come to clinical attention. As can be seen, the Core City sample contained almost as many alcoholics as all other prior samples combined.

In order to understand the etiology of alcoholism it is imperative to separate the antecedents of alcoholism from those of other unfavorable adult outcomes. As a first step, Table 2.2 presents the intercorrelations of important premorbid variables. All are described in detail in Chapter 7 and in the Appendix. Each variable might be expected to affect adult outcome. Irish and Anglo-American ethnicity were associated with parental alcoholism. I.Q. powerfully affected educational attainment, and itself appeared to be enhanced by childhood environmental strengths. Although quite independent of other items comprising the childhood environmental weaknesses scale, I.Q. was significantly negatively correlated with the variables in the scale that reflected inadequate *maternal* affection and supervision. Childhood strengths, boyhood competence, and childhood emotional problems—ratings that depended on many common factors—seem inextricably intercorrelated; but, like I.Q., boyhood competence and emotional problems seemed relatively independent of childhood environmental weaknesses per se. Alcoholism in a parent, not surprisingly, correlated very highly with the presence of childhood weaknesses but less dramatically with the absence of childhood environmental strengths. Presumably, an alcoholic parent *causes* childhood environmental weaknesses but does not preclude strengths being present in the same environment. In general, Table 2.2 lends support to the thesis that both innate and environmental emotional strengths may be more important than low I.Q. or external trauma to the adolescent outcome of the inner-city youth.

Table 2.3 presents the critical relationships between premorbid and outcome variables. The information in Table 2.3 is central to subsequent arguments made throughout this book. First, the table shows that parental social class correlates only in the most minimal way with a variety of adult outcome variables. (These variables are defined in detail in Chapter 7.) Second, as the McCords (1960) and the Gluecks (1950) predicted, multiproblem families, as reflected by the childhood environmental weaknesses scale, produced children who later were afflicted with sociopathy and alcoholism. (For the purposes of this table, alcohol use was assessed on a 3-point scale: 1 = asymptomatic drinking; 2 = alcohol abuse by the criteria of the DSM III (American Psy-

TABLE 2.2. Intercorrelation of the major premorbid variables.[a]

Variable	Education	I.Q.	Childhood weaknesses	Childhood strengths	Boyhood competence	Childhood emotional problems	Alcoholism in ancestors
Education	—						
I.Q.	.39	—					
Childhood weaknesses	-.18	*	—				
Childhood strengths	.24	.22	-.61	—			
Boyhood competence	.26	.22	-.25	.50	—		
Childhood emotional problems	-.12	-.17	.08	-.50	-.44	—	
Ethnicity[b]	*	*	-.15	.09	*	-.11	
Alcoholism in parents	*	*	.52	-.28	-.10	*	-.29

a. Pearson product-moment correlation coefficient was the statistic used. Significance: * indicates correlation statistically insignificant; $r = .08–.10$, $p < .05$; $r = .11–.15$, $p < .01$; $r > .15$, $p < .001$. Noteworthy correlations are in italics.

b. Ethnicity was arbitrarily scaled 1 = Irish, 2 = Anglo-American, 3 = Northern European, 4 = Mediterranean (Southern European). The rationale for this scaling will be presented later in this chapter.

TABLE 2.3. Relationship of childhood variables to adult outcome.[a]

	Adult outcome variables					
Childhood variables	Social competence	Social class (age 47)	Sociopathy	Mental health (HSRS)	% adult life unemployed	Alcohol use (DSM III)
Boyhood competence	.23	.28	−.22	.24	−.23	−.12
Childhood environmental strengths	.12	.21	−.19	.21	−.17	−.18
Childhood emotional problems	−.20	−.19	.13	−.19	*	*
I.Q.	.13	.35	*	.15	*	*
Childhood environmental weaknesses	*	.13	.18	*	.13	.15
Parental social class	*	.14	*	*	−.13	*
Alcoholism in heredity	*	*	*	*	*	.26
Ethnicity[b]	*	*	−.14	*	*	−.28

a. Pearson product-moment correlation coefficient was the statistic used. Correlations greater than .15 are significant at $p < .001$ and are in italic. Correlations greater than .12 are significant at $p < .05$; therefore, r's smaller than .12 ($p > .01$)

b. Irish = 1, Mediterranean = 4.

*Since hundreds of correlations were obtained, many by chance would have been significant at $p = .05$; therefore, r's smaller than .12 ($p > .01$) have been regarded as statistically insignificant.

chiatric Association 1980); 3 = alcohol dependence.) After 33 years, however, the effect of multiproblem family membership upon most adult outcome variables seemed attenuated. Third, measured intelligence, besides being highly correlated with adult social class through its effect on attained education ($r = .38$), was only modestly correlated with other outcome variables. In other words, parental social class, I.Q., and multiproblem family membership may be more important in cross-sectional studies than they are in studies with a lifespan perspective. The wounds of poverty appear less permanent than the wounds of lovelessness. This statement contradicts much that has been written about the consequences of poverty—but the Gluecks' research probably represents the first prospective lifetime study of the poor that has ever been undertaken.

Rather, it was the childhood variables to which Freud, not Marx, would have us pay attention that made the greatest difference. Success at working, the absence of emotional problems, and the presence of strengths rather than weaknesses in the childhood environment correlated most highly with adult outcome. Perhaps what is most striking about Table 2.3 is that, of all the childhood measures chosen, the boyhood competence scale, reflecting success at Erikson's Stage Four (Industry versus Inferiority), correlated most strongly with all the different facets of adult adjustment. The boyhood competence scale probably comes as close as any childhood variable in this study to that ineffable, platonic concept—ego strength. And ego strength undoubtedly is at the heart of what observers mean when they marvel at the "invulnerable child" who emerges seemingly unscathed from a multiproblem family.

As elaborated later in this chapter, alcoholism was most highly correlated with ethnicity and alcoholism in relatives, two premorbid variables that otherwise did not significantly predict adult outcome.

With this introduction to the relationship between the major premorbid and outcome variables, the etiology of alcoholism among the Core City men can be more systematically considered. The top section of Table 2.4 lists childhood antecedents in the lives of 71 Core City men who developed alcohol dependence that significantly distinguished them from the 260 Core City asymptomatic drinkers. The purpose of the next few sections of this chapter will be to determine which of the 11 variables in the table might be of primary etiological significance.

There were clear ethnic differences between men who became alcoholic and those who did not; there were also clear differences in the amount of alcohol abuse in their families. Men who became alcoholic were more likely

TABLE 2.4. Childhood differences and similarities between men who never abused alcohol and those who became dependent.

	Asymptomatic drinkers (n = 254 ± 6)[a]	Alcohol-dependent (n = 69 ±2)[a]
Differences		
Irish ethnicity	17%	30%
Italian ethnicity	35	6
Alcoholism in 2+ ancestors	9	21
Alcoholism in a parent	18	34
School behavior problems and truancy	2	13
Sociopath (5+ on Robins scale)	0.4	30
2+ times in jail	4	16
< 10 grades of education	28	42
Childhood environmental strengths ("warm")	26	13
Lack of cohesive family	40	51
Close relationship with father	30	13
Similarities		
I.Q. < 90	28	30
Parents in social class V	32	30
Multiproblem family	11	14
Warm relationship with mother	30	27
Inadequate maternal supervision	36	34
Childhood emotional problems	32	30
Boyhood competence (top quartile)	28	21

a. Of the 456 men in the study, 71 could be classified as alcohol-dependent and 260 as asymptomatic drinkers (1 or fewer problems with alcohol). Of the remaining 125 men, 62 had 2 or 3 alcohol-related problems; 49 were classified as alcohol abusers but not as alcohol-dependent; and 14 men were unclassified because of early death or lack of data.

to have been at risk for delinquency and less likely to have pursued their education. The childhood environments of the alcoholics were bleaker and less cohesive; and positive relationships between future alcoholics and their fathers were rare.

The findings of the bottom section of Table 2.4, however, focusing on childhood similarities rather than differences, are equally striking. Neither childhood emotional problems nor absence of boyhood competence, the harbingers of future mental illness in Table 2.3, markedly affected risk of future alcohol abuse. Warm mothers did not prevent, and multiproblem families per se did not greatly enhance, subsequent alcohol abuse. With the intent of examining apparent inconsistencies between the two sections of Table 2.4 and of isolating the primary premorbid factors that increase the risk of alcoholism, the next four sections will examine the variables in Table 2.4 in greater detail. For reason that will become apparent, Italian ethnicity, familial alcoholism, and school behavior problems will receive the greatest attention.

Cultural Factors

In Western societies one of the most obvious but least useful means of combating alcoholism has been to forbid drinking. With the exception of Moslem and Hindu countries, where social taboos against alcohol use have been successful, prohibition has rarely been an effective solution. As Will Rogers, the great American humorist, said, "Prohibition's only virtue was that it was better than no whiskey at all." Put differently, *proscriptions* against alcohol use have rarely been as effective as social *prescriptions* for alcohol use. First, cultures that teach children to drink responsibly, cultures that have ritualized when and where to drink, tend to have lower rates of alcohol abuse than cultures that forbid children to drink. Second, as Heath (1975) has demonstrated, how a society socializes drunkenness is as important as how it socializes drinking. For example, both France and Italy inculcate in their children responsible drinking practices; but, in fact, public drunkenness is far more socially acceptable in France than in Italy—and France experiences a higher rate of alcohol abuse.

Because of an abundance of confounding variables, cross-cultural obser-vations of this kind do not usually permit etiological conclusions. Cultures and countries differ from each other in many ways besides socialization of alcohol use. They differ enormously in their means of reporting alcohol abuse and in the kind of alcohol available and its price structure. There may be racial differences that affect metabolism; there may be alternative recreational drugs. Finally, many of the anecdotal differences used to illustrate alcohol differences in other countries are not based upon longitudinal study. For example, what really happens to the three-liters-of-wine-a-day French "social drinkers"? Does the "explosive relief drinking" by Finns *never* lead to future alcohol dependence? Answers to these questions are not yet known.

By chance, the Core City sample offered unique controls for many of the confounding variables. Virtually all of the Core City men lived in an urban environment (Boston) where alcohol was readily available and was the principal recreational drug of choice. The Core City men shared the same schools and legal system; and they shared the same ethnically diverse peer group. Where the Core City men differed from one another was in the cultural background of their parents. Sixty-one percent of their parents had been born in foreign countries, and ethnic intermarriage by their parents was rare.

Table 2.5 shows the dramatic effect of parental cultural background on the lifetime patterns of use and abuse of alcohol by the Core City men. In each ethnic group roughly 1 man in 5 used alcohol less often than once a month; these 80 men (20 percent) were classified as teetotalers. In comparison, 4 percent of the French population (Pittman 1967) and 50 percent of Protestant, middle-aged men in the rural southeastern United States (Cahalan et al. 1969) are teetotalers.

The Core City men whose parents had grown up in the Mediterranean cultures were far less likely than men from other ethnic groups to develop alcohol dependence. Compared to men from other ethnic groups, men of Anglo-Irish background were somewhat less likely to drink regularly without problems. Each group seemed equally at risk for problem drinking without dependence (about 1 in 10).

Contrary to popular belief, when boys from similar neighborhoods were examined, the Irish were not at higher risk for alcohol dependence than other Northern Europeans. As Table 2.6 illustrates, however, the Irish were more likely to manifest multiple alcohol-related problems. Compared with the Anglo-Americans, men of Irish extraction were almost twice as likely to have scores over eight on the Problem Drinking Scale. Yet they were no more likely to be diagnosed alcoholic, and the wives of Core City men of Irish extraction were rather less likely to be reported as objecting to their husbands' use of alcohol.

As a means of assessing the effect of culture upon alcoholism, ethnicity was numerically ranked according to the degree to which the parental culture sanctioned drinking and proscribed drunkenness. Thus, a rank of 1 was assigned to the Irish, who tend to forbid alcohol before age 21, to admire drunkenness among men, and to drink outside the home and apart from meals. A rank of 2 was assigned to men of American, Canadian, or English descent, and 3 was assigned to men of Northern European countries, who occupy an intermediate position. A rank of 4 was assigned to men from Italy, Portugal, Spain, Greece, Syria, and Armenia. In most of these cultures, children are taught to drink by their parents, drinking occurs with meals, and drunkenness is taboo. For the purposes of classification, the 6 Jews in the

TABLE 2.5. Use and abuse of alcohol among different ethnic groups.

		Alcohol use classification[a]		
Ethnic group	Abstainer (n = 80; 20%)	Asymptomatic drinker (n = 210; 52%)	Alcohol abuse without dependence (n = 40; 10%)	Alcohol-dependent (DSM III) (n = 71; 18%)
Irish (n = 76)	21%	43%	8%	28%
Old American (n = 35)	20	40	13	27
Polish, Russian (n = 17)	18	53	11	18
English, Anglo-Canadian (n = 98)	21	45	11	23
Northern Europe other (n = 20)	5	65	5	25
French Canadian (n = 26)	15	54	8	23
Southern Europe other[b] (n = 23)	30	57	9	4
Italian (n = 99)	18	70	8	4
Jewish (n = 6)	50	33	17	0
Chinese (n = 1)	0	0	100	0

a. Only the 401 men rated on the alcohol use scale are included here. Because there did not seem to be important ethnic differences in this subgroup, men with 2 and 3 on the PDS were included with the nonproblem drinkers.

b. Lebanon, Syria, Turkey, Greece, Portugal, Armenia.

TABLE 2.6. Ethnicity and reported drinking problems.

Problem	Irish (n = 76)	U.S., English, Canadian (n = 159)	Other Northern European (n = 37)	Mediterranean (n = 128)
Wife complains	22%	27%	32%	10%
Multiple medical problems	12	7	6	0
Clinical diagnosis of alcoholism	17	15	14	2
Multiple drunkenness arrests	26	17	14	5
Multiple hospitalizations for alcoholism	16	7	5	2
8+ problems on the PDS	26	16	17	3

Core City sample were also assigned to the Mediterranean group. While such an arbitrary classification is controversial and in individual cases may be misleading, the intent was to assess the probability that cultural attitudes toward alcohol might affect future problem drinking. Obviously, it would have been preferable to have obtained prospective data regarding parental attitudes rather than depending upon paternal ethnicity. (There was little intermarriage, and examining ethnicity in terms of maternal rather than paternal lineage did not alter the findings.)

Table 2.7 underscores the prognostic power of classifying men according to the extent to which their culture sanctioned childhood drinking and proscribed intoxication. Alcohol dependence developed seven times more frequently in the Irish than in those of Mediterranean descent. Late age of marriage has been postulated as enhancing the association between Irish ethnicity and a high incidence of alcoholism (Bales 1962); Bales believed that heavy drinking "with the boys" provided a substitute for marriage. However, in our sample Irish youth did not marry later than those in other ethnic groups. Drinking by Irishmen in Ireland, however, is undoubtedly different from that by Irish Americans in Boston.

Reviews by Pittman and Snyder (1962), Heath (1975), and Greely and McReady (1980) have shown that the interrelationships of drinking practices and culture are far more complex than can be encompassed by the reductionistic Table 2.7. But the table's findings nevertheless bear out observations made from much more detailed study of Irish (Bales 1962) and Italian (Lolli 1952) drinking practices. The Italians provide children with a long education

TABLE 2.7. Relationship between the culture in which parents were raised and the development of alcohol dependence in their sons.[a]

	Parents' culture		
Alcohol use classification (DSM III)	Irish (n = 75[c])	Other[b] (n = 195)	Mediterranean (n = 128)
No alcohol abuse	59%	58%	86%
Alcohol abuse without dependence	13	19	10
Alcohol dependence	28	23	4

a. Significance $p < .001$ (chi-square test).

b. Canadian, American, Northern European.

c. Total slightly different from Tables 2.5 and 2.6 because only 398 men could be rated on the DSM III rating for alcohol use.

in moderate alcohol use and encourage drinking with family members. They inculcate drinking practices that diminish the alcohol "high"; these practices include using low-proof alcohol and drinking alcohol with food. One Core City social drinker, whose Italian family had served him alcohol since he was 4, described how "my father gave me the 'look' when I once came home drunk."

In contrast, the Irish forbid children and adolescents from learning how to drink but they tolerate—and covertly praise—the capacity of men to drink large amounts of alcohol. Alcohol use is a guilty secret. An extreme example of this was the Core City alcoholic whose Irish mother had spoon-fed him whiskey at age 7 until he was drunk. The Irish prefer drinking in pubs where alcohol intake is carefully separated from the family dinner table and often from food intake of any kind (Stivers 1976). If in Italy low-proof wine has greater mystique than distilled liquor, in Ireland high-proof whiskey is more highly revered than low-proof beer. (A little reflection will bring to mind that the drinking practices that occur on many of our Native American reservations are an exaggeration of those in Ireland.)

Like any other form of education, teaching children to drink is not without risk. Unlike Ireland, Italy has a problem with alcoholism in children (Pittman 1967). Indeed, Italy is the only country of which I know that has an alcohol unit associated with a department of pediatrics! It is also probably true that the number of alcohol-related traffic fatalities increased when American states lowered the drinking age to 18 and that traffic fatalities have declined when states have raised the drinking age to 21. But adolescent automobile fatalities and occasional childhood alcohol dependence do not necessarily correlate with an increased total population risk for alcoholism. Besides, is not the best way to reduce adolescent traffic fatalities to raise the minimum age for teenage driving—not teenage drinking?

The comparison of French and Italian drinking practices is fascinating (Jellinek 1960; Pittman and Snyder 1962). Certainly, the French teach their children how to drink—a custom that probably diminishes the risk of alcohol abuse—but they tend not to encourage moderation in drinking, a failing that may increase the risk of alcoholism. To refuse a drink in Italy is quite acceptable; to refuse a drink in France may be construed as unpatriotic, or worse, ridiculous. In France, unlike Italy, public drunkenness is condoned. In the 1940s and 1950s Italy experienced a much lower rate of alcoholism than France. In the last 20 to 40 years, the average amount of alcohol consumed in Italy has gone steadily up with such a concomitant increase in the rate of alcoholism that the rate of death from cirrhosis in Italy now exceeds that in Ireland. In Italy, too, the price of wine relative to income has steadily declined, and as will be discussed later, the relative price of alcohol affects rates of alcoholism (Ornstein 1980). In the last 20 years, both the amount of alcohol consumed and the rate of alcoholism in France have gone down (Bruun et al. 1975); for France has become increasingly aware of its alcohol problem and through social policies is changing the way it regards drinking as a nation. Nevertheless, the average Frenchman still consumes four ounces of absolute alcohol a day (the equivalent of six to eight martinis); 7 percent drink more than three liters of wine a day (the equivalent of 18 martinis); and France still experiences the highest rate of alcoholism in the world.

Genetic Factors

In alcoholism, cultural background is but one of the many risk factors. More than 100 years ago it was noted that, to an extraordinary degree, alcoholism ran in families (Baer 1878). Since then there has been considerable controversy as to whether this familial transmission is caused by environmental or genetic factors. For 90 of the last 100 years, researchers have been stymied on how to disentangle nature from nurture. Thus, an enormous literature has accumulated that speculates upon the environmental transmission of alcoholism, but which fails to control for genetic transmission. Both Karl Menninger (1938), arguing from psychoanalytic evidence, and the McCords

(1960), arguing from what was at the time the best prospective study of alcoholism in existence, stated more or less categorically that alcoholism is not in any way a hereditary disorder. Simultaneously, because of the seemingly intractable and involuntary nature of alcoholism, a vast literature appeared purporting to show that alcoholism is an inherited disease of disordered metabolism (Jellinek 1960).

Over the past decade, however, evidence has accumulated to allow Goodwin (1979) to assert that genetic factors play a significant role in alcoholism, and Mendelson and Mello (1979) to assert that "it appears unlikely that individual or racial differences in alcohol metabolism can account for alcohol abuse." For example, there have been convincing studies showing that diverse Mongoloid populations, including Chinese with *low* rates of alcohol abuse and American Indian subgroups with *high* rates of alcohol abuse, share the same inborn metabolic intolerance of alcohol and its metabolites. Utne and colleagues (1977) have observed that although genetic factors control the rate of the metabolism of alcohol (Vesell et al. 1971; Seixas 1978), nevertheless alcohol elimination rates do not differ among the children of alcoholic and nonalcoholic parents. In other words, interindividual and interracial differences in alcohol metabolism exist; but they do not seem to be powerfully related to risk of alcohol dependence.

In the past ten years there has emerged an increasingly convincing body of evidence that if alcoholism is not a hereditary metabolic defect, neither is it primarily caused by alcoholism in the child's environment. From studies of cross-fostered children, Goodwin (1976, 1979) has persuasively marshalled evidence that the observed increased rate of alcoholism in the descendants of alcoholics appears to correlate with alcohol abuse in heredity, not in the environment. Certainly, parental alcoholism causes emotional pain and psychological disorders in the children of alcoholics; certainly, some children of alcoholics may model themselves on their parents; certainly, the family structure of alcoholics is peculiarly distorted to facilitate alcohol abuse. Nevertheless, there is no evidence that these factors statistically increase the risk of alcohol abuse in children if they are not biologically related to the alcoholic family member. Perhaps for every child who becomes alcoholic in response to an alcoholic environment, another eschews alcohol in response to the same environment (see Figure 2.1).

First, there have been four well-executed twin studies of alcoholism. In each study, identical twins exhibited much greater concordance for drinking behavior—and in some studies greater concordance for alcohol abuse—than did fraternal twins, who in theory shared the same family environment but not the same genes. Second, adoption studies, which are methodologically better suited than twin studies to separate nature from nurture, support the hereditary transmission of increased risk of alcoholism. There have been five adoption studies focusing on alcoholism. All but one, the least well executed, have pointed to the fact that while there was no significant relationship between alcohol abuse among adoptees and the foster parents with whom they lived, there was a consistent and significantly increased risk of alcoholism in adoptees (even if adopted at birth) if a biological parent had abused alcohol (Goodwin 1979).

The single contradictory adoption study was that done by Roe (1944) during World War II—a period of history when investigators were loath to identify hereditary factors in mental illness. Roe examined a small group of foster children of whom 21 were of "alcoholic" parentage. None of her subjects had developed problem drinking; but the sample was small and few men were followed past the age of 30.

The most elegant adoption studies were begun in 1970 (Goodwin et al. 1973). These studies involved interviewing the sons (average of age 30 years) of Danish alcoholics raised by nonalcoholic parents and a group of sons (average age 33 years) raised by their own alcoholic biologic parents. Paired with each of these two groups was a control group without alcoholic parents matched for age and, in the adopted group, for circumstances of adoption. Adoptees were included only if they had been separated from their biological parents in the first few weeks of life, and if they had been adopted by nonrelatives. Ratings of alcoholism were made by psychiatrists blind to the hypothesis of the study and to the parentage of the subjects. What is most impressive about Goodwin's study is the fact that the men whose biologic parents were alcoholics were four times more likely to be alcoholic than were the sons of nonalcoholic biologic parents. Conversely, there was no significant relationship between alcohol abuse in adoptees and the presence or absence of alcohol abuse in their adoptive parents. In another adoption study, Cadoret and colleagues (1980) confirmed that psychiatric and alcoholic problems in adoptive families did not predict alcoholism in unrelated adoptees. In a complex reanalysis of Bohman's (1978) original cross-fostering study, Cloninger and colleagues (1981) suggest that postnatal factors also played a role in the adoptees' alcoholism.

Third, in a cross-fostering study of half-siblings, Schuckit and colleagues (1972) also observed that children with an alcoholic biologic parent who were raised by nonalcoholic parents had a rate of alcohol abuse three times higher than children without alcoholic parents who were raised by an alcoholic step-parent or surrogate.

Within the Core City sample, the familial history of alcohol abuse was a potent predictor that the men themselves would abuse alcohol. Table 2.8 summarizes the relationship of family history of alcohol abuse with alcohol dependence and alcohol abuse in men themselves (defined by the DSM III criteria). At some point in their adult lives, 1 Core City man in 6 (18 percent) developed alcohol dependence. However, alcohol dependence occurred in only 10 percent of the 178 Core City men with no alcohol-abusing relatives but in 34 percent of the 71 men with several alcohol-abusing relatives—a threefold difference in risk. This relationship held whether alcohol abuse was measured by the DSM III criteria, by the PDS, or by the Cahalan scale.

The same relationship between family history and alcoholism held for the College sample. Of the 158 men with one or no alcoholic relatives, only 9 percent abused alcohol; 26 percent of the 46 College men with two or more known alcoholic relatives abused alcohol.

It was not possible to dissect the environmental contribution of alcohol-abusing Core City relatives from the genetic contribution of such relatives. Nevertheless, it was significant that when just the effect of alcohol abuse in ancestors (that is, in relatives who were not also part of the subjects' environment) was examined, men with several alcohol-abusing ancestors were twice as likely (29 percent) to become alcohol-dependent as were men (14 percent) with no known alcohol-abusing ancestors. It also seemed significant that the risk of encountering a few alcohol-related problems without dependence at some point in adult life did not seem affected by the number of alcoholic relatives.

The presence of alcoholic parents also greatly increased the risk of alcoholism in their children. Of the 244 men who grew up in households where neither parent nor parent surrogate abused alcohol, 11 percent became alcohol-dependent. In contrast, 28 percent of the men with alcohol-abusing fathers and 36 percent of the men with alcohol-abusing mothers (many of whom were also married to alcohol-abusing husbands) developed alcohol dependence. In order to interpret the significance of this observation, we must depend upon the previously cited cross-fostering studies by Goodwin and Schuckit which suggest that at least a significant fraction of the association between alcohol abuse in parents and in children is genetically rather than environmentally transmitted.

TABLE 2.8. Relationship between number of alcohol-abusing relatives and development of alcohol dependence among Core City men.

	Alcohol use and classification (DSM III)		
Scale of alcohol abuse	No alcohol abuse (n = 267)	Abuse without dependence (n = 60)	Alcohol dependence (n = 71)
Alcohol use in total sample (n = 398)	67%	15%[a]	18%
Alcohol abuse in heredity scale			
1 (no relatives) (n = 178)	78	12	10
2–3 (1–2 relatives) (n = 149)	60	20	20
4 (several relatives) (n = 71)	52	14	34[b]
Alcohol abuse in ancestors scale[c]			
1 (no relatives) (n = 213)	73	13	14
2–3 (1–2 relatives) (n = 133)	63	18	19
4 (several relatives) (n = 52)	58	13	29[b]
Alcohol abuse in parents scale			
Mother alcoholic (n = 36)	50	14	36[b]
Father alcoholic (n = 149)	58	14	28[b]
Neither parent alcoholic (n = 244)	75	15	11

a. As noted elsewhere, "alcohol abuse" as defined by the DSM III criteria was a somewhat more inclusive category than alcohol abuse defined by having 4+ symptoms on the PDS; thus this category included 15 percent of the men rather than 10 percent as in Table 2.5.

b. Significance $p < .01$ (chi-square test).

c. Excluding parents and siblings.

The fact that alcohol abuse was observed in so many of the families of the Core City men may seem surprising. In part, this high rate was because these men had been closely followed for 35 years; and as Cotton (1979) has noted, the observed rate of alcohol abuse in relatives appears to be a function of how well studied the samples are. In part, also, the Core City families—blue collar, urban, living in the Northeast—represented a population at high risk for alcoholism. In her review of major American studies of familial alcoholism, Cotton observed that one alcoholic in three is known to have a close alcoholic relative; but among the alcohol-dependent Core City men at least 76 percent had an alcohol-abusing relative, and so did 55 percent of the non-alcohol-dependent men. In Cotton's review, one alcoholic in four (27 percent) had an alcoholic father and one in 20 (5 percent) had an alcoholic mother. In our sample, more than half (60 percent) of the 71 alcohol-dependent men had an alcoholic father and one in six (18 percent) had an alcoholic mother.

In reviewing the relationship between family history of alcohol abuse and alcoholism in probands, Goodwin and others have suggested that *familial* alcoholism may be different from *acquired* alcoholism (Goodwin 1979; Cloninger et al. 1981). The former is thought to have a poorer prognosis and to begin at an earlier age. Implicit in this view is the belief that *familial* alcoholism, analogous to early-onset diabetes or process schizophrenia, is a more malignant subtype. The present data do not really support this point of view. It was true that alcohol dependence and experiencing many problems on the PDS correlated highly with the number of alcohol-abusing relatives and that alcohol abuse without dependence seemed to occur in roughly 15 percent of the men regardless of how many alcohol-abusing relatives they had. However, when the relationship between severity of alcohol abuse and heredity is examined in greater detail, the association becomes less clear-cut. Table 2.9 contrasts the 178 men with no alcohol-abusing relatives with the 71 men who had three or more alcohol-abusing relatives. As a group, alcohol abusers with many known alcoholic relatives were two or three times more likely to manifest any given symptom, but the symptom pattern of alcohol abusers with many alcoholic relatives did not seem very different from that of alcohol abusers with no known alcoholic relatives.

Contrary to Goodwin's hypothesis (1979), early onset of problem drinking in the Core City alcoholic men was not associated with alcoholic heredity. Half of the alcoholic men with no alcoholic relatives and only slightly more than half of those with many such relatives developed four or more alcohol-related problems before age 28. Indeed, among the Core City men, age of onset of alcohol abuse (four or more symptoms on the PDS) was insignificantly but, contrary to Goodwin's hypothesis, positively ($r = .02$) correlated with the number of alcohol-abusing relatives.

Although, compared to the Core City men, the modal College men lost control of their use of alcohol much later (age 39 as contrasted with age 28), College men with many alcohol-abusing relatives did not lose control of their use of alcohol at an earlier age than men without such relatives.

When examined closely, early age of onset of alcohol abuse among the Core City men appears more closely associated with family breakdown and number of antisocial relatives than with number of alcoholic relatives or

TABLE 2.9. Relation of alcohol abuse in heredity to specific drinking problems.

	Known alcohol-abusing relatives	
	No relatives (n = 178)	3+ relatives (n = 71)
4+ problems (PDS) before age 28	9%	24%
4+ problems (PDS) after age 28	9	20
4+ problems (PDS) ever	18	44
Ever diagnosed alcoholic	8	16
Wife complains	14	32
Blackouts	15	31
Alcohol-dependent ever (DSM III)	10	34
Morning drinking	12	32
Multiple arrests	8	28
Multiple job problems	5	16
Multiple medical problems	3	13

ethnicity. In a large study of problem drinkers in the navy, Frances and colleagues (1980) observed that alcoholic probands with many alcoholic relatives came from more disturbed families and were more antisocial and performed less well in school than alcoholic probands without familial alcoholism. Thus, the association of early-onset alcoholism and family history of alcohol abuse may possibly be mediated by environmental disruption by alcoholic parents rather than by genetic susceptibility.

At the present time, a conservative view of the role of genetic factors in alcoholism seems appropriate. Like cultural susceptibility, genetic susceptibility to alcoholism is but one of many risk factors and is most likely polygenic. Contrary to the assertion that alcoholics are sensitive or "allergic" to alcohol, the truth may be that (for polygenic reasons) many prealcoholics are less sensitive to alcohol than their social-drinking counterparts. That is, the person genetically at risk for alcoholism may be the individual with a "hollow leg"; the one who can drink his friends under the table without vomiting, losing his coordination, or suffering a hangover the next morning.

Before examining other etiological factors, I must address an important question. If 80 percent of the Irish subjects and only 35 percent of the Italian subjects had at least one alcoholic relative, are culture and family history of alcohol abuse really independent etiological factors or is one variable depend-

TABLE 2.10.   Ratio of alcohol-dependent to asymptomatic drinkers when both ethnicity and heredity are varied.

Ethnicity	No alcohol-abusing relatives	2+ alcohol-abusing relatives
Irish (n = 75)	1:2	1:2
Mediterranean (n = 130)	1:40	1:7
Other (n = 193)	1:5	3:4

ent upon the other? Put differently, do Irishmen abuse alcohol because of genetic susceptibility or does alcohol abuse only seem hereditary because Irish culture engenders alcohol abuse while Italian culture engenders drinking practices that tend to inhibit abuse? Table 2.10 portrays the ratio of alcohol-dependent men to asymptomatic drinkers when ethnicity and family history of alcohol are varied independently. For Irish subjects, the observed risk of alcohol abuse was not affected by familial prevalence of alcohol abuse. But a disproportionate number of Irish subjects with many alcoholic relatives were lifelong teetotalers. Men of American and Northern European extraction without alcoholic relatives were less likely than those of Irish extraction to become alcohol-dependent, but those with many alcoholic relatives were even more likely than the Irish to become alcohol-dependent. Italians with many alcoholic relatives were five times as likely to be alcohol-dependent as Italians without alcoholic relatives. In short, both culture and genes appeared to contribute to the causation of alcohol abuse among the Core City men.

〜 Genetic Factors Revisited

Since the original version of this book was written there has been considerable effort to explicate the genetic basis of alcoholism. While many initially promising leads have appeared, efforts to identify individual genes that are associated with increased risk of alcoholism have not been consistently replicated. Recently four out of six studies suggested that restriction fragment length (RFL) polymorphisms of the D_2 dopamine receptor gene were associated with alcoholism (Smith et al. 1992). Such evidence pointed toward a possible genetic association of the human D_2 dopamine receptor gene and alcoholism. More recently, however, Gelernter and colleagues (1993) have assembled convincing evidence that there is no association between alcoholism and the D_2 dopamine receptor locus.

Another still promising area of genetic investigation is that ethanol can profoundly affect the G protein adenyl-cyclase signal transduction pathway (Manji 1992). Abnormalities in G protein mediated effects on adenyl-cyclase second messenger systems have been suggested as a putative marker in alcoholism (Tabakoff et al. 1988).

Schuckit (1992) has recently reviewed efforts to identify biological differences that premorbidly distinguish individuals at risk for alcoholism from other individuals. While there have been many single reports of suggestive differences, most of these differences have not been confirmed or have proved insignificant. The most promising specific biological differences that have been replicated are the observations by Begleiter and Porjesz (1988) that the sons of alcoholics share the electrophysiologic abnormalities of their fathers. It has long been known that chronic alcoholics demonstrate certain functional aberrations in event-related brain potentials that may reflect a defect in certain aspects of anticipatory informational processing. The most striking defect is that, following a rare but anticipated sensory stimulus, alcoholics exhibit a diminished P300 (P3) component of the brain's event-related potentials. But such a defect could be the result of rather than a precursor of prolonged alcohol abuse. What is of interest is that Begleiter and his colleagues have demonstrated, and others have confirmed, that perhaps one-third of the *sons* of alcoholics *premorbidly* exhibit the same defect.

Of greater relevance may be the results from Schuckit's own laboratory that individuals at risk for alcoholism have greater tolerance to the effects of alcohol. This tolerance seems based on genetic factors as well as on heavy drinking. All of the investigations reviewed by Schuckit (1992) have demonstrated that, following modest doses of alcohol, despite identical blood alcohol concentrations, individuals with family histories of alcohol abuse have less intense subjective feelings of intoxication. Schuckit's own work has demonstrated that this less intense response to alcohol holds true not only for subjective intoxication but also for some motor performance tests as well as some hormonal and electrophysiologic responses to alcohol.

Still more important, Schuckit (1994) noted the subjective response to alcohol at age 20 of 32 men who by age 30 met criteria for alcohol abuse. He contrasted the response to alcohol of these 32 men with that of 107 men who on follow-up did not meet such criteria. There was little overlap between the two groups; premorbidly, future alcoholics manifested much less response to alcohol. Such lack of reactivity to alcohol also predicted which men with a family history of alcohol abuse would develop subsequent alcohol abuse. Such findings support the hypothesis that relative insensitivity to alcohol may be a cause, rather than merely a correlate, of alcoholism.

Childhood Environment

In 1940 Paul Schilder wrote that "the chronic alcoholic person is one who from his earliest childhood on has lived in a state of insecurity" (p. 290). Since then, in virtually all retrospective studies of alcoholics (Barry 1974) and in the two best prospective studies (McCord and McCord 1960; Robins 1966) unstable childhood has seemed to predict future alcoholism. Broken homes, irresponsible fathers, marital discord, and inconsistent upbringing seem most often implicated. However, as already mentioned, the subjects of both the McCords and Robins were drawn from underprivileged youths known to be at high risk for delinquency. In addition, Haberman (1966) compared the children of alcoholic and nonalcoholic parents and noted that the former, if they lived with their parents, were more likely to stutter, wet the bed, misbehave, and manifest phobias. Is, then, the disturbed childhood environment of alcoholics simply a function of parental alcoholism?

In a study of the more socially privileged, nondelinquent College men, childhood environment did not predict alcoholism (Vaillant 1980a). That was not because the ratings of childhood environmental strengths measured irrelevant variables, for, as Table 2.11 illustrates, the presence or absence of childhood environmental strengths significantly ($p < .05$) predicted which College men would take tranquilizers over their life span and which men 30 years later would require medicine for physical illness. Only alcohol abuse was independent of childhood environment.

In a large underprivileged but not particularly delinquent sample, what would be the relationship to alcoholism of the variables identified by the McCords and Robins? As illustrated in Table 2.4, raters blind to the Core City men's futures did judge premorbid family environment of alcohol-dependent Core City men to be significantly less "warm" and less cohesive. The future alcoholic was perceived as relatively distant from his father. But to what degree can these observed differences in childhood environment between future social drinkers and alcoholics be explained by differences in alcohol abuse by their parents?

Figure 2.1 provides an interesting analysis of the relationships among parental alcoholism, familial instability, and future drinking patterns. The association of childhood environmental weaknesses with future risk of alco-

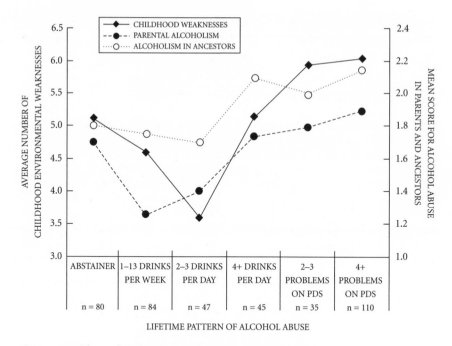

Figure 2.1 Evidence that the elevated frequency of childhood environmental weaknesses among alcoholics is a function of parental alcoholism.

hol abuse exactly paralleled the relation of parental alcohol abuse to the subject's future risk of alcohol abuse. The observed differences in environmental weaknesses are no greater than could be accounted for by the presence of an alcoholic parent in the subject's family. Put differently, of the 51 men who had *few* childhood environmental weaknesses but did have an alcoholic parent, 27 percent became alcohol-dependent. Of the 56 men with *many* environmental weaknesses but no alcoholic parent, only 5 percent became alcohol-dependent.

In contrast to men with alcoholic ancestors, Core City men with alcoholic parents were also significantly ($p < .01$) more likely to remain lifelong teetotalers. This observation helps to explain why the Irish subjects with many alcoholic relatives were not significantly more likely to abuse alcohol than Irish men with no alcoholic relatives. The men who best met the criteria for lifelong moderate social drinking had not only the most benign childhoods but also the fewest alcohol-abusing relatives.

TABLE 2.11. Relationship of adult drug and alcohol use to childhood environment in the College sample.

	Childhood environment[a]		
	Worst (n = 34)	Intermediate (n = 109)	Best (n = 41)
Problem drinking (ever)	18%	12%	17%
Regular use of prescription medications (recent)	36	10	2
Regular use of mood-altering drugs (ever)	18	14	7

a. This was the same scale used to measure childhood environmental strengths for the Core City sample.

Two conclusions may be tentatively entertained. First, the increased rate of familial problems in the childhood of the alcoholic men can be explained by parental alcoholism. Statistical confirmation of this observation is provided by Figure 2.1 and by the multiple regression analyses to be provided in Table 2.17. Second, while parental alcoholism is significantly correlated with both teetotaling and alcohol abuse, alcohol abuse in ancestors is associated with heavy drinking but not with teetotaling. In other words, if Schuckit and Goodwin suggest that the relationship of familial alcoholism to the subject's alcohol abuse is largely genetic, the association of parental alcohol abuse with teetotaling may be largely environmental.

Personality and Premorbid Emotional Stability

Three premorbid personality types have been repeatedly postulated to play an etiological role in alcoholism: the emotionally insecure, anxious, and dependent (Simmel 1948; Blane 1968); the depressed (Winokur et al. 1969); and the sociopathic (Robins 1966) and/or the minimally brain-damaged (Tarter 1981). Although early studies of prealcoholic personality have been seriously challenged (Syme 1957), more recent reviews of retrospective studies (Tahka 1966; Blum 1966) are in agreement that alcoholics premorbidly are passive-dependent, egocentric, latently homosexual, sociopathic, intolerant of psychic tension, lacking in self-esteem, and frightened of intimacy.

In 1960, when the McCords published the first real prospective study on the prealcoholic personality, these generalizations could be called into question. But even the McCords allowed retrospective hypotheses to come between them and their prospective data. They too suggested that heightened dependency was a cause of alcoholism: "We believe that the confirmed alcoholic increases his intake of alcohol because detoxification satisfies his dependency urges and obliterates reminders of his own inadequacies. We assume that his character is organized around a quest for dependency" (p. 156).

Not until several prospective studies were available could we seriously entertain the hypothesis that the "alcoholic personality" might be secondary to the disorder, alcoholism, and discard the alternative hypothesis that alcoholism merely reflected one symptom of personality disorder.

More recent prospective studies by Jones (1968), Kammeier and colleagues (1973), and Vaillant (1980a) all concur that premorbid traits of dependency do not increase the risk of alcoholism. Jones noted that future problem drinkers were rated by their adolescent peers as significantly more successful on items that reflected social engagement; they were described as being more outgoing and expressive and as being high in assurance, self-acceptance, and good spirits. Jones (1968, 1971) also observed that in junior high school future alcoholics were more often ($p < .01$) described by the following Q-sort items: rapid tempo, deceitful, undercontrolled, not overcontrolled, rebellious, pushes limits, and rejects dependency.

In the College sample, adult psychiatric outcome measures were derived between the ages of 20 and 47, and yet 58 percent of the men who became alcohol abusers did not lose control of their use of alcohol until after age 45. Thus, it was possible to determine if future alcoholics differed from non-alcoholics in young adulthood. The College alcohol abusers did not exhibit more premorbid evidence of dependent personality disorder than men who until age 60 continued to drink asymptomatically (Vaillant 1980a).

Results from the College sample revealed that bleak childhoods, childhood psychological problems, and psychological stability in college did not differentiate future social drinkers from future alcohol abusers; the same variables, however, predicted and presumably played a causal role in the development of "oral traits" (pessimism, passivity, self-doubt, and heightened dependency in adult life). As might be expected, men who displayed many such oral traits also showed evidence as young adults of personality disorders (a lifelong difficulty with loving, with perseverance, and with postponement of gratification). Such "oral-dependent" men were also more anxious and more inhibited about expressing aggression. Yet none of these traits assessed in young adulthood were significantly more common among the alcohol abusers. Once the College men began to abuse alcohol, however, oral-dependent traits were very common.

Prospective study of the College sample also allowed another personality difference that supposedly distinguishes alcoholics from nonalcoholics to be called into question. Using the Thematic Apperception Test (TAT), McClelland and colleagues (1972) had suggested that latent aggressive needs were a significant factor leading to heavy alcohol use. As with so many personality factors, however, this observation could not be confirmed prospectively. The TAT was administered to the College men at age 30, and they were scored for need aggression by a McClelland-trained rater. The scores did not predict subsequent alcohol abuse (Vaillant 1980a).

As adults, the Core City alcoholics appeared twice as likely to manifest psychological dysfunction on Luborsky's Health-Sickness Rating Scale and were six times as likely to be chronically unemployed. But as children, the men who became alcohol-dependent were only slightly more likely to come from multiproblem and welfare-dependent families, and they were no more likely to manifest childhood emotional problems (Table 2.4).

Thus, causal sequences are most important. When an alcoholic client complains that his wife left him for another man and that therefore he lost control over his use of alcohol, experienced alcohol counselors learn to respond with the question: "In the months before she decided to leave you, did your drinking sometimes annoy your wife?" Just so, social scientists must learn to appreciate that alcohol abuse creates dependency and interferes with personality stability more often than the reverse.

Anxiety and Alcohol Abuse

If premorbid personality instability and dependency do not lead to alcoholism, how can we explain the frequently observed association between anxiety and alcohol abuse? Cannot alcohol abuse be explained by alcohol's capacity to reduce tension (Masserman and Yum 1946)? Once again, our perceptions are often illusory. If alcoholism were just a symptom of emotional distress, we might expect that alcohol would be a good tranquilizer. Alcohol should achieve what the alcoholic insists that it does achieve; heavy alcohol ingestion should raise self-esteem, alleviate depression, reduce social isolation, and abolish anxiety. However, work by many investigators suggests that despite what alcoholics tell us, objective observation in the laboratory reveals that chronic use of alcohol makes alcoholic subjects more withdrawn, less self-confident, often more anxious, and commonly more depressed with increased suicidal ideation (McNamee et al. 1968; Tamerin et al. 1970; Nathan et al. 1970; Allman et al. 1972; Logue et al. 1978). Most often the "anxiety" that alcohol is most effective in relieving is the tremulousness, fearfulness, and dysphoria produced by brief abstinence in an alcohol-dependent individual.

Granted, the issue of tension reduction and alcohol use is very complex (Lipscomb et al. 1980). Small amounts of alcohol may briefly change mood for the better; larger amounts of alcohol may reduce guilt, release behavior usually suppressed by punishment, interfere with memory, and nonspecifically alter mental state. Granted, alcohol ingestion will relieve the dysphoric agitation and anxiety associated with physiological arousal; and as tolerance increases, the dose of alcohol needed to produce this effect will increase (Lipscomb et al. 1980). Granted, cross-sectional studies in social drinkers suggest that alcohol ingestion may increase in response to frustration (Marlatt et al. 1975), and alcohol ingestion may promote increased fantasies of power and personal competence (McClelland et al. 1972). Granted, the superego is notoriously "soluble" in ethanol. Any, or all, of these effects may become part of the learning paradigm that leads to alcohol abuse and to the illusion that alcohol is a tranquilizer. Nevertheless, in the treatment of anxiety or depression, such pharmacological effects would not make alcohol superior to barbiturates or to any "active placebo" (and the past 20 years of research have demonstrated that in the treatment of chronic anxiety and depression, barbiturates are no more effective than placebo).

The addict's verbal rationalizations for drug-seeking behavior are highly noticeable, while the actual pharmacological effects of the drugs are often less visible. These two facts distort our views regarding the etiology of drug abuse. For example, in a brilliant series of experiments, Shacter and others (1977) convincingly demonstrated that while smokers do smoke more during parties and under stress, the increase in smoking is not a function of either the social psychology of parties or the capacity of nicotine to relieve tension. Rather, the number of cigarettes that a cigarette addict smokes is in part a function of blood nicotine concentration. Both parties and stress acidify the urine, and acidified urine leads to a more rapid excretion of nicotine, which significantly lowers blood nicotine levels. If under double-blind conditions both party-goers and stressed subjects are fed bicarbonate to make their urine alkaline, then they smoke no more than under control conditions. In reviewing an analogous set of experiments, Marlatt and Rohsenow (1980) have assembled compelling evidence that the alleged relief of tension by alcohol has more to do with expectancy than with pharmacology. Prospective data from both the Core City and the College samples suggest that premorbidly anxious individuals were *not* at increased risk for alcoholism, but that alcohol-dependent individuals were unusually anxious.

〜 Anxiety and Alcohol Abuse Revisited

The last 15 years have somewhat clarified the close association that has been noted between alcoholism and anxiety disorders. Findings from the Epidemiologic Catchment Area studies (Robins et al. 1988) have confirmed that individuals with panic disorder are four times and individuals with phobic disorder are twice as likely as others to be alcoholics. These retrospective findings suggest, but do not prove, that the preexistence of either of these disorders, especially of panic disorder, renders the individual more susceptible to alcoholism. In addition, findings from Caroline Thomas's 40-year prospective study of Johns Hopkins physicians found that chronic anxiety in medical school doubled the risk of future development of alcoholism (Moore et al. 1990). Other reports of anxiety disorders predating alcoholism can also be found (Kushner et al. 1990). Finally, recent work by Higley et al. (1991) has found that monkeys separated from mothers at birth not only show clear biochemical evidence of chronic stress (higher blood and CSF metabolism of norepinephrine) but also voluntarily consume more alcohol than mother-reared controls.

These findings, however, must be tempered by findings from three important sources. First, the family studies of Merikangas and Weissman (Weissman et al. 1984; Merikangas et al. 1985) show that patients with anxiety disorders, *but without alcoholism,* do not possess an increased number of alcoholic relatives. In contrast, individuals manifesting both anxiety disorder and alcoholism do have more alcoholic relatives. These findings are more consistent with the hypothesis that anxiety disorders are often secondary to alcoholism than with the hypothesis that alcoholism is secondary to anxiety disorder.

Second, a careful review by Cappell and Greely (1987) of experimental studies of the relationship between tension reduction and alcohol use and abuse finds the relationship equivocal at best. In addition, the careful studies of air traffic controllers by Rose and colleagues (DeFrank et al. 1987) could not disentangle whether high ingestion of alcohol was the cause or the result of the increased stress.

Third, Brown and her colleagues (1991) studied the relationship between alcohol abuse and state and trait anxiety over time. For four months they repeatedly tested 171 hospitalized male alcoholics, 40 percent of whom reported significant state anxiety on admission. As would be expected, these alcoholics viewed themselves as chronically prone to anxiety and worry and perceived their drinking as a means of self-medicating anxiety. However, when they were given the State Trait Anxiety Inventory over time a clear pattern emerged. After two weeks of abstinence, state anxiety levels, markedly elevated on admission, had returned to normal. At three-month follow-up, if the men remained abstinent, both state and trait anxiety declined still further. Once in the community, if they relapsed, their anxiety levels were again elevated.

In conclusion, on the one hand, just as drugs like meprobamate and barbiturates have rarely been more effective than placebo in treating chronic anxiety states, just so alcohol is probably also not an effective means of self-medication for chronic anxiety. On the other hand, it seems clear that some facets of anxiety (for example, guilt and muscle tension) are effectively relieved by low doses of alcohol, and in some individuals preexisting panic disorder may play an etiologic role in the development of alcoholism.

Depression and Alcohol Abuse

How can we explain the close association between depression and alcoholism? Do not alcoholism and depression often occur in the same families? Yes, but for very complex reasons. Is not alcohol abuse often just a symptom of an individual's futile efforts to self-medicate depression? Perhaps, but this sort of alcohol abuse is often short-lived and would not meet the definitions of alcohol abuse used in this book. Goodwin and Erickson (1979) point out that alcohol ingestion may alter with mood and that mood may alter with alcohol ingestion, but neither fact necessarily leads to the syndrome of alcoholism or primary affective disorder.

There are five lines of evidence to suggest that depression is a symptom caused by alcoholism more often than the reverse. First, several laboratory studies documenting that alcohol ingestion increases rather than reduces depressive and suicidal ideation have already been cited in the discussion of anxiety. There is no good evidence that alcohol, or other sedative drugs for that matter, serve a useful pharmacological function in affective disorders.

Second, the rate of alcohol dependence among patients with bipolar affective disorder, a relatively rare condition, does not seem to be greater than the rate of alcoholism among other psychiatric patients (Woodruff et al. 1973; Morrison 1974). It is true that many bipolar patients when manic may drink excessively; but in an impressive 30-year follow-back study of the life course of over 1700 Scandinavian alcoholics, Sundby (1967) determined that occurrence of psychotic depression was, if anything, less than that observed for the general population.

Third, although Winokur and colleagues (1969) proposed genetic links between alcoholic and depressive disorders and documented that *some* cases of alcoholism may be variants of unipolar affective disorder, Morrison (1975) and Dunner and colleagues (1979) have presented evidence that, in family trees, alcoholism and bipolar affective illness are transmitted independently. Goodwin and Erickson (1979) found that as adults, daughters of alcoholic parents were unusually susceptible to clinical depression if their parents had raised them; but daughters who had been raised by foster parents experienced no more depression than controls.

Fourth, perhaps the most telling argument that alcoholism is not a symptom of primary depressive disorder is derived from recent work by Schlesser and colleagues (1980). Using the dexamethasone suppression test—a test that differentiates most genetically transmitted depression from most purely environmentally induced (secondary) depression—they examined individuals with secondary unipolar depression and individuals with depressive spectrum disease (DSD) (those individuals who met the DSM III criteria for primary depression and had a first-degree relative with antisocial disorder or alcoholism, but none with bipolar disease). They compared both these groups to individuals with bipolar depressive illness and unipolar depression with relatives who also showed depression (FTDD). Ninety-three percent of 41 patients with DSD and 100 percent of 42 patients with secondary unipolar depression, but only 20 percent with FTDD or bipolar depression, showed depression of serum cortisol on the dexamethasone suppression test. The implication is that the depressed relatives of alcoholic and antisocial probands resemble both patients with so-called neurotic depression and patients who are depressed secondary to medical illness. Thus, the depressed relatives of alcoholics may be unhappy not because of a common gene pool but rather because of the slings and arrows of outrageous fortune—for example, living for years with an antisocial or alcoholic relative.

Fifth, as discussed later (Chapter 7) and in an earlier account of the College sample (Vaillant 1980a), alcoholics do not premorbidly manifest either the personality traits or the childhoods known to be associated with secondary depression. Rather, there is compelling prospective evidence that the prolonged abuse of alcohol causes rather than alleviates depression (Kammeier et al. 1977; McLellan et al. 1979).

It is important to keep in mind that anxiety and depression are likely to make any disorder worse. Mental illness and especially depression exacerbate most chronic medical conditions. Coincidental depression will worsen an alcohol abuser's short-term prognosis and increase the likelihood that he will come to clinical attention. The purpose of this chapter is not to deny emotional illness any etiologic role in alcoholism but only to stress that there are other etiological variables that are more specific to alcoholism.

∼ Depression and Alcohol Abuse Revisited

The last 15 years have seen increasing clinical interest in the management of patients comorbid for alcoholism and other major psychiatric disorders. In the case of individuals with schizophrenia and with antisocial personality disorder who also suffer from alcoholism, it has often been clinically efficacious to focus upon the non-alcohol-related diagnosis first. For example, many young adults with antisocial personality disorder engage in drunkenness by decision; once they are mature enough to control their impulsive behavior, they are able to resume social drinking (Goodwin et al. 1971). Similarly, once their psychosis and living arrangements are controlled, many alcohol-abusing schizophrenics cease uncontrolled drinking (Drake et al. 1993).

However, the situation appears to be quite different for depressive disorder. Since the earlier version of this book was published there have been several important studies that support Schuckit's bold assertion that "For about 90 percent of the men and women who have symptoms of alcoholism and depression together, the primary diagnosis is alcoholism not affective disorder" (1986, p. 142).

In his thoughtful and comprehensive summary of the clinical literature Schuckit has summarized the evidence that in the general population alcohol use worsens rather than ameliorates depressive symptoms, and that in perhaps 30 percent of alcohol abusers alcohol abuse can lead to symptoms consistent with major depressive disorder. Such evidence contradicts the popular notion that depressed patients self-medicate with alcohol. It is true that mania is often associated with increased alcohol use, but in only a very small number of cases—Schuckit estimates 5 percent—does mania lead to sufficiently symptomatic drinking to qualify for diagnosis of alcohol abuse. In such cases, of course, lithium maintenance may be essential to controlling the mania and, secondarily, the alcohol abuse.

If alcoholism is but rarely the result of depression, it is often a major cause. For example, Brown and colleagues (1988) found that on admission 74 of 177 hospitalized alcoholics (42 percent) were clinically depressed (that is, had Hamilton Depression Rating Scale (HDRS) scores greater than 19), but that only 11 of these alcoholics (6 percent) exhibited HDRS scores that were still elevated four weeks later.

By reviewing their own work and that of others, Weissman and Merikangas (Weissman et al. 1984; Merikangas et al. 1985; Merikangas and Gelernter, 1990) have clarified the fact that alcoholism and major depressive disorder are genetically quite separate disorders. In a series of studies on the general population, Weissman and coworkers (1984) reported that alcoholism was no more common among the 2,003 first-degree relatives of 335 individuals with major depressive disorder than among individuals whose families were free of depression.

Similarly, Guze and coworkers (1986) conducted a careful family study of 500 representative hospitalized psychiatric patients. They noted that "primary" alcoholism was associated with antisocial personality, drug dependence, and "secondary" depression. Careful study of the first-degree relatives of these patients suggested that the association of alcoholism with drug dependence and antisocial personality occurred for environmental reasons rather than because the three diagnoses represented different facets of a single genetically transmitted disorder. In addition, the relatives of alcoholic patients with "secondary" depression did not show an increased prevalence of either anxiety or affective disorder, but depressed patients with so-called secondary alcoholism did have more alcoholic relatives. Such evidence militates against "secondary" alcoholism being simply due to self-medication.

Recent findings from my own prospective study of the College sample support Schuckit's position that alcohol abuse is usually horse to the cart of depression. At first glance there appeared to be a strong association between major depressive disorder and alcohol abuse in the College sample that contradicted Schuckit's findings. Alcohol-abusing College men were five times more likely than those who did not abuse alcohol to report being severely depressed. This meant that of the 31 men who at some point appeared to manifest major depressive disorder, 14 (44 percent) also manifested alcoholism. After following these men for 25 years, I had the subjective impression that many of the 14 abused alcohol in order to relieve their depression.

However, when the evidence was subjected to blind analysis, my clinical impression proved to be an illusion. One psychiatrist, blind to age of onset of depression, reviewed each man's entire record and estimated the year he first manifested evidence of DSM III alcohol abuse. A second psychiatrist, blind to age of onset of alcoholism, reviewed each man's record and determined the age of onset of major depressive disorder or probable major depressive disorder. In 4 of the 14 cases the psychiatrist looking for evidence of primary depression believed that the depressive symptoms could be entirely explained by alcohol abuse and that the patient did not merit a diagnosis of even secondary depression. In 6 cases the rater noted that the first episode of major depressive disorder had occurred 2 to 33 years (mean 12 years) *after* the patient met the DSM III criteria of alcohol abuse. In only 4 cases had a man's depression actually preceded his alcoholism. Given the prevalence of alcoholism and affective disorder among the 268 men in the College sample, primary alcoholism and primary depression could have occurred together in 6 men by chance alone.

Why, then, do alcoholism and depressive disorder seem to occur together so frequently in clinical settings? I believe there are four major reasons. First, as the findings from the Epidemiologic Catchment Area studies (Regier et al. 1990) indicate, alcoholism and major depressive disorder are the two most common psychiatric disorders. Thus, over a lifetime, chance alone produces frequent comorbidity of alcoholism and depression.

Second, in any series of clinical cases, patients with two disorders are likely to be oversampled. By this I mean that a patient with *mild* depression and *mild* alcohol abuse might go unnoticed if he or she only had one disorder. Again, individuals with two relapsing disorders have roughly twice the chance to be readmitted as patients with one such disorder. Thus, in any clinical series of consecutively admitted patients, patients comorbid for alcohol abuse and depression will be overrepresented.

Third, both alcoholism and depression lead to poor self-care, and poor self-care increases the likelihood of relapse for both alcohol abuse and depression.

Finally, and most relevant, alcoholism is a major *cause* of depression—both for alcohol-abusing individuals and for their close relatives. Summing up the available literature, Merikangas and Gelernter (1990) note: "In general, alcoholic patients with 'secondary' depression appear more similar to alcoholic patients without depression than they are to depressed patients without alcoholism" (p. 619). However, these authors correctly caution that given the heterogeneity of both depression and alcoholism, there may be subtypes of both disorders that share etiologic factors. The most obvious common factor shared by some depressed, alcoholic patients is environmental abuse from an alcoholic parent. For example, half of the children who come to child guidance clinics—most of whom have symptoms of depression—have an alcoholic parent. In contrast, alcoholics who come to alcohol clinics do not have significantly more depressed parents. Investigators often fail to differentiate the genetic from the environmental risks of having a family history positive for alcoholism. For example, because for daughters of alcoholic parents *environmentally* induced depression precedes *genetically* induced alcoholism,

Deykin and colleagues (1987) erroneously conclude that alcoholism reflects self-medication for depression rather than being a result of alcoholic heredity.

This reassessment of causation is highly relevant to treatment strategies for patients comorbid for alcoholism and depression. On the one hand, there is very little evidence that the administration of either tricyclic antidepressants or lithium (pharmacological treatments that are effective in reducing the relapse rate for primary depression) alters the course of alcoholism (Viamontes 1972; Halikas 1983; Dorus et al. 1989). On the other hand, there is abundant evidence that abstinence from alcohol abuse alleviates depression. The most obvious examples are the prospective studies by Brown and colleagues (1988) and by Pettinati and colleagues (1982), which both observed that after one to four years of sobriety many patients formerly comorbid for alcohol abuse and depression are no longer depressed.

A small fraction of alcoholics will also have primary depressive disorders that will benefit from pharmacotherapy, but effective treatment may be jeopardized unless their alcohol abuse is addressed first. If a patient is concurrently abusing alcohol, the maintenance of stable lithium levels is next to impossible, and the risk of a fatal overdose of tricyclic antidepressants will be increased by concurrent alcohol abuse. In short, if a patient is afflicted with both alcoholism and primary affective disorder, it will usually be appropriate to focus on the alcohol abuse first and most forcefully.

Sociopathy and Alcohol Abuse

Is antisocial personality of etiological importance to alcoholism? Robins (1966) and the McCords (1960) found the antecedents of alcoholism and sociopathy to be very similar; but, as already mentioned, both studies were limited by their focus upon a relatively antisocial group of schoolchildren. In such studies, the interweaving of alcoholic heredity and environment with sociopathic heredity and environment could not be unraveled.

In the Core City sample, too, separating alcoholism from sociopathy was not easy. Each of the three scales used to measure alcoholism correlated with the men's sociopathy scale score at an r of .6 or above. This section will test the hypothesis that sociopathy, when it precedes alcoholism, is a result of a nonspecifically unstable and unhappy childhood environment, and that alcoholism, when it precedes sociopathy, is associated with unstable, unhappy childhoods only if such childhoods are a consequence of familial alcoholism.

For the Core City men, who were chosen because they were *not* already antisocial in junior high school, Table 2.12 begins to tease apart the relationships among premorbid personality, alcoholism, and other facets of adult outcome. The table highlights differences in the premorbid antecedents of alcoholism, sociopathy, and poor adult mental health. The first four premorbid variables—childhood environmental strengths, boyhood competence, childhood emotional problems, and I.Q.—all predict poor adult mental health (that is, increased risk of depression, anxiety, and personality disorder). However, these four variables predict sociopathy less well and are only marginally useful in predicting alcoholism. As will be shown, if one controls for familial alcoholism and culture the apparent association between absence of childhood environmental strengths and alcoholism disappears entirely.

The next three variables in Table 2.12—childhood environmental weaknesses (multiproblem families), antisocial parents, and poor infant health—predict sociopathy better than they do either alcoholism or mental health. Recall from Figure 2.1 that the correlation of childhood environmental weaknesses and future alcoholism is a function of parental alcoholism. Our own data and those of the McCords and the Gluecks (1950) all demonstrate that criminal fathers and rejecting mothers correlate more highly with sociopathy than with alcoholism. In Table 2.12 antisocial parents predict sociopathy but not alcoholism, and alcoholic ancestors predict alcoholism but not sociopathy. In separating sociopathy and alcoholism, Bohman's (1978) careful cross-fostering study is suggestive but not conclusive. Bohman studied criminality and alcoholism in 2000 adoptees and in their biological parents. There was a strong association between alcohol abuse in biological parents and alcohol abuse in adopted-away children; but there was not a strong association between criminal behavior in parents and criminal behavior in their adopted-away children. Admittedly, Bohman's findings are opposed by earlier cross-fostering studies (Schulsinger 1972; Crowe 1974; Hutchings and Mednick 1975), which noted a disproportionate number of "criminal" children even if they were separated from their "criminal" parents at birth. In the genesis of sociopathy, it is likely that both nature and nurture play important roles and that the critical experiments remain to be done.

The next four variables in Table 2.12, variables already discussed in the preceding sections, are significantly associated with adult alcoholism but only minimally with sociopathy and not at all with poor mental health. This book argues that alcoholism may usefully be conceptualized as a unitary disorder. Thus, it is significant that the association between alcoholism and the premorbid variables in Table 2.12 was not affected by whether alcohol abuse was

TABLE 2.12. Childhood variables predicting poor adult mental health, sociopathy, and three definitions of alcoholism.[a]

	DSM III (1980) (n = 398)	Cahalan (1970) (n = 399)	PDS (Vaillant 1980a) (n = 442)	HSRS (Luborsky 1962) (n = 378)	Sociopathy (Robins 1966) (n = 430)
Mental health predictors					
Childhood environmental strengths	-.18	-.15	-.14	.21	-.17
Boyhood competence	-.12	-.14	-.11	.24	-.22
Childhood emotional problems	*	*	*	-.19	.13
I.Q.	*	*	*	.15	-.10
Sociopathy predictors					
Childhood environmental weaknesses	.15	.16	.14	-.10	.18
Antisocial parents	*	*	*	-.10	.13
Poor infant health	.11	.10	.09	-.12	.17
Alcoholism predictors					
Alcoholism in parents (1945)	.20	.17	.20	*	.10
Alcoholism in ancestors	.14	.15	.10	*	*
Alcoholism in heredity (1978)	.26	.28	.23	*	.11
Cultural background (Irish= 1, Mediterranean = 4)	-.28	-.25	-.27	*	-.12
Truancy and school behavior problems	.20	.20	.19	*	35
Hyperactivity	.10	.10	.09	*	.12

a. Pearson product-moment correlation coefficient was the statistic used. Significance: * indicates r not significant; r = .08–.10, p < .05; r = .11–.15, p < .01; r > .15, p < .001.

defined according to the medical model of the DSM III or the social deviance model of Cahalan.

The last two variables in Table 2.12, truancy and school behavior problems and hyperactivity, bring us to the heart of our dilemma. Since truancy was one of the 19 items on the Robins scale, it is not surprising that it correlated with the overall Robins score. But truancy was also significantly correlated with each of 13 of the other 18 individual items that made up the Robins scale, and also correlated very significantly with alcoholism. Hyperactivity, regrettably very crudely assessed, was weakly correlated with both alcoholism and sociopathy. The Core City men's scores on the PDS correlated with their score on the Robins scale of sociopathy with an *r* of .67.

Table 2.13 places the importance of premorbid antisocial behavior to alcoholism in a more realistic perspective. The Core City men who at age 14 were truant and exhibited school behavior problems were almost four times as likely as their peers to develop alcohol dependence. Since only 2 of these 16 men clearly abused alcohol before the age of 18, alcohol abuse could not be cited as the cause of their school misbehavior. Equally significant, however, from the viewpoint of etiology, is that serious truancy and school behavior problems were noted in only 9 of the 71 Core City men who became alcohol-dependent. In other words, many sociopaths later abuse alcohol as part of their antisocial behavior; but most alcoholics are not premorbidly sociopathic.

Schuckit (1973) has succinctly summarized the etiological possibilities that link alcoholism and sociopathy. The three possibilities are (1) that sociopaths abuse alcohol as but one symptom of their underlying antisocial personality; (2) that alcoholics manifest sociopathic symptoms as a consequence of their primary alcohol dependence; and (3) that there may be a common factor that underlies both alcoholism and sociopathy.

How one selects one's sample will determine which of Schuckit's three possibilities seems correct. The Robins sample was selected from a child guidance clinic where a majority of the male clients were referred for anti-social behavior; in such a sample, it is not surprising that one in four of the boys later received a sociopathic diagnosis and only one in 12 was diagnosed as a "primary" alcoholic. Seventy percent of Robins's "primary" alcoholics also met her criteria for sociopathy. In such a sample, sociopathy must often be the horse to the cart of alcoholism.

In contrast, among the middle-class College sample sociopathic behavior was almost always a consequence of alcohol abuse (Kammeier et al. 1973;

TABLE 2.13. Relationship of premorbid antisocial behavior to development of alcoholism.[a]

| | Truant or school behavior problems | |
| | Absent | Present |
Alcohol use classification (DSM III)	(n = 381)	(n = 16)
No alcohol abuse	263 (69%)	5 (31%)
Alcohol abuse	58 (15%)	2 (13%)
Alcohol dependence	60 (16%)	9 (56%)

a. Significance $p < .001$ (chi-square test).

Vaillant 1980a). In this second sample, Schuckit's second possibility seems more tenable. In samples selected solely for hyperactivity (Cantwell 1972; Morrison and Stewart 1971), in which both future alcohol dependence and sociopathy appear common, Schuckit's third possibility appears likely.

The Core City men, however, represent a more heterogeneous sample. They were selected in childhood for *not* being antisocial; but, nevertheless, at follow-up, the sample contained a significant number of men who met Robins's criteria for sociopathy. But, in the Core City sample, one in four were later diagnosed as alcohol abusers and only one in 12 (32 men) met Robins's criteria for sociopathy; 7 met the criteria for sociopathy but not for alcohol dependence. For 13 of the 25 Core City men who met Robins's criteria for both sociopathy and alcohol dependence, alcoholism was probably the cause and antisocial behavior merely a symptom. But for the other 12, both Schuckit's first and third possibilities deserve serious consideration.

For the Core City men, Tables 2.14 to 2.16 try to tease apart sociopathy and alcoholism as separate syndromes. The tables contrast the sociopaths (five or more symptoms on the Robins scale) and the alcoholics in Robins's premorbidly antisocial sample with the sociopaths and the alcoholics in the Core City nondelinquent sample. Robins's "primary" alcoholics resemble the Core City alcoholics, and the antisocial symptom patterns of the Core City sociopaths resemble those of Robins's more numerous sociopaths.

As Table 2.14 shows, the alcoholics from both samples were almost as likely as the sociopaths to manifest the Robins scale items of being reckless, promiscuous, belligerent, drug abusing, and often arrested. As a consequence, many alcoholics met the criteria for sociopathy. But there were also differences in many of the Robins items that are congruent with the view that sociopathy

TABLE 2.14. Similarities and differences between sociopaths and alcoholics.

	Sociopaths		Alcoholics	
	Robins *(n = 94)*	*Core City* *(n = 32)*	*Robins* *(n = 33)*	*Core City* *(n = 70)*
Similarities				
5+ symptoms of sociopathy	100%	100%	70%	30%
Heavy drinking	72	91	100	100
Repeated arrests	75	91	58	57
Physical aggression	58	59	49	30
Poor military record	22	25	15	13
Truancy	71	22	73	13
Drug abuse	14	12	6	13
Differences				
Poor work history	83	66	48	29
Public welfare	79	75	27	26
Poor marital history	81	47	46	16
Lack of friends	56	44	30	19
Impulsive behavior	67	34	30	13
Vagrancy	60	34	32	10
Suicide attempts	10	19	6	6
Aliases	29	3	9	1
Pathological lying	16	0	3	0

but not alcohol abuse is a primary personality disorder. Table 2.14 illustrates that compared to alcoholics, both the Robins and Core City sociopaths more often were socially isolated (friendless, dependent on public care, multiply divorced) and lacked a sense of self (demonstrating vagrancy, use of aliases, pathological lying, and inability to work). Had the Core City alcoholics and sociopaths been divided into mutually exclusive groups, these differences might have been still more dramatic.

Another feature that distinguished the Core City sociopaths from the Core City alcoholics was that the sociopaths manifested alcohol abuse at a much earlier age. Fifty-five percent of Core City sociopaths began drinking before age 17 and abusing alcohol by age 21. Only 22 percent of alcohol abusers who did not also meet the criteria for sociopathy began to use alcohol before age 17 and met the criteria for alcohol abuse by age 21.

However, as Table 2.15 illustrates, besides an earlier and more antisocial onset, the pattern of alcohol abuse that developed in Core City sociopaths

TABLE 2.15. Frequency of symptoms of alcohol abuse in Core City sociopaths and alcoholics.

Alcohol-related problem	Alcohol-dependent (n = 71)	Sociopaths[a] (n = 32)
Employer complains	50%	69%
Multiple job losses	41	71
Family/friends complain	93	93
Marital problems	71	63
Medical problems	68	82
Multiple medical problems	30	42
Diagnosis by clinician	56	71
Alcohol-related arrest	76	93
3+ alcohol-related arrests	61	85
Single hospitalization, clinic, or AA visits	59	71
3+ visits to clinics	37	56
2+ blackouts	80	81
Going on the wagon	79	74
Morning tremulousness/drinking	76	63
Tardiness or sick leave	55	62
Admits problem with control	90	71

a. Of these, 21 are included among the 71 men classified alcoholic-dependent by the DSM III criteria.

did not significantly differentiate them from those men who met only the criteria for alcohol dependence. Consistent with the sociopaths' impaired capacity for self-care, they showed a greater tendency, on the one hand, to deny that they experienced problems controlling alcohol use and, on the other, to manifest *multiple* arrests, job losses, hospitalizations, and medical complications.

What is the evidence for Schuckit's third possibility, that a common factor underlies both disorders? Could hyperactivity or minimal brain damage (MBD) prove a common link? Certainly, there are several studies, albeit flawed by retrospective design, which note the tendency for hyperactivity in childhood and sociopathy and alcoholism in adulthood to occur together in the same families (Cantwell 1972; Goodwin et al. 1975; Tarter et al. 1977; Morrison and Stewart 1971). Tarter (1981) asserts that alcoholics who lose control at an early age are truant and easily frustrated as children. He maintains that alcoholics with suggestive evidence of MBD should be regarded as "essential" or "primary" alcoholics and that those with late onset and no school behavior difficulties should be regarded as "secondary" alcoholics. One difficulty with these studies is that they run the risk of labeling premorbid sociopaths the "real" alcoholics. A second problem is that they use recollected symptoms (such as restlessness and impulsivity) and not signs (such as electroencephalographic, psychometric, or soft neurological signs of brain damage) to identify hyperactivity and MBD. Like studies that link alcoholism with unhappy childhoods, these studies fail to control for the alcoholic's distorted memory. Like the studies that suggest links between depression and alcoholism, these studies fail to control for the effects of each of these illnesses upon environment. For example, it is documented that children who grew up with alcoholic parents may be badly behaved, restless, and impulsive as a result of their family's disorganization (Haberman 1966). Without a careful prospective design, and without biologic indicators like dexamethasone suppression tests or neurological signs, nature cannot be separated from nurture.

Unfortunately, the present study of the Core City men manifests equally serious, if rather different, methodological flaws. Its prospective design is cleaner, but the Gluecks' data on which the hyperactivity scale is based were inconsistently gathered, depended largely on schoolroom ratings, and came from youths of roughly age 14, past the age of the maximum risk of hyper-activity. The childhood of each of our subjects was rated for symptoms of hyperactivity drawn from the modification of Wender's Temperament Ques-tionnaire (Wood et al. 1976) that is described in Chapter 7. Such hyperactivity as could be identified after the fact was significantly ($p < .01$) correlated with neglectful mothers, bleak childhood environments, emotional problems, tru-ancy, and sociopathy. However, it was correlated not at all with parental alcoholism and only minimally with the development of alcoholism in the subjects themselves ($r = .10$).

From the Core City data the most rigorous test that could be made of Schuckit's third possibility was to use multiple regression to examine premor-bid variables that might serve as a common etiological factor linking alco-holism with sociopathy.

Multiple regression is a statistical technique that can be used to estimate the unique association of each of two or more interrelated predictor variables (such as childhood weaknesses and parental alcoholism) with a target variable (such as adult alcohol abuse). Regression yields two estimates of the strength of association between each predictor and the target: the *percentage of ex-plained variance* and the *beta weight*. Predictors are entered seriatum into the regression, which assesses the amount of covariance between each predictor and residual variance in the target not accounted for by all predictors previously entered into the analysis. For example, if parental alcoholism is entered first into the analysis, then the association of childhood weaknesses with adult alcoholism disappears—because childhood weaknesses explain no variance in adult alcoholism not already accounted for by parental alcoholism. In multiple regression, therefore, the association of each theoretically causative variable with a target variable can be examined in turn. A variable whose etiological effect on outcome is primary and cannot be explained by its association with other variables will explain "additional variance" even if entered last in the analysis.

Unlike the explained variance, the beta weights for each variable are not affected by the order in which the variables are entered into the multiple regression analysis. The result of a multiple regression analysis can be expressed as a linear equation in which the value of the target variable is predicted from a weighted sum of the predictor variables. Regression techniques select a set of beta weights for each variable that permit the best prediction. Roughly speaking, the greater the beta weight associated with each independent (predictor) variable, the greater its predictive value. As with any correlational technique, multiple regression assesses association, not causation. It allows us to tell how strongly a particular set of (appropriately weighted) variables is associated with alcoholism. It does not tell us why.

The unique contributions of nine variables in Table 2.12 that were most highly correlated with alcoholism and/or sociopathy are examined in Table 2.16. To compensate for the fact that ethnicity was not ranked on a numerical scale, absence of Mediterranean ethnicity was treated as a dichotomous or "dummy" variable. The nine variables were entered into the equation in the order shown in the table.

The remote antecedents of sociopathy and alcoholism appear to be quite different; these differences militate against the possibility of a unifactorial common etiology. Four variables—antisocial parents, poor boyhood competence, multiproblem family membership, and maternal recollection of the subject's poor infant health (being "cranky, nervous, fretful as an infant") accounted for 8.1 percent of the observed variance in the adult Robins score but only 1.7 percent of the variance in the PDS. Excluding truancy, which was an item used to construct the Robins scale, the other four variables when combined explained only 4.5 percent additional variance in sociopathy. Such evidence at least suggests that the etiological variables that distinguish sociopathy from alcoholism are variables related to familial cohesion.

TABLE 2.16. Multiple regression analysis of premorbid variables that were correlated with both alcoholism and sociopathy in the Core City men.

	Sociopathy scale		Problem drinking scale	
Premorbid variable	Explained variance	Beta weight	Explained variance	Beta weight
Absence of Mediterranean ethnicity	2.3%	.11	8.1%	.22
Antisocial parents	1.4	.03	0.1	−.02
Alcoholism in heredity (1978)	0.5	.06	3.4	.20
Hyperactivity	1.7	.03	1.3	.06
Boyhood competence	3.5	−.12	0.5	−.04
Poor infant health	2.0	.17	0.6	.09
Childhood environmental weaknesses	1.2	.06	0.5	.05
Childhood environmental strengths	0.0	−.02	0.0	.00
Truancy/school behavior problems	7.7	.30	2.3	.16
Total explained variance	20%		17%	

Note: Italic type indicates the most significant variables.

In contrast, absence of Mediterranean ethnicity and number of alcoholic relatives explained 11 percent of the observed variance on the PDS, and even when entered last in the multiple regression analysis these variables explained 10.1 percent of the variance. When absence of Mediterranean ethnicity and alcoholic heredity were entered last in the examination of sociopathy, they explained only 1.6 percent of the variance. Such evidence suggests for alcoholism the unique etiological variance had more to do with cultural and genetic factors that directly affected subsequent alcohol use.

It is worth noting that hyperactivity (crudely measured) appeared to explain an equal amount of variance for alcohol abuse and for sociopathy. Certainly, existing studies (Robins 1966; Tarter 1981; and especially Goodwin et al. 1975) suggest that alcoholics are premorbidly more likely to be viewed as hyperactive and as daydreamers. Data from Jones (1968) and from the College sample also suggest that rapid tempo and being undercontrolled in late adolescence characterized many of the College men who went on to become problem drinkers. Table 2.17 displays the premorbid assessment of the personality traits of the College men. On the positive side, prealcoholic College men were less shy, inhibited, and self-conscious than future nonalcoholics and were just as likely to be viewed as sociable, sensible, and vital. One-third of both groups were given the highest rating for future psychological stability (Vaillant 1980a). On the negative side, the prealcoholic College

TABLE 2.17.   Premorbid personality traits that distinguished alcohol abusers from asymptomatic drinkers in the College sample.

Premorbid personality trait	Alcohol abusers $(n = 30)^a$	Asymptomatic $(n = 222)^a$
Different		
Self-driving	3%	16%
Shy	3	21
Inhibited	7	21
Self-conscious	13	27
Lack of purpose and values	37	20
Incompletely integrated	37	12
Same		
Asocial	7	10
Practical, organizing	30	39
Friendly	23	22
Vital affect	23	20
Just so	10	14

a. The sample here includes all 252 of the original 268 men whose premorbid personality traits were rated. Only 204 men were reported in the published account (Vaillant 1980a) of the etiology of these men's alcohol use.

men were significantly more likely (but still in only one-third of the cases) to be seen as "incompletely integrated" (that is, as erratic, unreliable, and manifesting poor judgment) and as "lacking in purpose and values" (that is, as drifting and unenthusiastic). In part, these data may be explained by the heavy college drinking of 5 of the future alcohol abusers, but the data are also consistent with the observation in Table 2.4 that a disproportionate number of future Core City alcohol abusers dropped out of school before the tenth grade.

The data presented in this section suggest that in premorbid personality the majority of alcoholics may be no different from nonalcoholics and that, at least for the Core City men, there was no common etiological factor underlying both sociopathy and alcoholism. It seems doubtful that Schuckit's third possibility, a major common factor underlying sociopathy and alcoholism, will be identified. However, the childhood data on the Core City men were gathered two decades before the syndrome of hyperactivity was recognized; and this variable deserves further scrutiny as a premorbid variable that may contribute to *both* sociopathy and alcoholism.

What seems clear is that both of Schuckit's first two possibilities are important. Thus, even if sociopathy and alcoholism have complex and in many respects quite different multifactorial etiologies, as soon as one disorder is present the second is likely to follow. On the one hand, sociopaths are very unhappy people who seek to alter the way they feel by abusing many kinds of drugs—one of which, in Western society, is likely to be alcohol. On the other hand, as a result of the pharmacological effects of alcohol, individuals who become habituated to alcohol are likely to violate enough social canons to meet diagnostic criteria for sociopathy.

∿ Sociopathy and Alcohol Abuse Revisited

Zucker and Gomberg (1986) sharply criticized the etiological conclusions in this chapter, suggesting that they "dismissed childhood effects out of hand." In their critique, Zucker and Gomberg underscored what I have also acknowledged: that the Core City sample of nondelinquents did not adequately reflect the contribution of "antisocial personality" to alcohol abuse. They noted that prior studies had observed that higher levels of activity and difficulties in school achievement characterize the childhoods of future alcoholics. They pointed out that in the Core City sample, too, even controlling for I.Q., future alcoholics did have lower educational attainment than their nonalcoholic peers. However, Zucker and Gomberg admitted that such personality attributes could not be separated from the premorbid attributes of antisocial disorder *per se.*

In reviewing their criticisms, I believe that in part Zucker and Gomberg simply could not believe the paradigm shift created by prospective studies, which rule out childhood personality as a principal cause of alcohol dependence. The illusion produced by poorly controlled, cross-sectional studies was too compelling. As Lindström (1992) points out, "investigators were often so convinced that alcoholism must be a symptom of underlying personality disorder that it simply did not occur to them that it might be an affliction with a life of its own and with other antecedents than poor mental health" (p. 72). Earlier investigators simply could not believe that the association between parental and child alcoholism might be more hereditary than environmental. Thus, like the McCords, Zucker and Gomberg preferred to ignore genetic factors and to place the blame for subsequent alcoholism on the child's distance from the father, on marital conflict, and on disrupted childhood families. They failed to be impressed by the fact that Core City youth who grew up in intact families but with alcoholic biological parents were at four or five times greater risk of developing alcoholism than those who grew up in severely disrupted families but did not have an alcoholic biological parent. In other words, parental conflict is associated with greater risk of alcoholism *only* when that conflict is an indicator of parental alcoholism.

Zucker and Gomberg also failed to cite work by Beardslee, a dynamically oriented child psychiatrist, who in an effort to demonstrate the importance of environmental and personality variables conducted careful blind reviews of the childhood data gathered on the College sample (Beardslee and Vaillant 1984) and on the Core City sample (Beardslee et al. 1986). Although Beardslee focused on putative environmental familial contributions to alcoholism, such as those suggested by Zucker and Gomberg, he was unable to distinguish future alcoholics from matched controls at better than chance levels. By way of contrast, he was able to identify, on the basis of disrupted childhoods, those subjects who in the future would be classified as mentally ill for reasons other than alcoholism.

The best argument for the influence of childhood personality upon alcoholism comes from work by Bohman and Cloninger (Cloninger et al. 1988a) in their reanalysis of 431 children (233 boys and 198 girls), half of whom were adopted in infancy. The children's personalities were studied intensively at age 11, and they were studied for alcoholism at age 27. But when examined closely, the data from this study merely support the already clear association between antisocial personality and alcohol abuse.

In their conclusions Cloninger and coworkers suggest that boys who were high in harm avoidance and low in novelty seeking (that is, neurotic, obsessional, overcontrolled) as well as boys low in harm avoidance and high in novelty seeking (that is, antisocial) were at high risk for alcoholism. Although the researchers used complex, statistically sophisticated techniques, their conclusions can be challenged. For as with the arguments of Zucker and Gomberg, once antisocial youth and alcoholic parents are controlled for, other childhood personality variables seem unimpressive. For example, if one looks more closely at Cloninger and Bohman's actual numbers, only 2 of their 13 high-harm-avoidance youth became alcoholic (Cloninger et al. 1988a, table 13), the same proportion as would have been expected by chance. In contrast, 16 (28 percent) of the 57 high-novelty-seeking youth were registered with Temperance boards, had arrests for drunkenness, or had been treated for alcoholism. Another difficulty with Cloninger's data is that in a youthful population identified in this way, transient misbehavior in antisocial youth due to drunkenness can be confounded with alcohol dependence. Longer follow-up is needed.

Finally, Cloninger and his colleagues, like Zucker and Gomberg, fail to distinguish *hereditary* personality traits from *environmental* personality traits that are secondary to being raised by alcoholic fathers. For example, in a careful study of 127 male and 87 female adoptees, Cadoret and colleagues (1985) were able to separate environmental from genetic influence. Alcohol abuse in adopted men and women was not increased by their having first-degree relatives with antisocial problems and, by inference, traits high in novelty seeking and low in harm avoidance. Nor did increased antisocial behavior occur in adoptees whose biological relatives had been alcoholic. The conclusion that may be drawn from Cadoret's data is that high-novelty-seeking, low-harm-avoidance personality traits may be transmitted genetically from antisocial relatives or acquired for environmental reasons in a disrupted family environment.

Failure to separate heredity from environment has also led to what, I believe, is the misleading distinction between Type 1 and Type 2 alcoholism. In the last ten years this dichotomy has received increasing notice (von Knorring et al. 1985, Cloninger, 1987a; Nordstrom and Berglund 1987a). Type 1 alcoholism is believed to affect both sexes and to have a relatively late onset (after age 25). Alcohol-related problems are relatively mild and rarely involve antisocial activity. Female alcoholic relatives are common. Type 1 alcoholics are thought to demonstrate the personality trait of high harm avoidance; thus, they are cautious, inhibited, more likely to worry, and to feel guilt over their alcoholism (Cloninger 1987b). They are unlikely to manifest the personality trait of seeking out novel and challenging events. Instead, they are postulated to use alcohol for its antianxiety effects and to be prone to binge drinking.

Clinically, the hypothesized Type 2 alcoholic is a man with an early onset of alcoholism (before age 25). He manifests a history of violence and illegal activity both with and without alcohol use and is more often a polydrug abuser. He is hypothesized to demonstrate the personality traits of low harm avoidance (little need for social approval and a lack of inhibition) and high novelty seeking (Cloninger 1987a). Thus he uses alcohol for its euphoric effects, and he is more likely to develop alcohol dependence. He is thought to be more likely to have male than female alcoholic relatives.

A hypothesis closely related to the Type 1/Type 2 distinction is the older "process/reactive" hypothesis (Levine and Zigler 1973), which posits that the course of alcoholism primarily due to genetic predisposition may be different from that of alcoholism that is primarily a result of environmental factors. As already noted, other studies (Tarter et al. 1977; Goodwin 1979; Cloninger et al. 1981) have suggested that alcoholics with heavy genetic loading may reflect "primary" alcoholism and may be analogous to individuals with juvenile-onset diabetes or process schizophrenia. This hypothesis is based on the clinical observation that alcoholism in individuals with many alcoholic relatives begins earlier, has a worse prognosis, and is more severe. In contrast, alcoholism that occurs in individuals without known alcoholic relatives has a relatively good prognosis, begins later, and is less severe. It has been suggested that the latter form of alcoholism is "secondary" to depression and other environmental risk factors and that Type 1 alcoholism is analogous to reactive schizophrenia and adult-onset diabetes.

But before the Type 1/Type 2 hypothesis can be believed, it first must be tested in a relatively normal community sample. Second, the environmental effects of alcoholic parents must be distinguished from the genetic effects of alcoholic parents. And third, the age during which the alcoholics are being studied must be controlled.

Certainly, if one studies young, antisocial, socially disadvantaged alcoholics, they tend to have alcoholic fathers, become alcoholic early, and show low harm avoidance. In contrast, late-onset, middle-class alcoholics often have better social adjustment and manifest less risk-taking behavior, and may have grown up without identified alcoholic parents. The difficulty with most such studies is that they are not drawn from homogeneous community samples and fail to control for antisocial personality disorder, a syndrome associated with, but genetically and environmentally distinct from, "primary" alcoholism (Bohman 1978, Vaillant 1983).

A second difficulty with the Type 1/Type 2 dichotomy is that it is reductionistic. Investigators who have concluded that genetic factors are responsible for alcohol abuse that begins earlier and is associated with greater social deviance have conducted studies in which the environmental contribution of alcoholic parents was ignored. (Goodwin et al. 1971; Buydens-Branchey et al. 1989; Cloninger et al. 1981). In placing the distinctions between Type 1 and Type 2 alcoholism on a genetic basis Cloninger (1987a) failed to control for the important environmental variables emphasized by McCord and McCord (1960), Robins and colleagues (1962), and Zucker and Gomberg (1986) as important in shaping alcoholic symptomatology.

Third, individuals alleged to manifest Type 1 and Type 2 personalities must be contrasted with others of the same age. The personalities of most people, including alcoholics, change between ages 16 and 46. By this I mean that many novelty-seeking, harm-ignoring adolescents grow up into novelty- and harm-avoiding parents.

In studying a multifactorial illness like alcoholism, rather than focusing on different alcoholic typologies, it may be more useful to focus on the relative contribution of different risk factors—for example, environment *and* heredity—to a unitary disorder. To assess the validity of the Type 1/Type 2 hypothesis, therefore, I have taken advantage of the two socioeconomically (that is, environmentally) very divergent Core City and College samples. *Within* each sample there were good data on both alcoholic heredity and alcoholic environment. The alcohol-abusing members of these two cohorts experienced very different ages of onset and alcoholic careers, but rather similar patterns of alcoholic heredity.

Among the 38 identified alcohol abusers within the College sample for whom we had data on alcoholic relatives, 16 (42 percent) had two or more alcohol-abusing relatives. The mean age of onset of alcoholic abuse in these men was 40.1 years. Eleven (29 percent) of the College alcohol abusers had no known alcoholic relatives. Their mean age of onset of alcoholism was 43.5 years, not significantly different from the age of onset of the men with several alcoholic relatives. However, of the 4 College men who became alcoholic by age 20, 2 grew up living with an alcoholic father and a third with an alcoholic mother. In other words, age of onset seemed predicted by environmental, not genetic factors.

Among the 150 identified alcohol abusers within the Core City sample, 85 (57 percent) had two or more known alcohol-abusing relatives. Their mean age of onset of alcoholism was 29.2 years. There were 43 (29 percent) Core City alcohol abusers with no known alcohol-abusing relatives; their mean age of onset was 29.3 years. In short, although the two samples did not differ significantly in their number of alcoholic relatives, the age of onset of alcohol abuse was 11 years earlier for the socially disadvantaged men *without* alcoholic relatives than for College men *with many* such relatives. This finding contradicts the Type 1/Type 2 hypothesis and suggests a role for environment in determining age of onset of alcohol abuse. For example, the Core City men were roughly ten times as likely as the College men to have come from multiproblem families, to exhibit multiple traits of sociopathy, to have criminal parents, and to have spent time in jail.

Tables 2.17A and 2.17B, which look at the Core City men in greater detail, confirm that age of onset of alcoholism seems more influenced by environmental than by biological factors. Table 2.17A suggests that from the point of view of biology and of clinical course the 40 Core City men who met DSM III criteria for alcohol abuse when young were very similar to those

TABLE 2.17A. Association of "biological" factors with age of onset of alcoholism in the Core City sample.

	n	9–21 n = 40	22–34 n = 69	35–57 n = 40
		Age at onset of alcoholism		
No alcoholic relatives	43	12 (30%)	20 (29%)	11 (27%)
2+ alcoholic relatives	95	21 (53%)	40 (58%)	24 (60%)
Alcohol-dependent (ever)	77	22 (55%)	38 (55%)	17 (43%)
Stable abstinence (age 60)	47	13 (33%)	22 (32%)	12 (30%)
Chronic alcoholism (age 60)	44	11 (27%)	15 (22%)	18 (45%)
Hyperactivity (age 12–14)	16	7 (18%)	4 (6%)	5 (13%)

Note: None of these relationships is significant.

who developed the disorder in midlife. Early-onset Core City alcoholics had no more genetic loading than Core City men with late onset; they were no more likely to meet criteria for alcohol dependence and no less likely by age 60 to achieve stable abstinence. In addition, in contradiction to the hypothesis that early-onset antisocial alcoholism is transmitted through male genetic linkage (Cloninger et al. 1981), the mean age of onset of the 14 Core City alcoholics with alcoholic mothers was 28.2 years; it was 29.4 years for Core City alcohol abusers whose mothers were not also afflicted.

The within-cohort comparison of the Core City men in Table 2.17B confirms the between-cohort comparison noted previously: namely, that men with early-onset alcoholism were much more likely to have grown up in disrupted families. The cause of such disruption was often, but not always, associated with parental alcoholism. In addition, men with early-onset alcoholism were more likely to be antisocial *before* (that is, to have had behavior problems in junior high school) and *after* (that is, to have manifested 5+ sociopathic traits) their development of alcoholism. While early-onset alcoholics were no more likely to meet criteria for alcohol dependence, they were twice as likely to conform to the definition of Cahalan's socially deviant "problem" drinker. In addition, binge drinking, a symptom that on theoretical grounds has been classified as a "loss of control" Type 1 trait (Cloninger et al. 1988a), actually occurred more often in the early-onset antisocial than in the late-onset Core City alcoholics.

The conclusions to be drawn from Table 2.17B are that genetic loading is an important predictor of *whether* an individual develops alcoholism and that

TABLE 2.17B.   Association of "environmental" factors with age of onset of alcoholism in the Core City sample.

	n	Age at onset of alcoholism		
		9–21 n = 40	22–34 n = 69	35–57 n = 40
"Multiproblem" family	25	10 (25%)	11 (16%)	4 (10%)
Warm childhood	63	12 (30%)	31 (45%)	19 (48%)[a]
Alcoholic caretaker	79	30 (75%)	32 (46%)	17 (43%)[a]
Abuse from alcoholic caretaker	38	15 (38%)	16 (23%)	7 (18%)[a]
Delinquent parent	52	15 (38%)	27 (39%)	10 (25%)
5+ sociopathic traits	27	15 (38%)	10 (14%)	2 (5%)[b]
Ever in jail	26	10 (25%)	14 (20%)	2 (5%)[a]
Binge drinker	68	26 (65%)	31 (45%)	11 (28%)[b]
School behavior problems	13	8 (20%)	4 (6%)	1 (3%)[a]
"Problem" drinker (Cahalan Scale)	70	28 (70%)	29 (42%)	13 (33%)[b]
Multiple alcohol-related arrests	54	20 (50%)	28 (41%)	6 (15%)[b]

a. $p < .05$
b. $p < .01$

an unstable childhood environment is an important predictor of *when* an individual loses control of alcohol.

The above findings underscore that the Type 1/Type 2 hypothesis ignores three important facets of alcoholism: first, that most individuals with antisocial personality disorder abuse alcohol in their youth; second, that alcoholic parents affect their children's environment as well as their heredity; third, that symptoms of alcoholism, like those of all chronic illnesses, are affected by an individual's age.

Let me discuss these three facets one at a time. In a series of linked papers (Schuckit and Irwin 1989; Irwin et al. 1990; Schuckit et al. 1990) the authors have called into serious question both the Type 1/Type 2 hypothesis and the relation to alcoholic heredity of the tridimensional personality questionnaire score (Cloninger 1987b) on which the hypothesis is based. They suggest that the Type 1/Type 2 hypothesis is seriously weakened if individuals with antisocial personality are removed from the sample. Through a careful literature review, Schuckit and Irwin (1989) note that the Type 2 pole of alcoholism cannot be distinguished from antisocial personality (high novelty seeking and low anxiety over harm and punishment). In addition, they also point out that von Knorring (von Knorring et al. 1985, 1987), whose work is often cited as supporting the Type 1/Type 2 distinction, found that neither personality nor age of onset consistently distinguished alcoholics classified Type 2 from those classified Type 1.

Cloninger's own data, when examined closely, do not hold up when antisocial subjects are excluded. Cloninger and colleagues (1988a, 1988b) stress that their larger sample size justifies their multivariate and complex statistical procedures. However, as already noted, once one excludes these antisocial youth, Cloninger's numbers do not support his statistics. Littrell (1988) has also criticized Cloninger's statistical analysis on other grounds.

Second, discussions of the etiology of alcoholism often fail to distinguish the effects of parental environment from those of heredity (Searles 1988). It is well known that an unstable childhood family environment leads to delinquency (Rutter 1992), that delinquents abuse drugs of many sorts, and that they are more likely than nondelinquents to manifest many symptoms shared with alcoholics (Vaillant 1983; Earls et al. 1988). Thus, it is not surprising that alcoholics who developed alcoholism when young were eight times as likely to manifest several sociopathic traits as late-onset alcoholics who had just as many alcoholic relatives. Put differently, of the four premorbid risk factors that contributed unique variance to whether a Core City youth would eventually develop alcoholism (heredity, ethnicity, hyperactivity, and school behavior problems) only school behavior problems—which also predicted delinquency—predicted the age of onset of alcohol abuse. When Beardslee and colleagues (1986) reanalyzed the contribution of genetic loading and the environmental disruption produced by having an alcoholic parent, they could discern no effect of the number of blood relatives on the age of onset of alcoholism or on its severity. Family history of alcoholism only affected whether the men developed alcohol dependence. In contrast, an unstable familial environment in itself did not predict *whether* a man subsequently lost control of alcohol, only *when* he developed alcoholism and whether he would be severely symptomatic and antisocial. In their study of male alcoholics subtyped by family history and antisocial personality Hesselbrock and colleagues (1985) also found that number of alcoholic relatives predicted *whether* dependence on alcohol would occur and having antisocial relatives predicted *when* such dependence would occur.

Third, the Type 1/Type 2 hypothesis may be in part an artifact of adult development. Certainly, the later the onset of any chronic illness (such as diabetes or schizophrenia), the more likely it is to have a relatively benign course. In addition, adolescents who are high in novelty seeking and low in harm avoidance may in midlife display personalities that seem quite the reverse. In their studies of monozygotic and dizygotic twins Pickens and colleagues (1991) underscore that in contrast to alcohol dependence, periods of "insobriety" were strongly age-graded and relatively independent of genetic factors. In a youthful population when alcoholism is diagnosed as it was by Bohman and Cloninger through misbehavior associated with alcohol use, the state of drunkenness can be confounded with the trait of alcohol dependence. Longer follow-up of Cloninger and Bohman's sample is needed to identify which of their temperance board registrants will meet the criteria for alcohol dependence.

A Case Example

The case history of "James O'Neill" illustrates the difference between the sociopath who abuses alcohol and the alcoholic who develops sociopathic behavior. In light of O'Neill's behavior when drinking, the reader will find it difficult to believe that O'Neill—prior to his alcohol abuse—had been judged by the College Study staff in 1950 to belong "in the unqualified group in terms of ethical character," and that the director of the health services had described O'Neill as a "sufficiently straightforward, decent, honest fellow, should be a good bet in any community."

James O'Neill came to psychiatric attention in 1957, 17 years after joining the College sample. His veteran's hospital chart revealed a 36-year-old man, a father of four, and a former assistant professor of economics who was being admitted to a psychiatric hospital for the first time. He complained of being a "failure at his marital and professional responsibilities because of drinking and missing teaching appointments." His admission note stated, "present symptoms include excessive drinking, insomnia, guilt and anxiety feeling." The diagnosis was "behavior disorder, inadequate personality."

Over an eight-month hospital stay, the following history was obtained: "According to the patient's statement, his drinking and gambling began in the summer of 1948, when he became depressed because he did not do well on his Ph.D. generals and was refused entrance into a fellowship organization. The patient at this time began to drink during the day, and to miss teaching appointments; however, he continued to teach and to keep his family together." He obtained his Ph.D. without difficulty, and in 1955 he transferred from the faculty of the University of California at Berkeley to the University of Pennsylvania.

In psychiatric interviews in 1957, O'Neill showed little emotion,

> although he clearly expressed his suspicions and anger through the people that he talked about. His pattern of drinking, sexual infidelity, gambling and irresponsible borrowing led him to recognize from his reading that it adds up to diagnosis of psychopathic personality—especially since he has experienced no real remorse about it. Since he gave some books to his son to sell, and among them were four books from the university library, he was accused of stealing books and shortly afterwards discharged for moral turpitude. He claims he did not sell university books knowingly.
>
> During all of the time he was frequenting bars, contacting bookies and registering in hotels to philander, he always used his own name. It's interesting when he was carrying on his nefarious pursuits, he got considerable satisfaction out of it being known that he was a professor . . . There is a difference between his relationship with women and his relationship with men. First of all, when his mother died in 1949, he felt no remorse at her death. He did not remember the year of his mother's death, and in view of the fact that he dates his extracurricular activities as beginning about nine years ago, this confusion is probably significant. He speaks warmly of his two sons, feeling that they like him—although he's not much of a father. His oldest son has none of his boy scout badges, because he has not been able to come to his father for help.
>
> On admission the patient was placed in group therapy twice a week. During his eight-month hospital stay the patient was taken into individual therapy three times a week. In therapy, the patient was able to work out a great deal of feelings toward his family, in particular toward his mother and also toward his wife. The patient felt quite hostile and anxious about the fact that he was an Army brat and *never* had a normal childhood and that his parents were always very cold and grown-up toward him. He harbored many feelings of hostility toward his wife whom he feels does not appreciate the fact that she's married to such an intelligent college professor, and all she wants is to have money and bigger homes.

The discharge diagnosis was "anxiety reaction manifested by feelings of ambivalence about his family and his parents and his work." The precipitating stress was considered to be "death of the patient's mother and a long history of drinking and gambling and going into debt." His predisposition was considered to be "an emotionally unstable personality for the past 20 years." A diagnosis of alcoholism was never even considered.

Fortunately for our investigation, James O'Neill had been one of the College sample chosen as a college sophomore for psychological health. In college, he had undergone several psychiatric interviews, psychological tests, and a home interview of his parents. Thus, there was in existence prospectively gathered information about James O'Neill.

A child psychiatrist blind to O'Neill's life after age 18 was asked to compare his childhood environment with those of his College sample peers. His childhood fell in the top third. The rater summarized the raw data on his family as follows:

> O'Neill was born in a difficult delivery. The mother was told not to have more children. His parents were reliable, consistent, obsessive, devoted parents. They were relatively understanding; their expectations appear to have been more non-verbal than explicit. The father was characterized as easy to meet, the mother was seen as more quiet; no alcoholism was reported. Warmth, thoughtfulness and devotion to the home were some of the comments. The subject spoke of going to his father first with any problems, and of being closer to his mother than to his father. His peer relations were reported to have been good, and little or no conflict with his parents was reported.

The child psychiatrist wrote that she would predict that "the young student would develop into an obsessional, hard-working, non-alcoholic citizen, whose work would be related to law, diplomacy and possibly teaching. He would rely on his intellect and verbal abilities to help in his work. He would probably marry and be relatively straight with his children. He would probably expect high standards from them."

Before O'Neill was 30, other observers had summed him up equally favorably. In college the dean's office ranked his stability as "A"; the internist of the college study described him as "enthusiastic, whimsical, direct, confident, no grudges or chips, impressed me as an outstanding fellow." The staff psychiatrist was initially greatly impressed by O'Neill's "combination of warmth, vitality and personality," and put him in the "A" group. Later, the same psychiatrist commented that the subject was "not too sound, showed mood fluctuations and hypomania." However, upon his college graduation the Grant Study staff consensus was that O'Neill should be ranked in the top third of this group of sophomores already preselected for psychological health. When O'Neill was 23 his commanding officer wrote that O'Neill gave "superior" attention to duty and that the officer "particularly desired him."

When he was 21, O'Neill married his childhood girlfriend. He had been in love with her since age 16, and in 1950, six years after they married, the marriage still seemed solid.

From the prospective record, it was also possible to record a more accurate sequence of O'Neill's feelings about his mother's death. The child psychiatrist from the prospective record had called their mother-child relationship among the best in the study. In 1950, six months after the death of his mother, a study observer had said that the subject felt the loss of his mother deeply. At the time of her death, his mother's physician had remarked that O'Neill "was devoted and helpful during the illness." It was only seven years later during his V.A. hospital admission that O'Neill reported having no feelings toward his mother and blamed her alleged coldness for his current unhappiness. Over time alcoholics develop excellent collections of "resentments."

It was not until 22 years later that O'Neill brought the study up to date on the progression of his alcoholism. He began drinking heavily in 1948 and by 1950 had begun morning drinking. By 1951 his wife's uncle, an early member of Alcoholics Anonymous, had suggested the possibility of alcoholism. However, the same year his own university's health services diagnosed him as having "combat fatigue," and his wife insisted to the College Study that he was not abusing alcohol. O'Neill admitted to me in 1972 that between 1952 and 1955 he had written his Ph.D. thesis while chronically intoxicated, and that he had regularly sold books from the university library in order to support his drinking. By 1954 his wife began to complain about his drinking; by 1955 it was campus gossip. In his 1957 and 1962 hospital admissions, the diagnosis of alcoholism was still not made, and O'Neill himself did not understand the cause-and-effect relationship.

Indeed, in October 1972 O'Neill described himself to me as having been "a classical psychopath, totally incapable of commitment to any man alive." I felt much more that he was a loner but a kindly man. In appearance he was balding and sported a distinguished mustache and elegant, if worn, clothes. At first during the interview he had a lot of trouble looking at me and seemed terribly restless. He chain-smoked, walked back and forth, lay down first on one bed and then on the other. Although he avoided eye contact, however, there was a serious awareness of me as a person and I always felt he was talking to me. He behaved like a cross between a diffident professor and a newly released prisoner of war, rather than like a person truly frightened of human contact.

I never got the feeling that O'Neill was cold or self-absorbed. If anything, he suffered from hypertrophy, not agenesis, of the conscience. His mental status revealed an energetic man who kept a tight rein on his feelings. As he put it to me, "I'm hyper-emotional; I'm a very oversexed guy. The feelings are there, but it's getting them out that's hard. The cauldron is always bubbling. In Alcoholics Anonymous, I'm known as Dr. Anti-Serenity."

In 1970 O'Neill became sober and a member of Alcoholics Anonymous. In his interview he made frequent reference to AA, which, besides his wife, was now clearly the most important relationship in his life. I asked him what his dominant mood was, and he said "incredulity . . . I consider myself lucky, most people in Alcoholics Anonymous do."

As I was leaving O'Neill's apartment I noted several books related to gambling on his bookshelf and wondered if this remained an interest. O'Neill said that he had now sublimated his interest in gambling by becoming a consultant to the Governor of Massachusetts in setting up the state lottery in Massachusetts—a considerably more profitable occupation than frequenting racetracks. In other words, with the remission of alcoholism, O'Neill's ego functioning had matured. Instead of acting out his compulsive gambling, he had harnessed that interest in a socially and personally constructive way.

In closing, O'Neill told me he could not agree with Alcoholics Anonymous in calling alcoholism a disease. "I think that I will the taking of a drink. I have a great deal of shame and guilt and remorse and think that's healthy." I heartily disagreed; I suspect that his shame had facilitated his denial of his "disease" for two decades.

Frank Moore, the vagabond protagonist of Robert Strauss's fascinating monograph *Escape from Custody* (1974), whose career as a skid-row alcoholic is painstakingly followed from age 39 to age 70, serves as a foil for James O'Neill. Between the ages 43 and 60, Moore spent almost 90 percent of his time in prison or in hospital settings, and his diagnosis of alcoholism was never in question. Frank Moore, however, did not begin as an alcoholic. His mother had been the unhappy daughter of his unhappy grandmother. His grandmother wished her grandson, Frank, would die when he was in the uterus of her 18-year-old daughter. Frank's father, discharged from the navy on psychiatric grounds, committed suicide five months after Frank's birth. Then, before Frank was 2, his mother abandoned him to a cold, disinterested grandfather, only to return to care for him herself when he was 12. Having repeated the ninth grade, Frank dropped out of school at 15 and at 16 ran off to the navy. Before Frank ever touched alcohol, he had already received a dishonorable military discharge and been sent to Alcatraz. He probably was imprisoned over a hundred different times; and since he spent nine-tenths of his middle adult life in institutions, he probably spent only a very small fraction of his adult life actually intoxicated. Yet the clinical diagnosis of this premorbid sociopath was alcoholism. Homeless, he learned to use this diagnosis as a ticket for shelter. Strauss documents that Frank Moore, the sociopath, was counted in literally hundreds of alcoholic admission statistics. His life would have kept a small alcohol detoxification ward busy for a year and surely convinced them that alcoholics are untreatable. Frank Moore, however, was nearly as crippled when sober as when drinking. Thus, Moore was a sociopath who was often diagnosed alcoholic; O'Neill was an alcoholic erroneously diagnosed a sociopath.

Other Etiological Factors

This chapter has focused largely on childhood risk factors. There are, however, many adult etiological factors that also affect the probability that an individual will develop alcohol dependence. Several of the most important demographic predictors of heavy drinking—religion, social class, community size, and sex—exert their effect so indirectly (Cahalan 1970) that they will not be considered here. Indeed, the effects of such broad demographic variables may be largely mediated through the more discrete factors to be cited in this section. Because alcoholism occurs less often in women than in men, many have speculated that alcoholism in women may be different (Schuckit et al. 1969; Winokur et al. 1971). Certainly, among women who abuse alcohol more etiological risk factors are usually present and in greater severity (Hesselbrock 1981), and alcohol metabolism is affected by sex differences (Camberwell Council on Alcoholism 1980). However, several recent studies suggest that in most respects female alcohol abusers do not differ from their male counterparts (Cahalan et al. 1969; Reich et al. 1975; Eshbaugh et al. 1980; Chatham et al. 1979).

The most important factor in alcoholism, of course, is the fact that alcohol can produce physiological and psychological habituation. However, the use—without abuse—of alcohol is endemic throughout much of the world. Thus, in the attempt to understand why alcohol use evolves into a disorder, appreciation of host resistance becomes more important than appreciation of the fact that alcohol is addicting. Most of us are exposed to the primary cause of alcoholism—alcohol—and yet we do not become dependent. Why?

For example, in the nineteenth century when a large number of children were accidentally given a massive inoculation of live tuberculosis bacilli, one-third died, one-third became ill and recovered, and one-third manifested only superficial skin lesions (Vaillant 1962). Why? To understand the etiology of tuberculosis, we must do more than understand germ theory; we must pay attention to host resistance. We must do the same for alcoholism.

In other studies, at least six factors have been well documented that significantly affect host resistance to alcohol dependence. The first factor is the rapidity with which alcohol reaches the brain. The rate at which a mood-altering drug is absorbed from the intestine and the rate of onset of its pharmacological effects upon the central nervous system alter both its capacity to produce a subjective "high" and its potential for abuse. Thus, cultural patterns that encourage consumption of low-proof alcoholic beverages or that direct that alcohol be drunk only with food—which delays intestinal absorption of alcohol—reduce the likelihood that an individual will develop dependence (Jellinek 1960). In contrast, drinking practices that encourage high-proof alcohol to be ingested in the absence of food (for example, in inner-city bars and in the gin mills at the perimeter of Indian reservations) increase the likelihood of alcohol dependence. Fasting is known to slow the metabolism of alcohol and prolong elevated blood alcohol levels (Mendelson 1970). Indeed, any cultural or familial custom that preferentially encourages consumption of high-proof distilled spirits over low-proof fermented beverages will tend to increase the risk of alcohol abuse.

Second, occupation is an important contributing factor (Plant 1979)—especially occupations that break down the time-dependent rituals that help to protect "social" drinkers from round-the-clock alcohol consumption. Occupations like bartending and the diplomatic service put an individual in close contact with alcohol during the day. Similarly, unemployment and occupations, like writing and journalism, that deprive an individual of the structure of the working day and therefore facilitate drinking at odd times are associated with increased rates of alcoholism. However, alcoholism may also affect occupational choice. Certain occupations that are free of excessive supervision and structure—traveling sales, roofing, housepainting—often attract individuals who already have well-established drinking problems.

The third factor is often related to the second. The drinking habits of an individual's immediate social group powerfully affect how the individual uses or abuses alcohol (Bacon 1957; Cahalan and Room 1972; Jessor and Jessor 1975; Plant 1979). It has been consistently shown that the heavy-drinking adolescent can be distinguished from his or her more abstemious peers by social extroversion, adventurousness, mild deviance, dependence on peer-group pressure, independence from parental or religious-group pressure, and social involvement in heavy-drinking peer groups (Jessor and Jessor 1975; Margulies et al. 1977; Fillmore et al. 1979). Schmidt and Popham (1975) point out that the ways in which peer-group drinking practices affect alcohol abuse can be very complex. They point out that *how* a peer group drinks (for example, while carrying guns or in moving cars) may be just as important in determining whether one's drinking leads to problems as *how much* a peer group drinks.

A common reason for the young men in the Core City group to shift from a pattern of heavy, prealcoholic drinking to "social" drinking was marriage and a concomitant shift in social network. Despite a vast literature implicating nonalcoholic spouses as the *cause* of their partners' alcohol abuse (Paolino and McCrady 1977), a careful study by Orford and Edwards (1977) indicates that alcoholic spouses create unhappy marriages far more often than unhappy marriages create alcoholic spouses. However, the "modeling" of alcohol abuse by a spouse or a lover may lead to alcohol abuse in the partner.

A dramatic example of the effect of peer pressure upon alcohol abuse was the Father Matthews abstinence movement in Ireland. Father Matthews was a charismatic priest who in 1837 began an extraordinarily popular abstinence movement whose numbers went up geometrically, until by 1844 5 million Irishmen had taken the pledge of abstinence and annual liquor production had fallen from 12 million gallons of distilled spirits in 1838 to only 5 million in 1844. The abstinence movement and its reduction of alcohol consumption died with Father Matthews, although the Great Famine of 1846 may also have played a role in its death. By 1856 the whole social phenomenon was only a memory.

A fourth factor is legal availability, age limits, and time and location of alcohol sales, which exert a limited effect upon alcohol abuse. This effect is most clearly seen in Moslem countries, where law is supported not only by alternative mood-altering drugs and social mores but also by agricultural and climatic patterns that inhibit production of crops from which alcohol may be cheaply produced. In contrast, the greatest lesson of Prohibition in the United States was the futility of trying to use laws alone to combat alcohol abuse. From 1919 to 1932, the Volstead Act produced a modest reduction in alcohol production and consumption in the United States. The overall problems arising from alcohol consumption were by no means ameliorated by Prohibition; but between 1919 and 1932 the risk of death from cirrhosis did decline to a statistically significant degree (Terris 1967), and a 30 percent reduction in per capita alcohol consumption endured until 1940 (Haggard and Jellinek 1942). The overall failure of Prohibition, however, illustrated that in the absence of cultural support legal proscription of alcohol per se will be an ineffective remedy.

The fifth factor affecting alcohol abuse is the cost of alcohol. The extent of alcohol abuse appears to bear a direct relationship to the per capita consumption of alcohol (de Lint and Schmidt 1968; Schmidt and Popham 1978). Thus, to the extent that social policy and price structure affect alcohol consumption, these factors will also influence alcohol abuse. At the present time, the evidence that the consumption of distilled spirits is affected by price relative to disposable income appears incontrovertible (Lau 1975; Bruun et al. 1975; Special Committee of the Royal College of Psychiatrists 1979; Ornstein 1980). Indeed, the reduction in U.S. per capita alcohol consumption from 1933 to 1940 may have had as much to do with the Depression and reduced discretionary income as with the aftereffects of Prohibition. In the laboratory, Mello et al. (1968) observed experimentally that when alcoholics were working for alcohol on an operant apparatus, blood alcohol of the alcoholic subjects was directly related to the number of responses (the behavioral "cost") necessary to produce a reinforcement of beverage alcohol.

The effect that price and social policy would have had upon wine consumption seems more uncertain. It is noteworthy, however, that in the 1970s, when the State of California mounted a media campaign for moderating the ingestion of wine, the California wine industry insisted that the media campaign be stopped. Price manipulation appears to have the least effect upon beer consumption (Ornstein 1980).

A vivid illustration of the relationship between alcohol abuse and social policy comes from the epidemic of gin abuse that affected London in the mid-eighteenth century (Coffey 1966). The number of alcoholics in England had increased parallel to the English production of gin, which went from half a million gallons in 1685 to 11 million gallons in 1750. This increase in gin production reflected improved distilling technology and the economic need to find a profitable use for excess grain. The concomitant increase in the abuse of gin also reflected the effect of introducing a new rapid-acting mood-altering drug into a community that had not evolved social controls for its use. The result of increased consumption of gin was an appalling rise in public drunkenness and an associated increase in mortality. In 1751 a bill was passed to tax and to control the distillation of gin. Gin consumption dropped by 90 percent to a million gallons by 1790, and alcohol abuse in London declined equally dramatically. Coffey suggests that "the rise and decline of gin drinking can be related directly to taxation and legislation" (1966, p. 673). Would that subsequent alcohol legislation could have been as effective! As Moore and Gerstein (1981) have convincingly demonstrated, reducing alcohol abuse by manipulating social policy is a very difficult process.

A sixth factor is social instability, which in itself has a powerful effect upon host resistance to alcohol abuse (Pittman and Snyder 1962; Leighton et al. 1963). In illuminating the profound effects of social factors upon host susceptibility to environmental disease agents, Cassel (1976) provides a classic review of the effects of the social environment upon host resistance. He points out that it is social demoralization, not crowding per se, that is bad for health. The citizens of both Hong Kong, a crowded city, and Holland, a crowded country, enjoy excellent health. But when individuals are involved in any rapidly changing social environment, they become more susceptible to endemic diseases of all kinds. Thus, social support networks become an individual's chief buffer against the deleterious effects of social change. If either social stability or support by friends is absent, the individual is at risk.

Alcohol is an addicting substance; and, to some degree, all alcohol users are at risk for dependence. Where societies are stable and have evolved rituals for social drinking, alcohol abuse is lower; where societies break down and individuals become demoralized and societal control over alcohol ingestion is diminished, alcohol abuse is higher.

Alcohol *use* is widely spread around the world, but alcohol abuse appears peculiarly a Western disease. Alcohol abuse is a concomitant of the destabilization that accompanies the impact of a modern industrial society upon one less industrialized. Edwards (1974) points out that the use of any mood-altering drug results in behavior that reflects a dynamic equilibrium between the culture and the drug's effects. According to Edwards, ritualized controlled social drinking will break down when any of three conditions are met: when the culture itself is changing and loosening its control over individual members, when the sudden introduction of a substance with high dependence-inducing properties imposes a particular threat to an unprepared society, or when individuals, unresponsive to cultural influences, use addicting drugs.

One need only examine the interface between Western industrialized cultures and those of developing countries to appreciate that societal change and alcohol abuse often go hand in hand. The disorganizing impact of the industrial revolution in eighteenth-century London undoubtedly also contributed to London's gin epidemic, and to its motto "drunk for a penny, dead drunk for tuppence." Similar epidemics of alcoholism may be seen in the aboriginal communities at the fringe of modern Australian cities, at the interface of American Indian communities and white settlements, and in the new African cities with their sudden mix of tribal and European ways. All offer grim testimony that a society's safe use of alcohol depends upon the painstaking elaboration of societal rituals to constrain alcohol abuse. Such rituals often require generations to develop.

While unambiguous data to support these generalizations are not available from the Core City study, an incident reported by Rosenberg et al. (1973) concerning Boston alcoholics of the same age and social class as our subjects is instructive. Twenty-nine men were living in an inner-city halfway house for alcoholics. Their social supports were tenuous or they would not have been living in a halfway house. Nevertheless, in a structured environment, the men's average abstinence was seven weeks. Then the halfway house burned down. Within two weeks, 50 percent of the men had relapsed to active alcohol abuse, most within 24 hours. The 50 percent who relapsed had been abstinent virtually as long as the 50 percent who continued to abstain. The effect of loss of social support upon alcohol abuse appeared incontrovertible.

When earlier in this chapter I compared Italians and Irish in Boston, I was not just comparing cultural attitudes toward alcohol, but also differences in cultural cohesion. Whatever their special themes and permissions, integrated cultures and communities provide each member with enduring collective representations of benign strength, with ritual means of calling upon those representations, and perhaps with means for transforming alcoholic gratification either into Celtic guilt or into Latin self-esteem.

In the etiology of any illness, host and agent and environment—like the three corners of a triangle—all play critical and interactive roles. Alcoholism is no different. When the agent, alcohol, is either readily accessible (inexpensive and/or available at sales outlets that are numerous and often open), or when alcohol is available in rapid-acting forms, then abuse will increase. Whenever the host is demoralized, ignorant of healthy drinking practices, or susceptible to heavy-drinking peers, or whenever the host has a high genetic tolerance for alcohol's dysphoric effects, values altered consciousness, or is poorly socialized into the culture, then alcohol abuse will increase. When the environment makes alcohol the recreational drug of choice or fails to structure healthy drinking practices or places no taboos on alcohol problems or is disorganized, then alcohol abuse will increase. In the causation (and the treatment) of alcoholism, biology, psychology, sociology, and economics are inextricably entwined.

Conclusions

In summarizing the four sections on the contribution of culture, heredity, childhood, and premorbid personality to alcoholism, it seems useful to apply Occam's razor. What is the smallest number of variables that will explain all the others?

The independent contribution of all the major premorbid variables from Chapter 7 to mental health (HSRS), to sociopathy, and to total number of alcohol-related problems was assessed by multiple regression, shown in Table 2.18. At best, multiple regression is a crude approximation, which can suggest but never prove causation. The order in which variables are entered in the regression equation affects the percentage of explained variance but not the beta weights. For each of the three outcome variables in Table 2.18, the putative causative variables were entered in the same order. Boyhood competence, childhood environmental strengths, I.Q., and HSRS variables made the greatest independent contribution to mental health. (Had childhood environmental strengths been entered first, it would have explained 4.2 percent of the variance.) Poor boyhood competence, truancy, multiproblem family membership (childhood environmental weaknesses), and poor infant health appeared to contribute the most to sociopathy. Lastly, as this chapter has underscored, alcohol abuse was predicted by a set of variables depending on culture and family history of alcohol abuse that were different from those predicting mental health and sociopathy.

Although the correlations of .2 and .3 between premorbid and outcome variables (Tables 2.3 and 2.12) are small, and although the ability of this study to explain only 13.5 percent of variance in adult mental health (Table 2.18) may not appear impressive, it must be remembered that 33 years separated the two sets of ratings and that the ratings themselves reflect imperfect measurements which further reduce correlations. In reviewing correlations between personality variables observed across two decades or more, Kohlberg and colleagues (1972) noted that correlations of .3 were about as high as were commonly observed. Childhood variables can never be expected to "explain" the bulk of observed variance in adult outcomes. Or, put differently, students of life-span development are increasingly impressed at how modest is the effect of childhood upon middle life. Of equal interest, however, is the suggestion in Tables 2.12 and 2.18 that the things that go right in our lives *do* predict future success and that the events that go wrong in our lives do not forever damn us.

TABLE 2.18.   Independent contributions of major premorbid variables to mental health, sociopathy, and alcoholism.

Variable	HSRS		Sociopathy		PDS	
	Variance explained[a]	Beta weight	Variance explained	Beta weight	Variance explained	Beta weight
Boyhood competence	6.1%	.15	5.7%	−.14	1.2%	−.07
Childhood environmental strengths	0.9	.00	1.5	−.02	1.1	−.08
Childhood emotional problems	0.2	−.04	0.0	.04	0.3	.09
I.Q.	1.0	.07	0.1	−.02	0.0	.01
Childhood environmental weaknesses	0.0	.05	2.0	.02	0.4	.20
Parental social class	0.9	.10	0.4	−.08	0.0	−.02
Alcoholism in heredity	0.1	−.00	1.4	.07	5.8	.15
Absence of Mediterranean ethnicity	0.0	−.01	1.0	.11	5.0	.23
School problems and truancy	0.0	−.02	6.9	.27	1.8	.13
Poor infant health	0.9	−.04	2.1	.14	0.8	.08
HSRS variables[b]	3.4	−.22	0.1	.04	0.0	.01
Total explained variance	13.5		21.1		16.6	

a. Italic type indicates childhood variables that appeared to contribute most independently to the adult variable in question. Beta weights usually, but not invariably, reflect the importance of a given variable. (Inclusion of the composite item "HSRS variables" minimized the beta weight of the important contribution to HSRS of childhood environmental strengths.)

b. HSRS variables refers to the sum of 8 dichotomous clinical judgments assessed by the Gluecks (1950) that were observed to be significantly and negatively correlated with HSRS. These variables were chosen ex post facto to construct an additional explanatory composite variable. The 8 items were: inadequate maternal discipline, few joint family activities, poor infant health, impractical, restless, feels inadequate, lacks common sense, emotionally disturbed father.

Concerning the multiple etiologies of alcoholism, several findings from this study of the Core City sample bear directly upon prevention and upon treatment. First, retrospective studies of the etiology of alcoholism appear to have badly misled us. In the future, insistence upon prospective design will avoid many erroneous causal conclusions.

But even prospective studies of alcoholism can mislead our attention. Although their data pointed elsewhere, previous studies have generally favored psychodynamic explanations, rather than viewing alcoholism as an affliction with a life of its own (McCord and McCord 1960; Lisansky-Gomberg 1968; Jones 1968; Hoffmann et al. 1974). Thus, after reviewing all of the earlier prospective studies, Hoffmann could write: "Alcoholism might be viewed as a lifestyle chosen by a person to cope with his own needs and the pressures of his environment" (Hoffmann et al. 1976, p. 352). His co-workers chose to interpret the same data differently (Kammeier et al. 1973; Loper et al. 1973) and to perceive alcoholism as a causal agent rather than a symptom. Like Hoffmann, the McCords could not quite believe their data and editorialized about their findings as follows: "Conflict over dependency desires is basic to alcoholism" (p. 105); "In our view, interpersonal relationships within the family are the key to alcoholism" (p. 87); and "Alcoholism is a response to stress or anxiety" (p. 54).

In a sense, the McCords were victims of history. Jellinek did not popularize the disease concept of alcoholism or the value of Italian drinking practices until the same year the McCords wrote their monograph. The only cross-fostering study of alcoholism extant at that time (Roe 1944) was negative for heredity, and in 1960 multiple regression techniques were not readily available.

Thus, the McCords suggested that dominant fathers, immigrant Catholics, and the lowest social class produced the fewest alcoholics, but they failed to note that in Cambridge and Somerville, Massachusetts, in 1940 such individuals were predominantly first- and second-generation Italians. Although the 51 alcoholic fathers and the 15 alcoholic mothers in their study parented a disproportionate number of alcoholic children, the McCords wrote: "The evidence for hereditary explanation of the disorder is unlikely" (p. 28). Instead, they emphasized the importance of poor conjugal relations, reliance on parental surrogates, and inconsistent parental discipline as leading to alcoholism.

Returning to Tables 2.16 and 2.18, the independent contribution of heredity, ethnicity, and premorbid antisocial behavior to the development of alcohol-related problems seems clear. Each premorbid variable made an important and independent contribution to the explained variance in subsequent alcohol problems. Depending on whether childhood environmental strengths or boyhood competence was entered first into the regression equation, one or the other made a small additional independent contribution. Irish ethnicity, as distinct from other non-Mediterranean cultures, made no additional contribution to the explained etiological variance.

As an independent check on the conclusions in Table 2.16, 113 psychosocial variables, originally coded by the Gluecks when the men were early adolescents, were examined for their value in predicting subsequent alcohol abuse. Six items—father's alcoholism, parental marital conflict, poor maternal supervision, many moves, no attachment to father, and no family cohesiveness—were very significantly ($p < .01$) correlated with subsequent development of alcohol-related problems in the Core City subjects. These six dichotomously rated Glueck items were almost identical to the variables identified by the McCords as having the greatest etiological significance in alcoholism; and these items were used to create a 7-point composite prediction variable. When this composite variable was entered first into the multiple regression matrix depicted in Table 2.18, it explained 7 percent of the observed variance in subsequent alcohol-related problems. However, when this variable was entered last in the regression and the contribution of parental alcoholism was controlled, it explained only 1 percent further variance.

What we learn about the etiology of alcoholism must affect our treatment. We must stop trying to treat alcoholism as if it were merely a symptom of underlying distress. We must learn to mistrust recent retrospective studies like Tyndel's, which after reviewing the charts of 1000 patients admitted to the medical unit of Toronto's Addiction Research Foundation decreed that "100 percent of alcoholic patients in an uncommonly large series of investigated cases lead to the conclusion that the development of the disease process of alcoholism is inconceivable without underlying psychopathology" (1974, p. 24). Instead, we must learn to heed an old Japanese proverb: "First, the man takes a drink, then the drink takes a drink, then the drink takes the man."

We must spot the fallacious etiological implication in Kissen's otherwise correct statement: "It is a truism that most alcoholics cannot cope. They cannot deal with the normal frustrations and irritations of the external world" (Kissen and Begleiter 1977, p. 31). They were not always so helpless! When after analyzing the MMPI's of alcoholics Hampton wrote, "The more maladjusted the individual is on the average, the more need he seems to show for alcohol as a crutch" (1951, p. 503) he was 180 degrees off course. A more accurate statement of his data and Kissen's generalizations might be: The more an individual abuses alcohol the more maladjusted and crippled he will appear.

A second conclusion is that if culture does play such an important role in the genesis of alcoholism, we must try to uncover ways of socializing healthy drinking practices, so that such practices will remain for a lifetime under an individual's conscious choice. Introducing children to the ceremonial and sanctioned use of low-proof alcoholic beverages taken with meals in the presence of others, coupled with social sanctions against drunkenness and against drinking at unspecified times, would appear to provide the best protection against future alcohol abuse. Within reason, altering price structure can sometimes affect alcohol use; governments should experiment with ways of reducing overall consumption, especially of high-proof alcohol, by price manipulation and education. Society must learn to recognize the health consequences and to appreciate the long-range dangers of providing cheap alcohol as a fringe benefit in military PX's. The reader may argue that Italy has a higher rate of alcoholism than Ireland and that price manipulation has only limited efficacy. I would offer a threefold reply. First, the etiology of alcoholism is multifactorial, and in order to demonstrate the value of cultural drinking practices one must hold other confounding factors constant. Second, recommendations of this kind demand experimental proof, and providing such proof should be a focus of future research. Moore and Gerstein (1981) offer a superb discussion of the complexities that are involved. Third, the dream that some etiological factor will be identified that will allow the eradication of alcohol abuse, or even a major subtype of alcohol abuse, is likely to remain just that—a dream.

When investigators focus only upon one class of data in a multifactorial problem, the results can range from misleading to preposterous. I have listened to Nobel Laureates and famous biochemists discuss the dream that the morbidity of alcoholism would be cured if one could protect the hepatic alcohol transaminase and thereby prevent cirrhosis. Apparently traffic fatalities, battered wives, and the despair of a life spent on skid row escaped their attention.

Finally, if genetic factors play an important etiologic role in alcoholism— and I believe that they do—individuals with many alcoholic relatives should be alerted to recognize the early signs and symptoms of alcoholism and to be doubly careful to learn safe drinking habits. They should appreciate that alcohol abuse, like cigarette abuse, reflects an ingrained habit that cannot occur overnight. The present prospective study offers no credence to the common belief that some individuals become alcoholics after the first drink. The progression from alcohol use to abuse takes years; this fact is a major focus of the next chapter.

3 ∼ The Natural History of Alcoholism

An examination of the life course and drinking patterns of the Core City men will illustrate a number of facets of the natural history of alcohol use. One such facet is the characteristics of men who have used alcohol in moderation all their lives. What distinguishes these men from those who chose never to drink at all? What differentiates "heavy" social drinkers from moderate drinkers? Do "heavy drinkers" have more in common with "alcoholics" or with "moderate drinkers"?

Second, what actually happens to alcoholics over time—not just to those who attend our clinics but to the whole constellation of treated and untreated alcoholics? How can the theoretical model of inexorable alcoholic progression—a model illustrated by Hogarth, retrospectively documented by Jellinek (1952), and believed as an article of faith by Alcoholics Anonymous—be reconciled with the unpredictable oscillations between use and abuse of alcohol observed in prospective studies of alcoholics (such as Polich et al. 1981; Orford and Edwards 1977; Clark 1976; Cahalan and Room 1974). Such short-term prospective investigations reveal that during any given month a majority of so-called alcoholics will be observed to be either abstinent or drinking asymptomatically. Since this can be said of neither cigarette addicts nor heroin addicts, is alcoholism best conceptualized as a state or a trait? As in Chapter 1, a goal of this chapter will be to clarify when the *state*, abuse of alcohol, becomes the *trait*, alcoholism.

Third, I shall discuss the course of alcoholics who come to clinics. How does the course followed by "treated" alcoholics differ from that of untreated alcoholics? To address this question I shall introduce a new longitudinal study

120

of 100 patients admitted to an alcohol detoxification unit and followed annually for eight years—the Clinic sample.

Finally, I shall examine the long-term effect of alcohol abuse upon physical health and the nontreatment variables that may affect the natural course of alcoholism.

In proposing such ambitions, I must repeat two caveats from the start of the book. First, this study of alcohol use and abuse by the Core City men is cohort-dependent. This study is not a prevalence study or a population study, in the sense, say, that Cahalan's group sampled the prevalence of alcohol use and abuse within the whole population of the United States. The data in this chapter derive from the peculiarities of the sampling procedures involved in selecting the Core City, the College, and the Clinic samples, and apply to white males living in one part of the country and during one period in history. The findings presented here may not be characteristic of other groups and must be regarded as complementary to cross-sectional studies of more representative samples. This caveat is necessary because perhaps no disorder is more a product of its social setting than addiction to mood-altering drugs. Drugs depend both for their desirability and for their effect on the milieu in which they are taken. Modes of and rationalizations for drug taking depend upon and usually create a subculture. Thus, in part, the natural history of alcoholism is like that of a society; parts of it must be rewritten every few years.

Second, this chapter sheds no light upon the life course of women alcoholics. In spite of a growing body of work on women alcoholics (Schuckit et al. 1969; Edwards et al. 1972; Gomberg 1976; and other studies reviewed by Robins and Smith 1980), our understanding of alcoholism in women is still extremely sketchy. For example, in the United Kingdom the male-to-female ratio of arrests for drunkenness is 14:1; for psychiatric hospitalizations for alcoholism it is 5:1; and yet for cirrhosis, the male-to-female ratio is 1:1. How are we to interpret such data? Recently, there has been suggestive evidence that the course of alcoholism in women (from first drink to loss of control to abstinence or death) may be accelerated compared to that in men (Fillmore 1975; Camberwell Council on Alcoholism 1980; Hesselbrock 1981). According to Robins and Smith, however, "It is clear from longitudinal studies that drug and alcohol problems often terminate spontaneously. The differences between the sexes do not appear to be very great" (1980, p. 219). More data are needed. Until we have good longitudinal follow-ups of alcohol use and abuse by women, our view of alcoholism will remain severely limited.

～ Alcoholism in Women Revisited

The last 15 years have seen important strides in understanding the natural history of alcoholism in women, including several important reviews of the subject (Wilsnack and Beckman 1989; Blume 1986; Schmidt et al. 1990; Gomberg 1991). In part, this progress is due to conscious efforts by investigators and granting agencies to redress decades of neglect and denial of alcoholism in women. In part the increased attention to alcohol abuse in women is due to the increasing prevalence of alcohol abuse among young women (Blume 1986; Dunn 1988) and the increased incidence and recognition of the fetal alcohol syndrome. Unfortunately, the last 15 years have still not produced adequate prospective longitudinal studies of alcoholism by which the relevance to women of the findings from the Core City and College cohorts might be tested.

Allowing for the greater denial of alcohol abuse by women, alcohol abuse in the United States is probably two and a half times more frequent in men than in women. The male/female ratio is probably still greater for older age cohorts, but alcohol abuse in these cohorts is more difficult to identify. For example, until their late 50s or 60s the men in the College sample were very reluctant to acknowledge that their wives had drinking problems. Only after 50 years of follow-up was it apparent that if alcohol abuse was at some time present in 20 percent of the 268 College men, it was present in 10 percent of their wives. The lower incidence of alcoholism among women seems independent of genetic factors (Guze et al. 1986).

There are two major gender differences that make the course of alcoholism in women somewhat different from that in men. On the one hand, women are metabolically less tolerant of alcohol than are men. Second, probably because there are more social taboos against heavy drinking in women, women who develop alcoholism have more risk factors present and experience a more rapid and clandestine course (Wilsnack et al. 1984).

First, women can drink less alcohol safely. As little as two to four drinks a day by women can lead to cirrhosis (Norton et al. 1987) and to brain atrophy (Jacobson 1986). In a study by Haver (1987) women whose total annual consumption averaged more than a pint of hard liquor a week or more (only 10–15 standard drinks) also met DSM III criteria for alcohol abuse. In contrast, as noted elsewhere in this book, many men can drink up to four standard drinks a day with relative safety. The reason for the lower tolerance of women to alcohol is not entirely clear. One reason why women may be more sensitive to alcohol than men is that they are more likely than men to be also taking sedative tranquilizers, especially benzodiazepines. A second reason is that women on average weigh less and have a smaller blood volume and a lower ratio of body water to body fat than men. Thus the ingestion of a given volume of alcohol will result in somewhat higher blood alcohol levels in women than in men (Blume 1986). More recent work, however, has revealed a third and more important reason for the difference in tolerance. In women there appears to be lower gastric oxidation of ethanol. After a given dose of alcohol the differences in blood alcohol level between men and women are much greater when alcohol is administered orally than when it is given intravenously. After controlling for weight, a woman's blood alcohol level after a fixed oral dose of ethanol is one and a half times as high as a man's (Frezza et al. 1990). Apparently, men detoxify almost 50 percent of orally ingested alcohol through their higher gastric alcohol dehydrogenase activity.

The second major reason for gender differences in the course of alcohol abuse is due to the stronger social sanctions against heavy drinking in women. For example, in popular literature and cinema, intoxication in men is considered a source of general merriment; intoxication in women amuses no one. Women who develop alcoholism develop it for the same reasons as men: premorbid antisocial personality, hyperactivity (Glen and Parsons 1989), heavy-drinking peers (especially spouses), alcoholic biological relatives, work environments conducive to heavy drinking, and being raised in cultures that forbid drinking and yet encourage drunkenness. But each of these factors, except for hyperactivity, is more likely to be present in women who eventually abuse alcohol than in men (Svanum and McAdoo 1991; Blume 1986).

Women alcoholics have more alcoholic relatives than do men (Gomberg 1991). They are more likely to be antisocial and demoralized (Schmidt et al. 1990), to be afflicted with other psychiatric disorders (Helzer and Pryzbeck 1988), to be socially isolated (Dahlgren 1978), and to have an alcoholic spouse (Jacob et al. 1987). Since men are far more likely to leave alcoholic wives than women are to leave alcoholic husbands, alcoholism in women is more frequently associated with broken families and lack of social supports. Suicide attempts are more frequent in alcoholic women (Blume 1986).

In addition, because alcoholism is more stigmatized in women (Schmidt et al. 1990), the diagnosis is more likely to be missed; and women face more barriers to obtaining treatment. Such denial by both women themselves and their caregivers increases the likelihood that they will be treated for secondary depression and anxiety rather than primary alcoholism. Therefore, alcoholism in women is more likely to be complicated by the secondary abuse of prescription drugs (Blume 1986).

Women, in general, are prone to the more fulminant course seen in antisocial men (Fillmore 1987). This is because the net effect of having more risk factors, more denial, and greater difficulty obtaining treatment puts women at greater risk for rapid progression of alcohol-related complications. Alcoholic women are more likely to die from cirrhosis and violence; and they experience more medical complications in general from alcohol abuse (Ashley et al. 1977, Blume 1986). Indeed, women who die from alcoholism and its direct sequelae do so an estimated 11 years earlier than their male counterparts (Krasner et al. 1977). Brenner (1967) followed 1,343 alcoholics for four to seven years after treatment and noted excess deaths from accidents to be six times the expected rate for men, but 16 times the expected rate for women. The single blessing to their accelerated course is that female alcohol abusers are not only more likely to develop dependence and to die but also progress more rapidly to stable abstinence (Ashley et al. 1977).

However, the similarities of alcoholism in men and women are greater than the differences (Kagle 1987). Thus, with the two exceptions noted above, most of the findings in this book should be equally applicable to women (Wilsnack and Cheloha 1987). In summarizing the course of alcoholism in ten U.S. surveys, Knupfer (1989) notes that high education is associated with more moderate alcohol abuse in both men and women, and that low education is associated with earlier onset of alcohol abuse in both men and women. Beverage choice between American men and women does not seem very different (Klatsky et al. 1990). As with men, alcohol abuse appears to be the cause of psychological problems in women, rather than psychological problems causing the alcohol abuse (Wilsnack 1979). For example, although women frequently state that alcohol abuse decreases their social anxiety with men, empirical study shows that women have more anxiety with men when drinking alcohol than when not drinking (Gomberg 1991). The best follow-up study of women, thus far, is a five-year study by Wilsnack and colleagues (1991). They found that, similar to the case with men in our study, after age 40 the course of alcohol abuse seemed relatively stable rather than progressive.

Patterns of Alcohol Use among the Core City and College Men

In order to assess lifetime alcohol consumption by the Core City men, we employed a 7-point alcohol-use scale derived from Cahalan's quantity-frequency-variability classification (Cahalan et al. 1969). This alcohol-use

TABLE 3.1. Average alcohol consumption among the Core City men, and by ethnicity.

Group	Alcohol use	n	Total sample (n=400)	Irish (n=76)	Anglo-American (n=159)	North European (n=37)	Mediter-ranean (n=128)
I	Abstainers	80	20%	21%	20%	11%	22%
	Moderate drinkers						
II	1–13 drinks/week	83	21	13	13	21.5	35
III	2–3 drinks/day	47	12	9	12	8	14
	Heavy drinkers						
IV	3–4 drinks/day	45	11	14	7	21.5	12
V	2–3 on PDS score	35	9	7	13	8	5
	Problem drinkers						
VI	Alcohol abuse						
	< 5 years	19	4	4	7	3	2
VII	Alcohol abuse						
	5 + years	91	23	32	28	27	10
	Total	400	100	100	100	100	100

scale, as used here, reflected the estimated peak 5–10 years of alcohol consumption by the Core City men during the preceding 30 years. As such, the scale represents a very crude and retrospective estimate. Although the alcohol-use scale is adequate to permit statistical comparison between groups, the lifetime alcohol use by some individuals is probably incorrectly classified.

If in their interviews at ages 25, 31, and 47 the Core City men reported that they had drunk less than one drink a month all their lives, they were classified as *abstainers*. A "drink" is defined as half an ounce of absolute alcohol and is equivalent to a shot (one and a half ounces) of 80 proof spirits or "hard" liquor, 6 ounces of wine, or one 12 ounce can of beer). As Table 3.1 illustrates, 80 men, most of whom drank only on ceremonial occasions if at all, were classified as abstainers (group I).

In group II were 83 men with no heavy drinking who averaged 1 to 13 drinks a week, and in group III were 47 men who consumed on the average two to three drinks a day and/or up to seven drinks at one sitting no more than once a week. These two groups were categorized as moderate drinkers. In group IV were 45 men who consumed on the average three to four drinks a day and/or more than that once a week but for whom there was no evidence of more than one alcohol-related problem on the PDS.

Group V was the most ambiguous group; it included the 35 men who had experienced from two to three problems on the PDS and who often drank more than six drinks a day. In the analyses in Chapters 1 and 2, Core City men who fell in group V were excluded from the category called asymptomatic drinkers. By the more liberal diagnostic criteria of the DSM III, 15 of these 35 men would have been classified as "alcohol abusers"; but by the modified Cahalan criteria used in this study, only one would have been classified as a "problem drinker." In terms of their number of known alcoholic relatives, this borderline group resembled the asymptomatic drinkers, rather than the men in groups VI and VII who were labeled by the PDS as alcohol abusers.

Group VI consisted of 19 men who manifested four or more symptoms on the PDS for only a brief period of their lives (more than one year and less than 5). In group VII were 91 men who met the criteria for alcohol abuse for more than five years; this last group included 65 of the 71 men classified as alcohol-dependent by the DSM III criteria.

Unfortunately, the greater the number of alcohol-related problems, the less reliable were estimates of quantity-frequency-variability and the more irregular was the pattern of consumption. Indeed, studies of severe alcoholics reveal that although alcohol abusers are fairly accurate in reporting alcohol-related problems, they tend to underestimate their alcohol consumption by more than 50 percent (Edwards and Grant 1980). Virtually all the men in groups V, VI, and VII had more than six drinks (more than half a pint of hard liquor) several days a week, but they did not necessarily drink every day. Nonetheless, the differences between the estimated total alcohol consumption of a group IV drinker and that of a group VII drinker were substantial. In a year, the average alcohol abuser, even if abstinent for half of that year, might consume the equivalent of 75 fifths of whiskey; whereas even drinking every day the average group IV drinker might consume 15–25 fifths of whiskey a year.

Table 3.1 also examines the relation of alcohol use to ethnicity. In general, the percentage of abstainers in the Core City sample did not differ across ethnic groups, but the reasons for abstaining probably did. Many of the men from Mediterranean countries, especially those from Syria and Lebanon, came from families that traditionally used little, if any, alcohol. In contrast, many of the Irish and Anglo-American abstainers had come from families with alcoholic parents; their abstention represented a reaction against alcohol abuse rather than identification with cultural mores.

Only one Irish-American in five was a moderate drinker, in contrast to almost half of those of Mediterranean descent. Heavy drinkers, those men in groups IV and V, seemed evenly distributed among ethnic groups; but the cells are too small to be meaningful. As already discussed in Chapter 2, sustained alcohol abuse was much less common among the men of Mediterranean heritage.

∼ Groups IV and V Revisited

If alcoholism is a "progressive" disease, the future course of the alcohol users in categories IV and V is worthy of study. Did their course support or challenge the idea that heavy alcohol use is a predictor of future alcohol abuse? Did the heavy users with a few symptoms of abuse progress inexorably to alcoholism?

Before I answer this question, let me make clear what I will be calling alcoholism in this revision of the book. Chapter 1 introduced four overlapping definitions of alcoholism. The first was a problem-based model defined as four or more items on the PDS. The second was a social deviance model defined as seven or more items on the Cahalan Scale. The third was the widely used statistical or case-finding model, the DSM III category of alcohol abuse. The fourth and most stringent definition was the medical model reflected by the DSM III category of alcohol dependence. Since the first publication of this book, three new "official" diagnoses of alcoholism have been devised by DSM III-R, DSM IV, and ICD-10. In this revision I am complicating the definition of alcoholism further by adding new cases of alcohol abuse identified during the 15 years that have elapsed since the data for the earlier version were gathered. Therefore, to reduce confusion, I will use only the DSM III definitions of alcoholism: alcohol abuse and alcohol dependence.

Table 3.1A summarizes why by age 60 the number of Core City alcohol abusers had increased from 120 men with four or more problems on the PDS to 150 men who met DSM III criteria for alcohol abuse. At age 47, 130 of these 150 had already been classified as alcohol abusers by DSM III criteria. Nine men developed alcohol abuse (n = 5) or alcohol dependence (n = 4) after age 47. Finally, there were 11 men who had originally been identified as meeting criteria for alcohol abuse on the PDS but who because of withdrawal or early death had not been interviewed at age 47. These men were not originally classified on the DSM III and alcohol-use scales.

As can be seen in Table 3.1B, using the DSM III rather than the PDS definition meant that 1 man who had been classified as a light social drinker (Group II), 4 as heavy social drinkers (Group IV), and 17 as Group V men who at age 47 had had less than four problems on the PDS still met DSM III

TABLE 3.1A.   Changes in lifetime DSM III diagnosis of alcohol abuse between age 47 and age 60 in the Core City sample.

	Age 47 DSM III diagnosis				
Age 60 DSM III diagnosis	Without abuse	Alcohol abuse	Alcohol dependent	Previously unclassified due to early death or withdrawal	Total
Without abuse	260	0	0	4	264
Alcohol abuse	5	59	0	9	73
Alcohol dependent	4	0	71	2	77
Total	269	59	71	15	414

criteria for "alcohol abuse." In addition, 8 men—those in parentheses in the table—met DSM III criteria for alcoholism *after* age 47.

In contradiction to the hypothesis that alcohol abuse is inexorably progressive, only 1 of the 8 "new" alcoholics came from the ranks of the 35 men in Group V who had already evidenced minimal evidence of problem drinking. In contrast, 2 men who were moderate social drinkers and 5 of the 45 heavy social drinkers (Group IV) developed alcohol abuse or dependence by age 60.

I believe that the paradox of less "progression" of alcohol use/abuse in Group V than in Groups III and IV can be resolved as follows. On the one hand, alcohol abuse and dependence can develop at any age. Alcohol abuse is most likely to develop among heavy drinkers, and it may progress to dependence. Thus, after age 47 some Group IV drinkers developed alcohol abuse. On the other hand, many men when young have problems resulting from transient heavy drinking and drunkenness. These behaviors resulted in their receiving two or three points on the PDS scale before age 40 but not a diagnosis of alcohol abuse. As these men matured, they learned from their mistakes and/or changed their social networks. By age 40 they had already cut down their drinking, and by age 47 they had achieved a pattern of stable social drinking.

As will be more clearly illustrated later in this chapter by the future course of the College alcohol abusers, alcohol use/abuse stabilizes by middle life. As with cigarette use and much obesity, progression in alcohol abuse occurs largely during the first decade or two of problem use.

But if the problem-drinking score at an earlier time in life did not predict late-onset alcoholism, risk factors did. What distinguished the new alcoholics from the heavy drinkers who did not progress and what distinguished the

TABLE 3.1B.   Average alcohol consumption of the Core City men at age 47 and their DSM III classification of alcohol abuse at age 60.

			Age 60 DSM III classification		
Group	Alcohol use ages 19–47	n	Without abuse n = 260	Alcohol abuse n = 65	Alcohol dependence n = 75
I	Abstainers	80	80	—	—
	Moderate drinkers				
II	1–13 drinks/week	83	82	1	0
III	2–3 drinks/day	47	45	1 (1)[b]	1 (1)[b]
	Heavy drinkers				
IV	3–4 drinks/day	45	36	7 (3)[b]	2 (2)[b]
V	2–3 on PDS score	35	17	14	4 (1)[b]
	Problem drinkers				
VI	Alcohol abuse < 5 years	19	0	16	3
VII	Alcohol abuse 5+ years	91	0	26	65
	Unclassified				
	Total	400[a]	260	65	75

a. At age 47, 4 men without abuse, 8 alcohol abusers and 2 alcohol-dependent men could not be classified on the alcohol-use scale.

b. Numbers in parentheses identify the men in each group who did not meet criteria for alcohol abuse at age 47 but who did by age 60.

Group V heavy drinkers who at age 47 met DSM III criteria for alcohol abuse from the Group V drinkers who did not was their relative number of risk factors. Hyperactivity, ethnicity, school behavior problems, and especially family history of alcoholism were about twice as common among the 27 Group IV and V men reclassified as DSM III alcohol abusers as among the 53 men who were not reclassified. Put differently, the "loss of control" inherent in the clinical concept of alcohol abuse bore as strong a relationship to hereditary factors as it did to reported quantity and/or frequency.

Comparison of the College and Core City Samples to a U.S. Sample

Table 3.2 contrasts the pattern of drinking by the College and Core City samples with broader population samples. Cahalan's more representative American Drinking Practices (ADP) Study (Cahalan et al. 1969) was derived

TABLE 3.2. Comparison of the drinking practices of the College and Core City men with those in the American Drinking Practices (ADP) Study.

Alcohol use	ADP			Core City		College
	Total sample (n = 2746)	N.E. U.S. (n = 280)	Age 40–49 (n = 114)	Current pattern (n = 400)	Lifetime pattern (n = 400)	Lifetime pattern (n = 186)
Rare or never (<1 drink/month)	47%	17%	32%	30%	20%	26%[a]
Light to moderate (1 drink/month to 2 drinks/day)	41	50	38	38	33	50
Heavy (3+ drinks/day)	12	33	30	32	47[b]	24

a. Less than one drink a day (almost none drink less than once a month).

b. This category included 190 men. At the time of the interview (age 47), 38 men (10 percent of the total 400) had been abstinent for at least a year. Forty-two more had returned to asymptomatic drinking, and about half of these (15 percent of the total 400) manifested a current pattern of light to moderate drinking.

from a national probability sample. Unlike the Core City and College samples, the ADP included women as well as men, young and old as well as middle-aged, and rural blacks as well as white city-dwellers.

The table suggests that if sex, age, and geographical distribution are controlled then the patterns of alcohol use among the samples studied in this book are not atypical for the United States as a whole. At first glance, the use of alcohol by the Core City men seems very unlike the national pattern. At some point in their lives, almost half of the Core City men (Table 3.2, column 5) met Cahalan's criterion for heavy drinking (3 or more drinks a day) as contrasted with only 12 percent of American adults as a whole (column 1). However, when alcohol use by a comparable subsample of Cahalan's cohort— white men in their fifth decade of life (column 3)—are compared with *current* usage of alcohol by the Core City men (column 4), alcohol use seems very comparable. Currently, many of the heavy drinkers among the Core City men have returned to a pattern of social drinking or, in order to control alcohol abuse, are now abstainers (almost 10 percent of the entire sample).

Compared to the national ADP sample, the College men were probably more atypical, in that they included no lifetime teetotalers and perhaps fewer sustained alcohol abusers than other samples. In part, the bias against abstinence in the College sample derives from its largely upper-middle-class Anglo-American cultural background; however, as the rest of this section will suggest, a disproportionate percentage of moderate drinkers might be expected in a sample selected, as was the College sample, for mental health.

⟿ Prevalence of Alcohol Abuse Revisited

Over the last 15 years (that is, since 1978) both definitions of alcoholism and estimates of lifetime prevalence of alcohol abuse have undergone revisions, but without necessitating significant alterations to the overall picture described in the original version of this book. The definitions of alcoholism have been revised by the National Council on Alcoholism and Drug Dependence (Morse and Flavin 1992), by the American Psychiatric Association (APA 1987; APA in press) and by the World Health Organization (WHO in press). Each of these changes is a little different from the others, but each change represents only fine-tuning of the definitions already presented.

For the College sample at age 70 the lifetime prevalence of alcohol abuse (using DSM III criteria) was 22 percent. This figure is based on the fact that at some time during their adult lives 52 of the 241 adequately studied College subjects met criteria for DSM III alcohol abuse. (The 64 men drawn from the Harvard classes 1939–1941 and excluded from the original version of this book are included in this revision to expand the n). The other 27 of the original 268 College men in the study were excluded for the following reasons: 6 died in World War II before age 30; 12 withdrew from the sample, but at least 2 of these are known to have been serious alcohol abusers; 7 died between ages 25 and 45 without evidence of alcohol abuse; and for 2 there was inadequate information.

For the Core City sample at age 60 the lifetime prevalence of alcoholism (DSM III criteria) was 36 percent. This figure is based on the fact that at some point in their adult lives 150 of the 414 adequately studied Core City men in the sample met criteria for alcohol abuse (Table 3.1A). The other 42 of the original 456 Core City men in the sample were excluded for the following reasons: 21 could not be classified at all owing to death before age 33 (13 men) or to inadequate information (8 men); for the remaining 21 men limited information regarding alcohol abuse was available. Of the latter 21 study members, 9 (8 withdrawals and 1 with incomplete data) probably met criteria for alcohol abuse; and 12 (11 withdrawals and 1 with incomplete data) probably did not meet those criteria. Thus, based on limited information, the prevalence of alcohol abuse of men who withdrew early from the two samples may be similar to the prevalence of alcohol abuse among those who remained active members.

An important new estimate of the lifetime prevalence of alcoholism in the United States using DSM III criteria has been provided by the Epidemiological Catchment Area study of 20,000 adults (Robins et al. 1988; Regier et al. 1990). This study put the lifetime prevalence of alcohol abuse among white middle-aged males at 24 percent, a figure that falls somewhere between the estimates for the College sample of 22 percent and for the Core City sample of 36 percent.

Patterns of Alcohol Abuse and Mental Health

Table 3.3 makes a point similar to the one made in Table 1.7. On the one hand, multiple alcohol-related problems, physiological dependence, and problems with control are rare in men who do not exceed an average of four drinks a day. On the other hand, at some time in their lives, many moderate drinkers may use alcohol to feel better (Cahalan's psychological dependency), they may be arrested once in their lives for drunken driving, or their relatives may believe they drink too much.

TABLE 3.3. Average alcohol consumption and alcohol-related problems among Core City men not called alcohol abusers.

	Average alcohol consumption				
Problem	Abstinent (n = 80)	1–13 drinks/week (n = 84)	2–3 drinks/day (n = 47)	3–4 drinks/day (n = 45)	PDS score >1 but < 4 (n = 35)
3+ problems on Robins scale	6%	2%	11%	9%	18%
3+ problems on Cahalan scale	0	1	6	16	70
Psychological dependence	1	12	17	50	67
Relative ever complained	0	7	17	36	76
Ever arrested for drinking	0	5	9	18	41
Admits problem with control	0	2	0	2	27
Met DSM III criteria for alcohol abuse	0	1	0	9	54
Met DSM III criteria for alcohol dependence	0	0	0	0	9
Received a diagnosis of alcoholism	0	0	0	0	0

Figure 3.1 introduces an interesting aspect of lifelong abstinence in a drinking culture. Although, as Chapter 2 suggests, alcohol abuse does not seem to be a result of premorbid psychopathology, the capacity for sustained moderate social drinking seems correlated with positive mental health. Only 23 percent of the 44 men with HSRS scores of less than 60 reported drinking in moderation, as contrasted with 82 percent of the 17 men with HSRS scores over 90. Core City lifelong abstainers seemed just as psychologically impaired as future alcohol abusers. The Greek philosophers who advocated the golden mean would nod approval.

The fact that the proportion of men who never used alcohol bore a direct, inverse relationship to the men's scores on the HSRS is intriguing. As Chapter

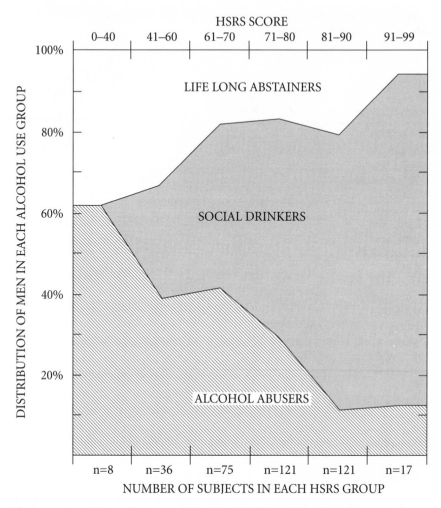

Figure 3.1 Association of poor mental health with lifelong abstention: the proportion of teetotalers, asymptomatic drinkers, and alcohol abusers within HSRS groups.

2 illustrates, alcohol abuse is often a cause of psychopathology; but there is no obvious reason why *abstention* from alcohol should cause psychopathology. Tables 3.4 and 3.5 examine the relationship between abstinence and psychological vulnerability in greater detail. Capacity to drink in moderation seems associated with a warm childhood and good premorbid ego function. As children, future abstainers exhibited significantly worse emotional and

TABLE 3.4. The childhood emotional vulnerability of lifelong Core City abstainers.

Childhood variable	Abstainers (n = 80)	Moderate drinkers (n = 130)	Heavy drinkers (n = 80)	Alcohol abusers (n = 110)
Childhood emotional problems	35%	27%	26%	30%
Poor childhood physical health	33*	14	24	31
Parent or surrogate with alcoholism	39*	24	41	55
Warm childhood environment	16*	35	16	14
Best boyhood competence	17*	37	23	19
Childhood social class V	25	34	26	30
Multiproblem family	10	10	11	15
I.Q. < 90	29	26	29	31
Many alcoholic relatives	10	13	18	29

*Abstainers significantly different from other asymptomatic drinkers: $p < .05$ (chi-square test).

TABLE 3.5. Evidence that capacity for sustained moderate drinking is associated with positive mental health.

Variable	Abstainers (n = 80)[a]	Moderate drinker (n = 130)	Heavy drinker (n = 80)	Alcohol abuser (n = 110)
Adult social class V	10%	0%	10%	21%
< $10,000/yr income	20	8	13	33
HSRS < 60	19	1	11	19
Never married	14	3	14	14
Least mature defenses	23	10	17	50
Regular use of mood-altering drugs	21	12	13	29
Ever received a psychiatric diagnosis	35	17	24	39
Never achieved independence	13	0	6	11
Adult social class I–II	9	18	6	1
HSRS > 80	35	56	32	15
Pastimes with friends	22	41	40	25
Takes enjoyable vacations	15	27	28	16
Best object relations	21	31	22	13
Most mature defenses	14	29	20	7

a. Abstainers were significantly different from other asymptomatic drinkers on all the variables listed here: $p < .05$ (chi-square test).

physical health and fewer family and emotional strengths than moderate social drinkers. All 44 of the moderate drinkers whose parents had been in social class V were socially upwardly mobile; this was not true of the abstainers. These differences were not due to abstainers' being less intelligent or more socially disadvantaged than men who were to become lifelong moderate drinkers.

One explanation for the childhood differences between abstainers and moderate drinkers depicted in Table 3.4 may be the association of lifelong abstention with the disrupting effect of an alcoholic parent within the home (see Figure 2.1).

A second explanation for the phenomenon illustrated in Figure 3.1 may be that the capacity for lifelong social drinking requires ego strengths, as does mastery of any instinctual drive.

Table 3.5 suggests that compared to the moderate drinkers, the abstainers, like the alcohol abusers, were twice as likely to use defenses associated with character disorder, to take tranquilizers, and to have received a psychiatric diagnosis from a clinician (one not associated with the study). Ten of the 80 abstainers never achieved an adult existence that was independent of their parents or some supportive institution, and 15 received HSRS scores of less than 60. This was true of only 1 of the 130 moderate drinkers. Undoubtedly, this U-shaped relationship between alcohol use and mental health is limited to cultures where moderate to heavy drinking is an entrenched social norm and where deviation may represent a failure in the socialization process.

For the College men, among whom complete abstention was virtually unknown, light drinking (once a month to twice a week) was positively correlated with mental health and with warm childhoods (Vaillant 1980a). However, when the 92 College moderate drinkers (1–3 drinks daily) were compared with 18 men who for many years drank 5–8 ounces (4–5 drinks) of hard liquor a day *without* problems, the findings were intriguing. Stoicism seemed to characterize heavy asymptomatic College drinkers. As Table 3.6 suggests, by age 53 these 18 College heavy drinkers never used mood-altering drugs and were not currently taking prescription medicine. Only 1 took five days a year of sick leave, and a disproportionate number of heavy social drinkers who also were heavy smokers had managed to stop smoking. By way of contrast, virtually none of the College alcohol abusers ever stopped smoking. Unlike alcohol abuse, heavy asymptomatic drinking in the College sample was not associated with poor health.

The numbers are small, but heavy social drinking by the College sample was negatively correlated with happy families. Almost half of the light drinkers and a third of the moderate drinkers enjoyed successful first marriages

TABLE 3.6.   Relationship between health and drinking practices in the College sample.

Characteristics of College men at age 50	*Lifetime drinking habits*		
	Moderate (1–3 drinks/day) (n = 92)	*Heavy (3–5 drinks/day) (n = 18)*	*Alcohol-related problems (n = 26)*
Excellent physical health	54%	55%	35%
Health deteriorated last 10 years	10	11	35
5+ days of sick leave/year	21	6	38
Regular prescription medicine	11	0	35
Regular use of mood-altering drugs	9	0	38
% of heavy smokers who stopped[a]	48	70	6
Poor college psychosocial adjustment	22	6	27
Clearly good marriage[a]	36	18	4
Adjustment of grown children excellent[a]	35	15	20

a. Since not all men were heavy smokers, were married, or had children over 15, these numbers are smaller than the total sample.

and children with good young-adult adjustment. This was true for less than a fifth of the heavy drinkers, although they, if anything, had been rated as better than the moderate drinkers in college.

Table 3.7 is congruent with Table 3.6. With the exception of a higher divorce rate, the heavy asymptomatic Core City drinkers also enjoyed relatively good psychosocial health. Although heavy Core City drinkers were more likely to get divorced than abstainers or moderate drinkers, two-thirds achieved stable second marriages; this was true for only one-sixth of the 36 divorced alcohol abusers. Compared to heavy social drinkers, Core City alcohol abusers were far more likely to be chronically physically ill, two-pack-a-day smokers, sociopathic, and chronically unemployed. The distinction between heavy drinking and alcoholism is not just academic.

Patterns of Alcohol Abuse and Physical Health

In the nineteenth century, Francis Anstie (1864) set three alcoholic drinks a day as the safe limit. As noted previously, a "drink" equals half an ounce of absolute alcohol—the amount in an average serving of beverage alcohol. In

TABLE 3.7. Relationship between health and drinking practices in the Core City sample.

Characteristics of Core City men	Abstainers (n = 80)	Moderate drinkers (n = 130)	Heavy drinkers (n = 80)	Alcohol abusers (n = 110)
School behavior and truancy	3%	2%	1%	11%
Many alcoholic relatives	10	13	18	29
Multiproblem family	10	10	11	15
4+ years unemployed	20	6	13	41
3+ injuries	5	7	11	15
5+ Robins scale symptoms	1	0	1	24
2+ months in hospital	5	4	3	10
50+ pack/years smoking	17	14	19	45
Divorce	10	12	22	33

recent years, estimates of the amount of alcohol that can be drunk each day in safety have varied enormously. On the one hand, Davies (1980) suggests that even one ounce of absolute alcohol or two drinks a day is dangerous, and Lundquist writes that "about 60g of alcohol (a little more than 2 ounces [sic] of whiskey or brandy) daily is, in many cases, a sign of being dangerously dependent" (1973, p. 334). In contrast, Armor and colleagues (1978) suggest that three ounces of absolute alcohol (seven drinks a day) can be construed as social or asymptomatic drinking.

Assuming a middle position, Schmidt and Popham (1975, 1978) and their colleagues at the Addiction Research Foundation in Ontario define "hazardous" drinking as 80 grams of absolute alcohol a day (six drinks, half a pint of whiskey, a 750 ml bottle of wine, or a six-pack of beer). A ten-year study of 1899 employees of the Western Electric Company confirmed this figure: "The results show essentially no increase in mortality with alcohol consumption until one reaches five or more drinks/day, at which point, the mortality rate essentially doubles" (Dyer et al. 1977, p. 1070).

The careful review of alcohol and mortality by Room and Day (1974) also agrees with this figure and suggests that not until daily consumption exceeds five drinks is alcohol use unequivocally hazardous. For evidence, Room and Day depended heavily upon the empirical data on alcohol consumption and morbidity derived from the 16-year prospective Framingham Heart Study and the nine-year Alameda County, California, Study. Room and Day examined five categories of alcohol use: abstinence, less than a drink a day, 1–2 drinks a day, 2–3 drinks a day, and more than 3 drinks a day (50+ ounces of absolute alcohol a month). Their review failed to demonstrate any convincing relationship between these categories of alcohol utilization and mortality except that "there is a consistent tendency for those who are currently abstinent to show a higher mortality than those who are currently moderately drinking" (p. 86).

The observed association between abstinence and increased mortality has sometimes been offered as evidence that a few drinks a day are good for one's cardiac health. To my knowledge, there is no good evidence for this theory. Two alternative explanations may be more accurate. First, in communities where drinking is the rule, the abstinent tend to manifest impaired mental health and interpersonal relations and as a consequence of these latter factors may experience greater physical morbidity. Second, as documented by Table 3.2, cohorts identified in cross-sectional study as abstinent may contain many severe alcoholics in remission; such individuals are observed to have almost as high a mortality as active alcoholics (Pell and D'Alonzo 1973).

∾ Coronary Heart Disease Revisited

Since the proceding paragraph was written, there has been continued controversy over whether the so-called U-shaped curve of cardiovascular disease in relation to alcohol use is illusion or clinical fact (Marmot et al. 1981). In the last five years, carefully controlled studies have rebutted the objections that I raised above and have consistently supported the hypothesis that use of alcohol in low doses (1–2 drinks) reduces the risk of coronary heart disease.

In 1988 a *Lancet* editorial still called the protective effect of alcohol a "myth," and the research on which such mistrust was based has been well reviewed by Shaper (1990). One major objection was that abstainers would be at higher risk for heart disease than social drinkers if the reason for their abstinence was prior alcohol abuse or preexisting health problems. Prior alcohol abuse would also put them at risk for higher smoking histories, poor self-care, and the residual effects of alcohol abuse on their myocardium. A second objection, which I have already raised above, is that in a drinking culture for a man never to use alcohol socially might indicate poor social skills, and those poor social skills might lead to the increased mortality that goes with social isolation and mental illness.

Another possible objection not raised by Shaper was that much of the early support for the protective effect of alcohol came from epidemiological studies of heart disease that had gathered inadequate data on alcohol use and abuse. For example, with regard to the Framingham Study, Gordon and Kannel (1983) acknowledge that "the questions about drinking in this study were included as a trivial part in a much larger examination" (p. 1373). In another well-known prospective study of heart disease, the Albany Study, Gordon and Doyle (1987) had such limited data on drinking that their estimates of alcohol use were uncorrelated with motor vehicle accidents.

More recently, however, these objections have been systematically answered. The first objection was addressed by an excellent study by Jackson and colleagues (1991) that showed that when moderate drinkers were compared with *lifelong* teetotalers, moderate drinkers had a significantly lower risk of coronary heart disease. They noted that controlling for blood HDL levels significantly reduced the association between moderate alcohol use and lower risk of coronary heart disease, supporting the hypothesis that the protective effect of alcohol was at least partially mediated by elevating blood HDL levels.

Two additional studies (De Labry et al. 1992; Boffetta and Garfinkel 1990) that also controlled for past illnesses showed a clear U-shaped curve, with the risk of coronary heart disease mortality being lowest for those consuming four drinks a day. The study by Boffetta and Garfinkel is especially revealing in that it noted that nondrinkers enjoyed many health advantages over moderate drinkers. Compared to no drinking at all, even one drink a day led to increased esophageal cancer, two drinks a day increased the risk of liver cirrhosis, three drinks a day increased the risk of cancer of the oral cavity, and six drinks a day increased the risk of accidental death.

My own objection to the U-curve hypothesis, based on the observation that the poor social skills of the Core City teetotalers were deleterious to physical health, has been refuted by studies noting that even in cultures in which lifelong abstinence is a social norm, teetotaling is associated with increased risk for coronary heart disease. For example, Marmot and Brunner (1991) noted that among Japanese-American males—half of whom were teetotalers—the nondrinkers exhibited a higher rate of coronary heart disease than did the alcohol users. In another study Stampfer and colleagues (1988) observed that one to three drinks a day reduced the risk of coronary heart disease in women, in whom teetotaling is an acceptable norm, to 50 percent of that of nondrinking controls. Recently, Marmot and Brunner (1991) have reviewed 17 studies, virtually all of which showed a decreased relative risk of coronary heart disease among moderate drinkers when compared to nondrinkers who were either lifelong teetotalers or at least not former alcohol abusers.

The most likely cause of the protective effect of alcohol in heart disease is that modest alcohol use increases blood levels of the high-density lipoprotein (HDL) cholesterol fractions that are known to be associated with reduced risk for heart disease (Castelli et al. 1977). Recently, Criqui (1990) has pointed out that one to two drinks of alcohol a day almost certainly increases the blood HDL fraction. Multivariate analysis suggests that elevation of the HDL fraction accounts for 50 percent of the reduction in risk by moderate alcohol use and that the rest of the variance may be explained by the fact that small doses of alcohol reduce blood coagulation. Criqui points out that drinking more than two drinks a day probably cancels out any further protective effects of alcohol upon coronary heart disease by increasing the risk of hypertension, arrhythmias, and cardiomyopathy.

To conclude, the evidence that two to four drinks of alcohol are protective against coronary heart disease remains inferential, but the data are so consistent and from so many different sources and the logical arguments for confounding variables have been so well controlled that it seems reasonable to regard the U-shaped curve as a clinical reality. Nonetheless, it must be borne in mind that any increase in alcohol use by a population increases the risk of other alcohol-related problems. Therefore, increasing the number of social drinkers is unlikely to increase a nation's overall health.

The Safe Limits of Alcohol Consumption

From this book's data, only the College sample sheds light on the limits of safe alcohol consumption. The men in the College sample have reported their alcohol use relatively accurately every 2 years for 40 years. Between the ages of 40 and 60, several men regularly recorded drinking six ounces (four drinks) of whiskey a day—or more than a gallon a month—for more than 20 years without problems. However, no man in our College sample reported drinking over five drinks a day without also reporting unwanted symptoms and concern over his capacity to control his drinking.

From this section, two tentative conclusions are possible. First, in the northeastern United States where there are no large religious or cultural groups that advocate total abstinence, moderate use of alcohol may be associated with good social skills and capacity for play, or what psychoanalysts term regression in the service of the ego. On the one hand, not drinking may represent a reaction against alcohol use as a result of having grown up in an alcoholic household—which itself may well have been injurious to childhood and adult adaptation. On the other hand, not drinking may also reflect a failure of socialization within the culture and a poor capacity to take chances or to trust oneself to be adventurous. Table 3.5 clearly illustrates that abstainers had far more difficulty with object relations, vacations, and pastimes than did heavy social drinkers. In addition, the abstainers included a disproportionate number of men who never really negotiated adolescence and separated from their families of origin.

Unlike the equally immature sociopaths, abstainers did not engage in antisocial activities. Perhaps, in some vulnerable individuals, alcohol use raises the specter of loss of control. In a study of abstainers in a Protestant congregation that discouraged drinking, Goodwin and his colleagues (1969) note, but do not remark upon, the fact that abstainers had lower incomes, were more likely to be single, and were more likely to have been treated for psychiatric illness.

A second major conclusion for this section is that, unlike abstinence, alcohol abuse and alcohol dependence *cause* poor psychological function rather than merely reflecting it. The fact that in Table 3.7 divorce, chronic physical illness, chronic unemployment, and multiple injuries occurred far more often among the alcohol abusers than among the equally psychologically vulnerable abstainers or among the often intoxicated heavy drinkers supports the distinction made in this book between alcoholism as a disease and heavy drinking under voluntary control as a variant of healthy drinking.

The Natural History of Treated and Untreated Alcoholism

In 1966, reviewing "the fate of the untreated alcoholic," Kendell and Staton could find only one study in the world literature that addressed the question: What is the life course of untreated alcoholism? The single paper was by Lemere (1953) who obtained information about the life course of 500 deceased alcoholics from their relatives. Lemere stated that before their death, one-fifth of these alcoholics had achieved remission. Of these, about half (one-tenth of the total sample) had become abstinent—almost all without any formal treatment; and the other half had returned to "normal" drinking or more commonly to "controlled" asymptomatic drinking. If with the passage of time, this fifth of Lemere's sample had seemed to do very well, another fifth had stopped drinking in later life simply because they were too ill to continue. Almost three-fifths were said to have abused alcohol until they died at the untimely average age of 52. Eleven percent of Lemere's sample died from suicide. Depending as it did upon the recollection of his psychiatric patients about their elderly alcohol-abusing relatives, Lemere's paper was too methodologically limited to be regarded as an accurate reflection of the life course of alcoholism. Kendell and Staton (1966) themselves reported a follow-up of 57 untreated alcoholics followed for 2 to 13 years (mean = 7 years). At time of last follow-up, 11 of these 57 had died; and of the 46 survivors, 20 percent had achieved stable abstinence. Equally important, 11 percent had returned to social drinking. These figures are somewhat more hopeful than those provided by Lemere; but the numbers are very small.

Two years later, in an often-quoted paper, Drew (1968) suggested that alcoholism might be a self-limiting disease. Using the Australian state of Victoria (population 3 million) as a demographic base, Drew noted that the frequency of first admissions for alcoholism increased until age 55. Such incidence figures however, did not result in a large number of elderly alcoholics. Rather, after age 50, Drew pointed out, the prevalence of active alcoholics in the population steadily declined. In reviewing the literature, Drew noted that the peak age for arrests for drunken driving was between 40 and 50. If the rate at which people developed alcoholism was steady, or increased between 25 and 50, why, with increasing age, should the number of alcoholics appear to decline instead of increase? On the basis of his literature review, Drew suggested that the treatment of alcoholism was sufficiently ineffective that successful clinical intervention per se could not account for the disappearance of alcoholics in older population cohorts. Rather, he concluded that alcoholism might be "a problem of young adulthood and middle age" and that "a process of 'spontaneous recovery' probably accounts for a quite significant proportion of alcoholics who cease to appear in alcoholism statistics as their age increases." Unfortunately, Drew failed to address seriously an alternative possibility, namely, that alcoholism was not a self-limiting illness, but rather as suggested by Lemere (1953), Alcoholics Anonymous, and Jellinek (1952), a fatal one. Few mongols or cystic fibrotics become middle-aged; the reason is their inexorable early mortality, not their spontaneous recovery. What, then, is the life course of untreated alcoholism?

The ten studies depicted in Table 3.8, each lasting for seven years or longer, attempt to address this question. In trying to present data in uniform fashion from ten idiosyncratically designed studies, I have taken certain liberties. First, the percentages of abstinent and currently asymptomatic drinkers have been based on total number of located survivors; therefore the figures in Table 3.8

TABLE 3.8. Ten long-term follow-up studies of alcohol abuse.

Study and nature of sample	Nature of treatment	Type and length of follow-up	Size of original sample
Voetglin and Broz 1949 Private inpatient; good prognosis; ages 30–50	Emetine aversion and follow-up	Mail 10 years	?
Myerson and Mayer 1966 Halfway house; skid row; ages 40–60	Supportive services only	Interviews 10 years	101
Sundby 1967 Clinic; poor prognosis; all classes; ages 30–55	Nonspecific	Record search 20–35 years	1722
Goodwin, Crane, and Guze 1971 Prison; alcoholic only by history; ages 20–35	Nonspecific	Interviews 8 years	c.111
Lundquist 1973 Inpatient; good prognosis; middle class; ages 30–55	1–4 weeks in hospital	Interviews 9 years	200
Bratfos 1974 Inpatient; poor prognosis; ages 30–60	3 weeks in hospital; group therapy and Antabuse	Record search 10 years	1179
Hyman 1976 Private outpatient clinic; good prognosis; ages 30–55	A few outpatient visits	Interviews 15 years	54
Clinic sample Inpatient; poor prognosis; public clinic; ages 30–50	Detoxification; AA-oriented; follow-up	Interviews 8 years	106
Ojesjo 1981 Community; good prognosis; age Σ46	Nonspecific	Interviews 15 years	96
Core City sample Community; good prognosis; blue-collar; ages 20–40	Nonspecific	Interviews 20 ± 10 years	120

TABLE 3.8. continued

Attrition (%)		Number of survivors followed	Outcome for survivors (%)		
Lost or refused	Dead		Abstinent	Asymptomatic drinkers	Still alcoholic
?	?	104	22%		78%
1%	20%	80	22		78
2	62	632	64		36
13	5	93	8%	33%	59
0	23	155	37		63
59	14	412	13	0	87
19	33	26	19	19	62
6	27	71	39	6	55
0	26	71	32		68
8	10	102	34	20	46

may not match the figures in the original papers. Many authors included the dead and/or the lost as part of the numerical base upon which their outcome percentages were based. Second, alcoholics who were institutionalized or chronically invalided because of alcohol abuse or whose alcohol-related problems had improved but had not fully remitted are categorized "still alcoholic" and placed among the unimproved. Third, several studies did not distinguish between abstinence and return to asymptomatic drinking. Thus, it is likely that Table 3.8 underrepresents the proportion of alcohol abusers who returned to "asymptomatic drinking" as defined by this book.

Without knowing the men's age at time of death, it is difficult to make sense of the percentage who died during the follow-up period; but this facet of the natural history of alcoholism will be elaborated in a later section. In general, at any age, the mortality of alcoholic samples was three times what would have been expected for a normal sample of the same age.

Excluded from Table 3.8 are a few other studies of exceptionally long duration. Gerard and Saenger (1966) report on 100 alcoholics followed for eight years, of whom roughly a quarter became abstinent and perhaps 5 returned to social drinking. A Canadian study by Gibbins referred to by Schmidt (1968) reported 23 percent of alcoholics abstinent after ten years, and a study by Beaubrun (1967) found 37 percent of 57 alcoholics abstinent after ten years. Unfortunately, the details of these three studies were never fully published; their rates of attrition are unclear, and their data do not allow an accurate assessment of how many in their samples may have returned to asymptomatic drinking. Because the 20-year follow-up by Fillmore (1975) addressed alcohol-related problems rather than alcoholism, it, too, is excluded. Finally, an ongoing ten-year follow-up of previously well studied alcoholics, by Griffith Edwards at the Institute of Psychiatry in London, is not yet published. This last-mentioned study is likely to shed much light on the natural history of alcoholism.

The studies presented in Table 3.8 include two studies from Norway, two from Sweden, and six from the United States. They reflect several different social groups of alcoholics including felons (Goodwin et al. 1971), members of the upper middle class (Voetglin and Broz 1949), and residents of skid row (Myerson and Mayer 1966), of small rural towns (Ojesjo and Hagnell 1982), and of large cities (the Core City sample). Unfortunately the data hardly encompass the total universe of alcohol abuse. The ten studies contained few women and no alcohol abusers from countries like Portugal and France where binge drinking and "loss of control drinking" are unusual.

Nevertheless, the overall outcomes of these ten studies bear remarkable similarity to the findings of the early groundbreaking study of 57 patients by Kendell and Staton (1966); roughly 2–3 percent of alcoholics become abstinent each year and another 1 percent return annually to asymptomatic drinking. The high death rate accounts for a significant but not a major proportion of those alcoholics who by 55 are no longer problem drinkers.

The first column of Table 3.8 characterizes the samples in terms of age, derivation of sample, and prognosis. (Prognosis was based on the work of Costello [1980] who after reviewing many outcome studies observed that employment and marital status at intake provided the most powerful predictors of outcome.) Prognosis was probably affected by the proportion of alcoholics in each study who were physiologically dependent.

With the exception of the study by Bratfos (1974), the rates of attrition (excluding death) of the studies average out to less than 0.5 percent per year. Such low attrition demonstrates that it is certainly possible to follow cohorts of alcoholics for long periods of time. Studies like the Rand Report (Polich et al. 1981) which report attrition of 4 percent or more per year should probably be considered methodologically unacceptable. The danger of high rates of attrition, of course, is that two very important subgroups of alcoholics are especially likely to drop from sight: those who die and those who do so well that they cease to appear in clinic or public records.

For most purposes, the results displayed in Table 3.8 reflect the natural evolution of alcoholism. Thus far there is no compelling evidence that any specific brief clinical intervention permanently alters the course of the disorder. Table 3.8 includes several samples both of persistently "treated" alcoholics (Voetglin and Broz 1949 and the Clinic sample) and several samples of essentially untreated alcoholics (Goodwin et al. 1971; Ojesjo 1981). As Drew would have predicted, the length of follow-up, not intensity of treatment, was most closely associated with a decline in the proportion of active alcoholics. The implication is that alcoholics recover not because we treat them, but because they heal themselves.

A moment's reflection, however, will reveal that in a longitudinal study a sharp distinction between "treated" and "untreated" alcoholics is not possible. For one thing, over time many initially "untreated" alcoholics became progressively impaired and obtain a wide variety of different "treatment" experiences. Second, over time many alcoholics originally selected for having been treated in some specific manner will relapse only to recover through some quite different sort of therapeutic intervention. Thus, after the first year of follow-up, efforts to compare a matched "treated" to an untreated cohort of alcoholics will become increasingly futile.

The first study in Table 3.8, by Voetglin and Broz (1949), was a follow-up of men who had been at Shadel's clinic in Washington state seven to ten years previously. In spite of the very high rates of remission that were originally reported by this clinic (Shadel 1944), only 22 percent of these patients on long-term follow-up were regarded as still in stable remission. The lesson to be learned is that assessment of stable remission requires a time frame of years, not months.

The study by Myerson and Mayer (1966) represents the first really careful long-term follow-up of alcoholic patients. Unfortunately, the authors study a very socially isolated skid-row sample whose members when first followed were relatively old. Thus, it is not surprising that the authors observed a relatively low rate of recovery.

In many respects, the study by Sundby (1967) of 1722 male alcoholics treated in Norwegian clinics between 1925 and 1940 provides the best picture that we have of the natural history of alcoholism. Because of the large size of the sample, and the fact that the authors believed that their sample was representative of Norwegian alcoholics in general, the follow-up represents an extraordinary effort. Unfortunately, the study depended largely on institutional records. The quality of remissions from alcohol abuse and the reasons for them remain uncertain. Like the authors of the preceding two studies, Sundby did not specify return to asymptomatic drinking as a clearly identified outcome.

The fact that after 20 to 35 years Sundby observed a 64 percent rate of abstinence is, in part, a function of the fact that 62 percent of his original sample, including many of the most afflicted alcoholics, had died. However, of his 1061 recorded deaths, Sundby estimated that 48 percent probably had died sober; and he suggested that 53 percent of his total sample reflected 5-year cures. On the one hand, insistence upon five years of abstinence is a very conservative criterion for good outcome; on the other hand, Sundby's dependence upon institutional records may have inflated the number of apparent good outcomes. Nevertheless, Sundby's data support Drew's rather than Lemere's, view of the disorder; if alcoholics can but survive, they will often recover.

A fascinating finding from Sundby's study was that only 2 percent of the sample were ever diagnosed schizophrenic and only 0.35 percent were ever diagnosed as suffering from affective psychosis. The finding suggests that if alcoholism is often observed in psychotic patients it is because such patients repeatedly present themselves for clinical attention rather than because alcoholism is an important correlate of functional psychosis.

The eight-year follow-up by Goodwin and colleagues (1971) is noteworthy because it reflects the lowest death rate and the highest rate of return to asymptomatic drinking. That was because the felons who made up the sample were very young (average age 27). Unlike the men in most of the other samples, they had not sought treatment for alcohol dependence; but rather, when they were interviewed in prison, they had merely reported a past history of alcohol-related troubles. Thus, Goodwin's study is heuristically important because it underscores a fundamental principle involved in the reversibility of alcohol abuse. By inadvertently selecting alcoholics who had abused alcohol for only a short time and with little physiological dependence, Goodwin and his co-workers were able to identify a rather large number of "alcoholics" who were to return to asymptomatic drinking.

The most common reason given by the felons for returning to asymptomatic drinking was marriage and/or increasing family responsibilities. Marriage was also the reason most often given for returning to asymptomatic drinking by those Core City men who between the ages of 20 and 30 had experienced only two or three of the problems on the PDS. The implication is that if young problem drinkers in whom no dependence has occurred alter their peer group, they can often reverse their pattern of alcohol abuse and chronic progressive alcoholism does not occur.

Bratfos (1974) came to very different conclusions from those of Goodwin, Crane, and Guze, but he studied a very different sample. In a ten-year study of 412 Norwegian alcoholics, Bratfos observed no return to asymptomatic drinking. Instead, he viewed alcoholism as a "chronic progressive disease." This conclusion may result from both his failure to interview more than a small fraction of his original sample and the fact that on entrance to his study, 87 percent of his sample were both middle-aged and estimated to be gamma (physiologically dependent) alcoholics. In noting the bleakest results in any of the ten studies summarized in Table 3.8, Bratfos also employed the strictest definition of abstinence—four to ten years.

The study of Ojesjo (1981) represents, with the exception of the Core City study, the only longitudinal study of alcoholics derived from a relatively unselected community sample. Ojesjo began with a representative community sample of men drawn from the District of Lundby in Sweden. Twenty-five years before, Essen-Moller (1956) had selected 1312 men for an epidemiological study of mental illness. After ten years, Hagnell and Tunving refollowed up Essen-Moller's Lundby cohort with only 2 percent attrition (Hagnell 1966; Hagnell and Tunving 1972). Within the sample, they identified 96 alcohol abusers. The average age of the alcohol abusers was 47 years, and half of the 96 would have met the DSM III criteria for alcohol dependence. After the elapse of another 15 years, this sample was followed up again by Hagnell and Ojesjo; all but 4 of the 25 observed deaths among their 96 alcoholics occurred after age 65, and only 3 deaths occurred from suicide (Hagnell and Ojesjo 1975; Ojesjo 1981). Only two-thirds ever received clinical care for their alcoholism; no differential effect of treatment could be discerned. A third of the men who became abstinent cited ill health as the reason.

Only in the Clinic sample (to be discussed in a later section) and the Core City sample were subjects reinterviewed by multiple times. Like the men in Sundby's study, less than half of the Core City alcoholics were still abusing alcohol at last follow-up. Indeed, it is no accident that the durations of these two studies which report the highest rates of recovery were twice as long as the other studies cited. In summary, then, Drew's hypothesis that eventually alcoholics recover appears at least partly vindicated, and the natural rate of stable remission from alcoholism is perhaps 2 to 3 percent a year.

∽ The Natural History of Alcoholism Revisited

The last 15 years have seen additional progress in understanding the natural history of alcoholism, and as predicted, one of the most significant studies has come from Griffith Edwards and his coworkers at the Maudsley Hospital, who have followed their original (Orford and Edwards 1977) treatment group for 20 years (Edwards et al. 1983; Marshall et al. 1994; Taylor et al. 1985).

Work by Edwards and colleagues (1983) has supported the DSM III distinction between alcohol abuse and alcohol dependence. The authors underscore the paradox that in alcohol abuse the best long-term outcomes occur, on the one hand, among individuals with minimal alcohol abuse and good social stability, and, on the other hand, among individuals with the most severe alcohol dependence. In reviewing his data Edwards (1984) has also made the important distinction between the *natural history* of alcoholism (that is, the progression of alcohol abuse as a "disease" with a life of its own) and *drinking careers* (that is, how individuals use alcohol and respond to the consequences of abuse in an idiosyncratic fashion). This distinction is analogous to the distinction between the role the host plays and the role the bacteria or virus plays in shaping the symptomatology and course of an infectious disease. In an illness like alcoholism, characterized by relapses and remissions, the style of an individual's patterns of abstinence, controlled drinking, and alcohol abuse can vary greatly depending on the individual's personality, culture, and social environment.

Indeed, there have been several community studies pointing out the distinction between adolescent drinking careers, which may be characterized by voluntary episodic drunkenness, and the natural history of adult alcohol abuse, which is less under conscious control. In a 12-year follow-up of 384 junior high school students, 18 percent of whom were "problem drinkers" at 16, Jessor (1987) found that only 50 percent of the men and 26 percent of the women were still problem drinkers at age 26. In noting the "considerable discontinuity between adolescence and young adulthood" Jessor underscores the distinction between socially mediated drunkenness and the "alcohol dependence syndrome" as defined by Edwards (1986). The latter *is* far more common in middle life than in high school. Drunkenness and "problem drinking" at age 16 were more associated with loss of virginity, high social deviance, low church attendance, and low school performance than with continued problem drinking by age 26. Fillmore (1987) has also confirmed that chronicity of alcohol problems is highest in the middle years.

Two very important longitudinal studies of drinking habits of community samples (Glynn et al. 1985; Temple and Leino 1989) have helped to clarify a phenomenon noted by Cahalan (1970): that alcohol consumption and alcohol problems appear to decline after age 50. Common explanations of this phenomenon have been that heavy drinkers died young, that older heavy drinkers lied on questionnaires, and that problem drinkers "burned out." However, the most important reason for the apparent decline in alcohol consumption by the elderly appears to lie elsewhere. Temple and Leino (1989), in a 20-year follow-up of three staggered birth cohorts, and Glynn and colleagues (1985), in a nine-year follow-up of six staggered birth cohorts, found that the monthly consumption of alcohol and/or alcohol problems by a given birth cohort did not change appreciably over one or two decades. Rather, the reduced drinking behavior in older subjects appeared to be due more to generational changes (that is, birth cohort effects) than to growing older in itself. Glynn and colleagues noted that 20 percent of 106 30-year-olds but only 6 percent of 357 60-year-olds reported drinking problems—a threefold difference. Nine years later, however, the figures for the two samples were 19 percent and 7 percent respectively, an insignificant change. Temple and

Leino found that within a given birth cohort monthly consumption of alcohol did not change over 20 years, and that this stability seemed independent of response or nonresponse rate. Their findings raise the possibility that the greater prevalence of alcohol abuse noted previously among the Core City men, born in 1930, when contrasted to the College men, born in 1920, could represent a cohort effect rather than a product of lower socioeducational status.

However, Temple and Leino did observe that owing to abstinence among problem drinkers alcohol problems declined with time. Sixteen (16 percent) of the 103 subjects in their heaviest drinking group (more than 67 drinks a month) were abstinent or "infrequent" drinkers 20 years later. Twenty-four percent of their 538 men originally reported occasionally having 12 drinks or more at a sitting; 20 years later only 7 percent drank that heavily—a fall of almost two-thirds. Such findings are consistent with findings from the Study of Adult Development. First, a significant proportion of individuals with alcohol dependence become abstinent with time; second, and equally important, many alcohol abusers without dependence did *not* alter their drinking behavior over decades.

But, as Table 3.8 documents, both abstinence and mortality among alcohol abusers are important reasons for the decline in alcohol-related problems over time. Table 3.8A summarizes ten more recent studies that have followed alcohol-dependent individuals for 10 to 20 years. The first eight studies in Table 3.8A suggest that out of 675 alcoholic men and women followed for an average of 15 years until roughly age 60, only 169 (25 percent) were known to be still abusing alcohol at the end of the follow-up. These findings are similar to findings from the Study of Adult Development to be discussed below and fully congruent with the estimates of Drew and Lemere.

The findings from the two tables are from at least eight different countries and represent very diverse samples (for example, men and women, felons and individuals treated with controlled-drinking goals, and multiple ethnic groups); yet they paint a relatively uniform picture. Namely, the reason that alcoholism is relatively uncommon after the age of 60 is that roughly 2 percent of alcohol-dependent individuals become stably abstinent every year and after age 40 roughly 2 percent die every year. The tables also suggest that the findings from the Study of Adult Development may be representative of other populations.

Several of the individual studies in Table 3.8A deserve comment. The three studies with the lowest rates of alcohol abuse after ten years (Cross et al. 1990;

Finney and Moos 1991; O'Connor and Daly 1985) were all questionnaire studies, and all had high attrition rates. If their subjects dropped out because of sustained alcoholism, this would have inflated their recovery rates. The study by Längle and colleagues (1990) of 96 hospitalized German men and women is noteworthy for finding, by interview, 70 percent abstinent at ten years. Rates of controlled drinking were relatively high in two studies (McCabe 1986; Nordstrom and Berglund 1987) that on follow-up assessed drinking behavior on the basis of a few months rather than a full year. In other words, at any given time a significant number of alcohol abusers will appear to be using alcohol without problems. However, as Edwards (1989) notes, and as will be discussed more fully in Chapter 5, problem-free controlled drinking in former alcoholics is a very unstable category.

The study by Smith and colleagues (1983) is significant in that it is the only long-term follow-up of women. The authors noted that alcohol abuse shortened the average woman's life span by 15 years, and they found the death rate for women was four times what was expected. These excess deaths were divided fairly evenly between heart disease, cancer, violence, and cirrhosis.

The follow-up study by Finney and Moos (1991) is also noteworthy because it contrasts nondrinking behaviors like employment and social stability among alcoholics with similar behaviors among a sample of matched community controls. However, its findings are limited in that only 113 of the original 157 subjects were included for follow-up at the two-year point—a bias that may have excluded poor outcomes. The sample by Nordstrom and Berglund (1987) is also compromised by a very selective follow-up study. In order to identify "successfully adjusted alcoholics" they chose to follow up only 70 men who used very few sick days and 35 very ill alcoholics with disability pensions. Thus, not only was their sample not a community sample, it was not even representative of their clinic sample.

If after 20 years only 25 percent of the alcoholics are still drinking actively, what predicted chronicity? None of 25 intake variables chosen by Edwards and colleagues (1988) predicted outcome of drinking at ten years, including variables as promising as self-esteem, neuroticism, alcohol consumption, number of alcohol problems, alcohol-dependence score, social stability, and sociopathy. In part, this failure of predictive power is due to the fact, already noted, that alcohol abusers with the best prognosis come from two very divergent groups. Socially disadvantaged men with severe alcohol dependence are likely to become stably abstinent; they are also likely to die. Men with

TABLE 3.8A. Ten recent long-term follow-up studies of alcohol abuse.

Study and nature of sample	Nature of treatment	Type and length of follow-up	Size of original sample
Edwards et al. (1983) married, alcohol-dependent males age ca. 41	Outpatient Rx or advice	Interview 10 yr	99
Marshall, Edwards and Taylor (1994) Same sample as above	Same as above	Interview 20 yr	99
Nordstrom and Berglund (1987b) alcohol-dependent males age ca. 32; 70% excellent posthospital adjustment	Inpatient treatment	Interview 21 +/− 4 yr	105
O'Connor and Daly (1985) male voluntary first admission age ca. 48	Inpatient treatment	Questionnaire 20 yr	133
McCabe (1986) married, alcohol-dependent men and women age ca. 45	Inpatient treatment	Interview 16 yr	57
Pendry et al. (1982) alcohol-dependent male inpatients age ca. 40	Behavioral Rx to learn controlled drinking	Interview/ chart 10 yr	20
Finney and Moos (1991) high social stability men and women age ca. 40	Inpatient treatment	Questionnaire 10 yr	113 out of 157
Smith et al. (1983) alcohol-dependent women age ca. 44	Inpatient treatment	Interview 11 yr	103
Westermeyer and Peake (1983) Native Americans, severe dependence, men and women	Inpatient treatment	Interview 10 yr	45
Längle et al. (1993) alcohol-dependent men and women, age ca. 38	Inpatient treatment	Interview 10 yr	96
Cross et al. (1990) men and women, age ca. 48	Inpatient treatment plus AA	Questionnaire 10 yr	200

TABLE 3.8A continued

Attrition (%)		Number of survivors followed	Outcome for survivors (%)		
Lost or refused	Dead		Abstinent	Asymptomatic drinkers	Still alcoholic
13%	18%	68	28%	12%	60% n = 59
2%	43%	54	44%	30%	26% n = 14
21%	NA	84	18%	26%	56% n = 47
30%	40%	40	67%	15%	18% n = 7
4%	42%	31	26%	35%	39% n = 12
0	20%	16	38%	6%	56% n = 9
10% (35%)	17%	83	54%	24%	22% n = 18
11%[a]	31%	61	41%[a]		59%[a] n = 36
7%	20%	33	21%		79% n = 26
5%	22%	70	70%		30% n = 21
21%	22%	114	76%		24% n = 27

a. Estimated: text not clear.

excellent social stability and little dependence are likely to survive and to return to controlled drinking, but they are also very unlikely to achieve stable abstinence. Alcoholism is anything but unidimensional.

The Core City Sample

In order to bring the data from the Core City sample into sharper perspective, Figure 3.2 expands upon data from Table 3.8 and depicts a composite view of the use of alcohol by the Core City alcoholics over much of their adult life span. The figure was constructed by placing the lifetime patterns of alcohol use of 116 Core City alcohol abusers side by side and then estimating the percentage of men in any given category of alcohol use at five-year age intervals. The proportion of men in any category at any time is reflected by the area so shaded. The categories chosen in Figure 3.2 were social drinking, alcohol abuse, and remission from alcohol abuse either through stable abstinence or by return to asymptomatic drinking. As will be discussed later, the death rate of the relatively young alcoholics in community samples is very much lower than the death rate in older alcoholics in clinic samples. Thus, in Figure 3.2, the proportion of deaths from any cause is very modest.

The Core City men were interviewed at ages 25, 31, and 47, and their alcohol use was estimated from all data on their lives available to the study. Nevertheless, assembling the life charts summarized in Figure 3.2 necessitated dependence upon retrospective information. To compensate for this retrospective uncertainty, the two categories "? social drinking" and "? alcohol abuse" were devised. Not surprisingly, the percentage of the entire sample placed in these uncertain categories declined by the time of the age 47 interview. Although in any given year the judgment of a given man's alcohol use may be in error, the overall composite pattern depicted in Figure 3.2 is probably quite accurate.

For most of our subjects, the progression from asymptomatic social drinking to frank alcohol abuse to alcohol dependence occurred gradually over a span of 3 to 15 years. The retrospective study by Ullman (1953) and the testimonials of the Alcoholics Anonymous speakers, both of which suggest that alcohol abuse often begins after the alcoholic's first drink, were not confirmed in this prospective study. Rather, alcohol dependence appears very much to resemble tobacco dependence. Nobody "has to smoke" after a few weeks of cigarette use.

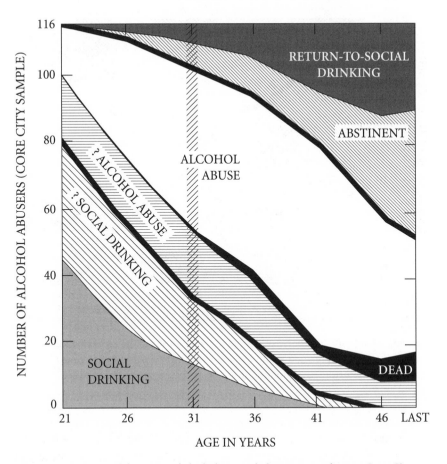

AGE IN YEARS

Figure 3.2 Composite life course of alcohol use and abuse among the 116 Core City men ever classified as alcohol abusers. Stippled area refers to the proportion drinking asymptomatically; lighter stippling indicates diagnostic uncertainty. Diagonal lines reflect men with 4+ symptoms of alcohol abuse; widely spaced diagonal lines indicate diagnostic uncertainty. The crosshatched line at age 31 is intended to accentuate differences in age of onset of alcohol abuse in the different samples in this and the following figures.

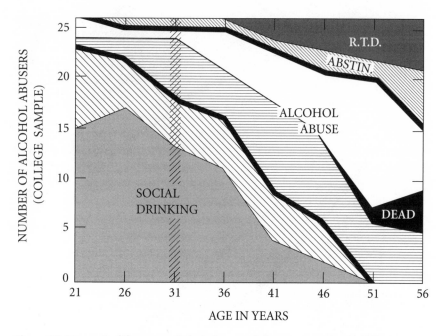

Figure 3.3 Composite life course of alcohol use and abuse among the 26 College alcohol abusers. Interpretation as in Figure 3.2. Abstin. = abstinence as defined in the text. R.T.D. = return to asymptomatic drinking after having met the criteria for alcohol abuse.

This gradual onset of alcoholism is made even clearer by Figure 3.3, which illustrates a composite life chart for alcohol use by the 26 alcohol abusers in the College sample. For these men, we had biennial questionnaire data regarding their use and abuse of alcohol. The onset of their alcohol abuse was even more gradual than that of the Core City sample. Many College alcohol abusers drank socially for as long as 20 years before their use of alcohol could be defined as abuse.

Admittedly, there is enormous individual variation in the evolution of alcoholism—both in the rapidity of onset of abuse and in the "progression" or eventual severity of alcohol dependence. Thus, compared to the alcoholism of the upper-middle-class, well socialized College sample, the alcoholism of the sociopaths in the Core City sample was a far more extreme disorder and one with a much more rapid onset. Figure 3.4 illustrates that many Core City sociopaths experienced onset in adolescence; the average PDS score of these

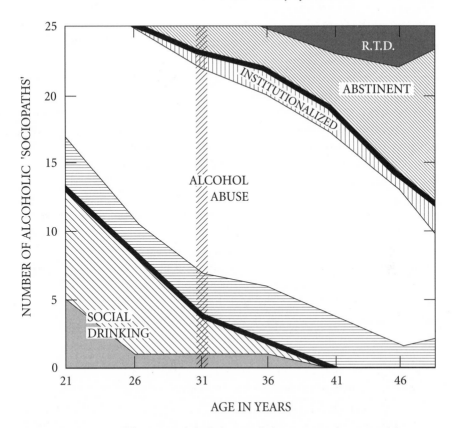

Figure 3.4 Composite life course of alcohol use and abuse among the 25 surviving Core City alcohol abusers who met Robins's criteria for sociopathy. Interpretation as in Figures 3.2 and 3.3. Note that a greater proportion of these men than of those in Figures 3.2 and 3.3 met the criteria for alcohol abuse unambiguously by age 31 and that fewer returned to asymptomatic drinking.

men was twice that of the College alcoholic. (However, the 3 College alcoholics who met Robins's criteria for sociopathy also had adolescent onsets and PDS scores over 14.) Thus, for the unhappy antisocial adolescent, the Alcoholics Anonymous testimonials may well be correct; alcohol was used from the beginning to alter consciousness, to obliterate conscience, and to defy social canons.

In short-term studies of alcoholism, sociopathy is often cited as a negative prognostic factor. However, contrasting the alcoholism of the College sample with that of the Core City sociopaths illustrates that, at last contact, a greater proportion of the sociopaths had achieved a stable recovery. In their eight-year study of felons, Goodwin and colleagues (1971) observed that neither the number of symptoms nor the severity of alcohol abuse correlated with the felon's eventual recovery from alcoholism.

Comparison of Figures 3.3 and 3.4 reveals yet another interesting point. It was only after many (10–15) years of severe alcohol abuse that most men achieved stable abstinence. Thus, one reason that more alcoholic Core City sociopaths than College alcoholics were in remission was that, although younger, the sociopaths had been severely alcoholic for a longer period.

Using Figure 3.2 as a point of reference, the course of alcohol use and abuse by the 456 Core City men may be summarized as follows. At some point, 160 Core City men were noted to experience one or more alcohol-related problems. Before reaching age 35, a quarter of these incipient alcohol abusers returned to asymptomatic drinking without "progressing" or incurring more than three known alcohol-related problems on the PDS. Some of these mild problem drinkers changed their peer group when they married; others "realized" that they had begun to lose control and reversed a habit while flexibility in their alcohol use still existed.

One hundred twenty Core City men went on to experience four or more symptoms of alcohol abuse on the PDS. Half did so after their 30th birthday; no more than half of the known alcohol abusers ever met the criteria for alcohol abuse at any given age. In other words, cross-sectional sampling cannot be expected to identify more than a fraction of the total members of a population who will ever develop alcoholism. From age 20 to 40 the proportion of the Core City men who were abusing alcohol at any given time waxed; then after 40, as Drew (1968) suggested, the rate of stable remissions exceeded the rate of new cases, and the proportion of active alcoholics in the entire sample waned. At 21, roughly 15 percent of the known Core City alcohol abusers met the criteria for alcohol abuse; by age 40, the proportion actively abusing alcohol was over 50 percent; at most recent follow-up the proportion had fallen to one-third. As might be expected, as the Core City men continue to be followed into their 50s, new cases of alcohol abuse and new remissions continue to be observed.

∾ The Core City Sample Revisited

Figure 3.4A depicts the course of alcohol abuse among the Core City men up to the age of 60. As already noted, the number of identified alcohol abusers

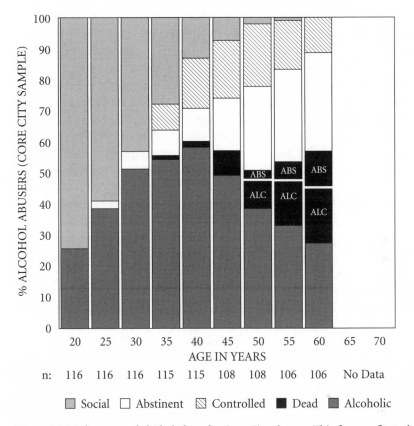

Figure 3.4A Life course of alcohol abuse by Core City abusers. This figure reflects the quinquennial alcohol-use status of the 116 Core City men who remained active in the study and met the DSM III criteria for alcohol abuse. The 8 men who because of brief duration of alcohol abuse and minimal symptoms were classified as "social drinkers" have been excluded. The proportion of deaths among men classified as alcohol abusers is indicated by the label ALC; the proportion among those classified as stably abstinent, by ABS.

was increased from 120 to 150 by the inclusion of all men who met the DSM III criteria for alcohol abuse and the 8 men who began alcohol abuse or dependence after age 47. Unfortunately, attrition also continued: 7 alcohol abusers had withdrawn from the study prior to interview at age 47 and 19 more had withdrawn by age 60. Eight other men, although meeting DSM III criteria for alcohol abuse, quickly returned to social drinking. Thus, Figure 3.4A includes only 116 men. In addition, there were 10 alcohol abusers who remained active participants in the study but for whom we did not have data on alcohol abuse at age 60. The National Death Index has been regularly searched for the entire sample so that our mortality data is virtually complete.

For both samples the follow-up method since age 47 has depended upon the men's answers on the biennial questionnaires to questions about problem drinking. On each questionnaire the men were asked four or more true-or-false questions designed to capture problem drinking. For example, "I wish I drank less alcohol. My relatives wish I drank less alcohol. My doctor advised me to use less alcohol. I have recently stopped drinking because. . ." They also were asked how much and how often they used alcohol, but this quantity-frequency data was usually unrevealing except to identify abstinence. Abstinence was defined as having less than one drink a month. If a subject with a prior diagnosis of alcohol abuse reported one or more alcohol-related problems in a year, he was regarded as an alcohol abuser for that year, and as a probable alcohol abuser for the preceding and following years. If a man did not respond to two consecutive questionnaires, data from recent physical exams was examined and a telephone interview was attempted.

The categories of alcohol abuse and abstinence are probably quite trustworthy. Most of the men categorized as abstinent in Figure 3.4A had been stably abstinent for a decade or more, and there was little reason to believe that men would report alcohol-related problems if these did not exist. The most problematic category was the former alcohol abusers who reported that they were now drinking regularly but without problems. For these men a face-to-face interview and information from relatives would have been more reliable.

Figure 3.4A is striking for several reasons. First, by age 60 only 27 percent (29) of the 116 men remaining in the study were still known to be abusing alcohol. This decline in alcohol abuse was due more to abstinence and mortality than to "burning out" or returning to social drinking. Almost one-third of the men (31) were no longer at risk for alcohol abuse because they were dead. Thirty-four men enjoyed stable abstinence and another 12 reported that they had returned to stable, asymptomatic drinking. (In addition, 8 men who had abused alcohol for less than five years in their youth were arbitrarily reclassified as social drinkers and excluded from the figure.) These men were all alcohol abusers by DSM III criteria but not by PDS criteria. Age 60 information was not available for the remaining 10 surviving men, but at last contact (ca. age 55) only 1 man had been stably abstinent and only 2 had unambiguously returned to asymptomatic drinking; thus as many as 7 additional men may have been abusing alcohol. Indeed, if the 26 men who withdrew from the study were included, and if the status of all 150 men were classified by when they were last heard from, 45 (30 percent) of the 150 men would be classified as still actively abusing alcohol.

Is Alcoholism a "Progressive Disease"?

Jellinek (1952) tentatively set forth a natural progression of the symptoms underlying the "disease" of gamma alcoholism. He derived his scheme from interviewing members of Alcoholics Anonymous. Since the publication of Jellinek's paper, the view of alcoholism as a progressive disease—proceeding inexorably from stage to stage in fixed sequence ending inevitably in abstinence or death—has become part of the enduring mythology of alcoholism.

In the past decade there has appeared a compelling and coherent body of empirical work, assembled by the Social Research Group at the University of California at Berkeley, that suggests quite the opposite. The evidence is based upon several well-executed epidemiological studies (Knupfer 1972; Cahalan and Room 1974; Fillmore 1975; Clark 1976; Room 1977; Roizen et al. 1978).

Summarizing much of this work, Clark and Cahalan write, "The common conception of alcoholism as a disease fails to cover a large part of the domain of alcohol problems and a more useful model would place greater emphasis on the development and correlates of *particular problems* related to drinking, rather than assuming that alcoholism as an underlying and unitary, progressive disease is the source of most alcohol problems" (1976, p. 251). They point out that Park's (1973) empirical effort to validate Jellinek's idea of progressive symptoms ended in failure: progression was found only for a small number of characteristic experiences, and then only by subdividing the alcoholics into more homogeneous groups. Clark and Cahalan suggest that no natural boundary exists between remission and nonremission from alcohol-related problems. Elsewhere, Clark restates the whole problem: "What is questioned is the usefulness of conceptualizing alcoholism as a progressive entity that is sufficiently different from other drinking problems to receive separate consideration" (1976, p. 1257).

In a four-year prospective study of alcohol use by a community sample of randomly selected white males, Clark and Cahalan (1976) found little evidence of "progression." Of particular interest, they noted that most respondents who reported loss of control also had alcohol-related problems, but that a majority of those who had an alcohol-related problem did not report loss of control. The symptoms of binge drinking, physical dependence, high alcohol intake, and loss of control tended to occur as a cluster; but otherwise, alcohol-related symptoms were remarkably independent of one another. Indeed, loss of control reported at the beginning of the observation period correlated with reported loss of control four years later with an r of only .13.

How can such findings be reconciled with Jellinek's concept of alcoholism as a progressive disease? How can such views be reconciled with the graphic and conceptual tidiness of Figure 3.2? In the figure, all the Core City men are dichotomized into alcoholics and nonalcoholics, into states of remission and disease. Clearly, methodological considerations become crucial. Contrasting the methodology used to study the Core City subjects with the methodology employed by Clark and Cahalan's group helps to reconcile the findings of these studies with those of Jellinek.

On the one hand, the course of a chronic relapsing disease may appear very unstable: if many mild cases are included, if data are gathered by questionnaire, if deaths are excluded, if periods of observation are short, if syndromes are broken down into individual symptoms, and if individual case histories are ignored. On the other hand, the course of a chronic disease may appear stable and progressive: if only severe cases are included, if data are gathered by skilled clinical interview, if all deaths are recorded, if symptoms—however individually unstable—are treated as a cluster, if long periods of observation are used, and if individual lives rather than statistical analyses are scrutinized. The first method is valuable to epidemiology and in understanding the behavior of heterogeneous populations. The second method is valuable to clinical medicine and in understanding population subgroups. Cahalan and his co-workers employed the first method; the Core City study employed the second method.

One difficulty with the first method is that, by depending upon statistical analyses of data derived from self-administered questionnaires, Cahalan and his co-workers lose the power of the clinical case history. For example, Clark (1976) reports that 18 out of 29 self-acknowledged binge drinkers reported no loss of control. Such an observation may seem reasonable enough in a computer analysis of the results of a self-administered questionnaire but might provoke incredulity in a clinician personally interviewing an informant. From a clinical vantage point binge drinking and loss of control occur together. It is no accident that sociological investigators who view a heterogeneous sample of drinkers from afar and who know their subjects only as data cards scoff at the idea of a progressive disease. For example, the Rand

Report (Armor et al. 1978) appeared to confirm the findings of the Berkeley Social Research Group that progression did not exist, but at first the authors of that report ignored the very significant fraction of their subjects who died—many as a result of alcoholism.

In contrast, a problem with the second method is that clinicians who follow the individual lives of severely ill alcoholics may become unduly entranced by small numbers of patients selected from biased samples and thus become too impressed by predictability and the progression of the life course of alcoholics.

I suspect that Clark and Cahalan may overstate their case when they suggest that problem drinking (six or more alcohol-related problems) is a very unstable phenomenon. Out of 786 men, they had relatively complete data on 521 men at two separate times four years apart (Roizen et al. 1978). Of these men, 59 had six or more alcohol-related problems at initial observation. Four years later, only 14 percent of these 59 men reported no problems at all—the proportion that Table 3.8 would predict if the remission rate is about 3 percent a year. The fact that 44 percent of these 59 men experienced fewer than six problems in the fourth year of follow-up conveyed to the authors that these subjects no longer met their criterion of problem drinking. But such a definition is idiosyncratic. Most alcohol *users* after all can drink for a year without *any* alcohol-related problems, and most alcoholics cannot. That is the crucial difference. Thus, in the study by Cahalan and his co-workers, although a majority of individuals who reported loss of control or evidence of physiological dependence ("symptomatic drinking") at one time, did not, by questionnaire, admit *that* particular problem four years later, more than three-quarters of such individuals continued to report *some* alcohol problem four years later, and therefore, met the criteria of this book for alcohol abuse.

Finally, it remains unclear how much the lack of correlation between alcohol abuse in Clark and Cahalan's sample in 1967 and four years later results from their 33 percent rate of attrition or from some alcoholic individuals who were abstinent in 1967 relapsing by 1972, or from severe problem drinkers in 1967 dying of their disease by 1972 and thus becoming lost to follow-up. For example, careful scrutiny of the apparent instability of alcohol abuse by a more completely studied community sample of alcoholics reveals that the absence of alcoholic progression that appears in statistical comparison of cross-sectional data may be more apparent than real. In studying 96 alcoholics at two separate times 15 years apart, Ojesjo (1981) categorized their subjects' alcoholism (in terms of increasing severity) as alcohol abuse, alcohol dependence, and chronic alcoholism (dependence with medical sequelae). Over time, these three categories seemed most unstable. Of 49 men categorized as alcohol abusers in 1957, only 4 were still categorized alcohol abusers in 1972. Of 29 men classified as alcohol-dependent in 1957, only 8 were still alcohol-dependent in 1972. Concealed in this apparent instability, however, was support for Jellinek's concept of progression. Among the 49 men who were counted as alcohol abusers in 1957, 17 were no longer alcohol abusers in 1972 because their alcoholism had progressed either to death or chronic alcoholism; another 25 had achieved stable remission. Of the 29 alcohol-dependent men, 13 had progressed to death or chronic alcoholism, 4 had achieved stable abstinence, and, as noted above, 8 remained alcohol-dependent. Thus, after 15 years, only 4 alcohol-dependent men contradicted the concept of progression by being reclassified in 1972 as alcohol abusers.

In making these criticisms of the work of the Berkeley Social Research Group, I must at the same time stress that their work has been invaluable in underscoring that a black and white medical model of alcoholism is untenable. In my allegiance to Jellinek and the medical model, both I and Figure 3.2 do oversimplify. Another advantage of the work of the Social Research Group is that it underscores the distinction between drunkenness and alcoholism. Aamark (1951) and Keller (1975) both elaborate the distinction between Cahalan's "problem drinker" and Jellinek's "clinic alcoholic." The modal "problem drinker" is aged 25 to 35 and is married and working. He (or she) has never been treated for alcoholism; and his use is markedly responsive to environmental factors and can, over time, become either more or less symptomatic. In such individuals, symptoms of alcohol abuse are likely to be "disjunctive," by which I mean that the presence of a given symptom of alcohol abuse in a given problem drinker will not significantly predict the presence of symptoms that Jellinek would suggest would theoretically precede it.

In contrast, the modal "clinic alcoholic" is ten years older, aged 35–45, and exhibits unstable marital and employment status. He (or she) may have sought treatment for alcoholism, and his use of alcohol is relatively insensitive to environmental variables. He often stops using alcohol entirely but is unable to use it asymptomatically for long periods. In such individuals the presence of a given symptom will be statistically associated with other earlier symptoms.

The two critical differences between the "problem drinker" and the "clinic alcoholic" are, first, that the clinic alcoholic is a subtype of the problem drinker and second, that the clinic alcoholic has been habitually using alcohol for a decade longer.

In her 20-year follow-up of college students, Fillmore (1975) found that only 20 percent of 50 serious college-aged problem drinkers still had problems 20 years later. She observed that blackouts in college correlated only .07 with severe alcohol problems 20 years later. Similarly, heavy college drinking in this book's College sample was a very poor predictor of heavy drinking at age 47. Indeed, within the College sample, midlife drinking habits bore a much higher relation to college smoking habits than they did to college drinking habits.

Thus, to Clark and Cahalan's assertion that "it is among young males rather than older males that the highest rate of almost all types of drinking problems are to be found" (1976, p. 258) must be added the clinical assertion that it is among older men, 35–50, that the greatest number of alcoholics—those for whom the notion of progressive disease model fits—will be found.

If I am to persist in my effort to discuss the natural evolution of alcoholism as a unitary phenomenon, I must follow Clark and Cahalan's suggestion of subdividing the alcoholics into more homogeneous groups. Table 3.9 reflects this effort. Although there have been efforts to classify alcoholics into categories—for example, the alpha, beta, and gamma categories of Jellinek (1960), the "reactive" and "essential" categories of Levine and Zigler (1973), and the "moderate" and "severe" categories of Cloninger and colleagues (1981)—there have been no systematic longitudinal follow-ups of such categories. Dynamic shifts in the unfolding of alcohol abuse make it difficult to defend any existing static definitions.

Table 3.9 outlines four broad life-course patterns into which I shall attempt to organize the unique life courses of the 110 best-studied Core City alcohol abusers. On the basis of the clinical interview, each Core City alcohol abuser was assigned to one of four patterns: "progressive" alcoholism, stable abstinence, return to asymptomatic drinking, or atypical (nonprogressive) alcoholism. These four patterns can be further condensed into two broad categories. The first category includes 73 men whose life course was consistent with Jellinek's view that alcoholism either continues to worsen or necessitates complete abstinence. The second category includes the 37 men whose *atypical* life course justifies the view of Clark and Cahalan that alcohol abuse is unpredictably episodic.

Table 3.9 makes it clear that the alcoholism of the alcoholics with a progressive course was more severe than that of the alcoholics with an atypical course. In terms of the three scales used to measure alcoholism, the alcoholics

TABLE 3.9.   Comparison of Core City men with different longitudinal patterns of alcohol abuse.

	Progressive course		Nonprogressive, atypical course	
	Progressive (n = 35)	Currently abstinent (n = 38)	Atypical (n = 19)	Return to asymptomatic drinking (n = 18)
Severity of alcoholism				
8+ problems on PDS	71%	61%	42%	11%
Dependent (DSM III)	74	74	42	33
7+ problems on Cahalan scale	71	71	47	39
Admits problems with control	71	89	58	72
Diagnosed alcoholic by clinician	56	51	32	6
50+ pack/years of smoking	53	57	37	28
Hospital or clinic visit	54	58	42	22
Risk factors				
1 + alcoholic relatives	69	79	63	67
Mediterranean ethnicity	17	11	11	22
Truancy or school problems	3	21	16	0
Consequences				
5+ on Robins scale	32	32	11	6
4+ years of unemployment	51	47	37	33
Social class IV-V	83	58	63	72
Alcohol-related medical problems	83	46	32	55
Chronic illness	44	43	37	21
10+ adult years unmarried	57	54	26	45
Psychological health				
HSRS > 80	0	26	17	17
Mood at interview "good"	28	68	72	39

whose drinking career conformed to the "disease" stereotype were more symptomatic; and they were more likely to be hospitalized and to be identified as alcoholic by clinicians. The most dramatic difference was that 65 percent of the progressive alcoholics had eight or more problems on the Problem Drinking Scale as contrasted to only 29 percent of the alcoholics with an atypical course. Thus, to some degree the concept of progressive alcoholism is a tautology. To experience many different alcohol-related symptoms requires that one's alcoholism progress.

There were other differences between progressive and nonprogressive alcoholics that are not spelled out in Table 3.9. The 18 men who returned to asymptomatic drinking used fewer mood-altering drugs, but they were just as likely as progressive alcoholics to have experienced difficulty with the law and to have gotten into alcohol-related fights. Consistent with Jellinek's model of progression, the men who returned to asymptomatic drinking had very rarely been fired or sustained chronic unemployment, and were far less likely to have engaged in binge drinking than men in the other three categories. Expressed differently, the alcohol abuser who comes to public attention because of barroom brawls or a single alcohol-related infraction is much less likely to be someone whose life will be ruled by alcohol than is the alcohol abuser who seeks help from clinics, who worries about his capacity for control, or who has job-related difficulties—events that Jellinek suggests occur later in the course of the disorder.

It is interesting, too, that severity of tobacco addiction paralleled alcohol addiction. In Table 3.9, the progressive alcoholics were twice as likely as the atypical alcoholics to be inveterate two-pack-a-day smokers. (Smoking was measured as the number of packs an individual smoked per day multiplied by the number of years he had smoked. Thus, someone who smoked 10 cigarettes a day for 20 years and someone who smoked two packs a day for five years and then stopped would both be referred to as ten-pack/year smokers.)

The many observers who believe that slums and anomie cause alcoholism and not the reverse have blamed the malignancy of progressive alcoholism on adverse social circumstances. However, in Table 3.9 poor social adjustment appears to be a result of the severity of alcohol abuse and not its cause. Originally there were no differences between the four subgroups of alcohol abusers in terms of I.Q., social class of parents, stability of childhood, or boyhood competence. In the past, the currently abstinent had experienced just as much antisocial behavior and unemployment as the men with the worst outcomes, but upward social mobility was most common among the currently abstinent. This finding suggests that low social class does not cause alcoholism as much as severe alcoholism causes low social class.

Alcohol-related medical problems were slightly more common among those who returned to asymptomatic drinking than among those who were abstinent; perhaps this was because the recognition of alcohol-related physical distress was often the critical confrontation that led such individuals to cut down on their drinking. One of the most dramatic differences in Table 3.9, however, is that *multiple* alcohol-related problems were twice as likely among the progressive alcoholics as among all other groups. Indeed, some clinicians believe that one of the defining characteristics of the chronic alcoholic is an unusually dense denial of the complications of alcoholism.

In the fourth category of Table 3.9, psychological health, there was a surprise. In recent years, some writers on alcoholism (Pattison 1968; Blane 1978), have decried the emphasis of treatment programs on abstinence rather than upon the less puritanical goal of return to moderate drinking. However, men who returned to asymptomatic drinking appeared no more cheerful to the interviewers than the men whose alcoholism was progressing. Although the numbers are admittedly small and halo effects were not controlled, the abstinent were the most likely to have been categorized as happy and as mentally healthy at interview.

~ Table 3.9 Revisited

Over the next 15 years significant changes occurred in the outcome categories presented in Table 3.9. By age 60 a third of the men in the table could be classified differently. In Table 3.9A the five outcome categories on the left-hand side include the category of "stable abstinence" which means that the men had been stably abstinent (less than one drink a month) for at least three years by time of death or by age 60 or at last contact, and that their abstinence was not a result of institutionalization. The category "continued alcohol abuse" refers to men who continued to meet the criteria for DSM III alcohol abuse at death or at last follow-up without experiencing a prolonged (more than three years) period of return to controlled drinking.

"Sustained return to controlled drinking" refers to men who had been able to continue to drink more frequently than once a month with no reported problems and had sustained this pattern for more than three years and until age 60, death, or last contact. The category "relapse from controlled drinking"

TABLE 3.9A.   Fate of 150 Core City men with different longitudinal patterns of alcohol abuse.

Longitudinal pattern at age 60	Longitudinal Pattern at age 47				
	"Progressive" alcoholism n = 35 (14)	*Currently abstinent* n = 38 (13)	*Atypical* n = 19 (2)	*Return to asymptomatic drinking* n = 18 (2)	*New cases* n = 40 (10)
Stable abstinence n = 48 (14)	4 (1)	30 (12)	2	4	8 (1)
Continued alcohol abuse n = 48 (19)	23 (12)	4	8	0	13 (7)
Sustained return-to-controlled drinking n = 18 (2)	6 (1)	1	4	6 (1)	1
Relapse from controlled drinking n = 7 (1)	0	0	0	6 (1)	1
Ever alcoholic; return to social drinking n = 8 (2)	0	0	0	0	8 (2)
Withdrew from study n = 21 (3)	2	3 (1)	5 (2)	2	9

Note: Numbers in parentheses indicate deaths.

refers to men who had established a clear pattern of asymptomatic drinking of three and usually more than five years but then had returned to alcohol abuse by the time of death or last contact. Finally, the small category "ever alcoholic; return to social drinking" refers to the 8 men who had met the category of DSM III alcohol abuse as young adults but who had not met the criteria for alcohol abuse used in the earlier version of this book (four or more alcohol-related problems on the PDS). All of these 8 men had fallen in alcohol use category V, had abused alcohol for less than five years, and had returned to social asymptomatic drinking for ten or more years and for the purposes of Figure 3.4A had been excluded. Evenly distributed through the four outcome categories at age 47 were 15 men who subsequently withdrew from the study.

Along the top of Table 3.9A are the same four age-47 categories that appear at the top of Table 3.9. As can be seen by the numbers in parentheses, 27 (37 percent) of the 73 Core City alcohol abusers who at age 47 fit the model of alcoholism as a "progressive disease" were dead by age 60, whereas only 4 (11 percent) of the 37 alcoholics with a less typical course at age 47 were dead.

Of the 35 men who at age 47 had manifested a pattern of progressive alcoholism, 23 had continued the pattern until age 60. But of these 23 chronic alcoholics only 11 were still alive. In addition, 2 of the "progressive" alcoholics had withdrawn from the study. Of the remaining 10 men, 4 had achieved stable abstinence and 6 reported trouble-free drinking. Thirty (79 percent) of the 38 men who were classified as stably abstinent at age 47 continued to be abstinent at age 60 or death. Over the intervening 15 years only 4 of these 38 abstinent men had relapsed. Only 3 had withdrawn from the study, and 1 had resumed controlled drinking.

The 37 men who did not originally conform to a model of alcoholism as a progressive disease clearly fared better than the men in the first two categories in the table in terms of mortality, but they did not enjoy a particularly benign course. At last contact 6 of these men had been abstinent for years, and 14 of the 37 had eventually conformed to a pattern of chronic alcohol abuse. Another 7 had withdrawn from the study, always a sign suggestive of poor outcome. Thus, of the 37 men with an atypical course at age 47, only 10 had continued to contradict the model of alcoholism as a chronic disease. Table 3.9A also illustrates the distribution of the "new" cases— those men not included in Table 3.9—among the age-60 outcome categories.

Table 3.9B examines the association of alcohol abuse outcome category at age 60 with the independent variables shown in Table 3.9. As noted by Edwards (et al. 1988), stable remission in alcohol abuse seems remarkably difficult to predict. It seems clear that the progress of alcohol abuse into stable abstinence or lifetime chronicity was predicted neither by severity nor by premorbid risk factors. Men from multiproblem families were no more likely to experience chronic alcohol abuse, and those who showed the best boyhood competence were no more likely to recover.

Men with an atypical course, however, while not as dramatically different as at age 47, did exhibit fewer risk factors and have lower mortality. Twelve of the 96 men with a "progressive" course (Table 3.9B) had manifested three or all four risk factors (northern European ethnicity, alcoholic heredity, hyperactivity, and antisocial behavior) prior to developing alcohol abuse, whereas only 1 of the 33 men who spent at least some time successfully

TABLE 3.9B. Comparison of Core City men with different patterns of alcohol abuse at age 60.

	"Progressive" course		Atypical or controlled drinkers $n = 33$	Drops $n = 21$
	Continued alcoholism $n = 48$	Stable abstinence $n = 48$		
Severity of alcoholism				
8+ problems on PDS	48%	42%	21%[a]	48%
Dependent (DSM III)	56	60	33[a]	52
Admits problems with control	56	78	64	56
Diagnosed alcoholic by clinicians	37	35	18	44
60+ packs/year of smoking	61	48	54	55
Hospital or clinic visit	38	44	27	38
30+ AA meetings	6	27	0	5
Risk Factors (premorbid)				
1+ alcoholic relatives	69	81	58[a]	76
Mediterranean ethnicity	15	6	21	14
Truancy or school problems	7	13	3	14
Hyperactivity	15	15	6	0
Best boyhood competence	19	23	9	19
Multiproblem childhood	19	13	18	24[b]
I.Q. < 90	25	21	36	43[a]
Concomitants (age 47)				
5+ on Robins scale	22	17	12	24
4+ years of unemployment	33	32	21	56[b]
Social class IV-V	64	57	64	80[b]
10+ years unmarried	50	43	55	37
HSRS > 85	5	18	12	7
Consequences (1994)				
Dead (1994)	44	31	15[a]	14
Chronic illness or dead (1994)	81	60	56	?

a. "Atypical" or "controlled drinkers" different from "progressive" ($p < .05$ chi square).
b. Drops significantly different from still participating alcoholics ($p < .06$ chi square).

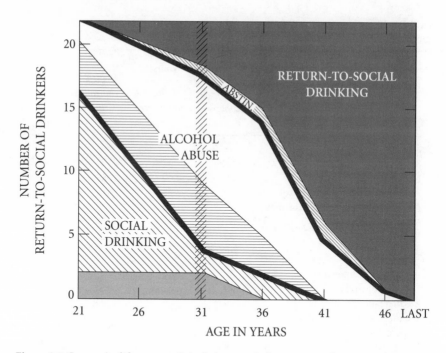

Figure 3.5 Composite life course of alcohol use and abuse among the 22 Core City return-to-social drinkers. Interpretation as in Figure 3.2.

returning to asymptomatic drinking had manifested that many risk factors. (These 33 were the men in Table 3.9A who ever returned to controlled (n = 25) or social (n = 8) drinking.

The men who dropped out of the study manifested the clearest evidence of relative social instability both premorbidly and postmorbidly. They were more likely to show low intelligence and to have had a multiproblem childhood; in adulthood they were more likely to be chronically unemployed, to be in the lowest social class, and to show multiple sociopathic traits on the Robins Scale of Sociopathy.

A Multifaceted Disease

When the lifespan drinking patterns of the 22 men in Figure 3.5 who had met one or more of this book's criteria for alcoholism and returned to asymptomatic drinking are compared to the drinking patterns of 42 men in

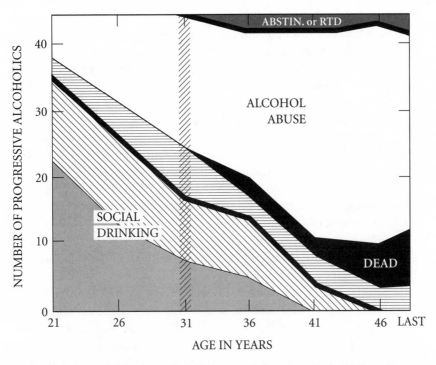

Figure 3.6 Composite life course of alcohol use and abuse among the 42 Core City progressive alcohol abusers. Interpretation as in Figure 3.2.

Figure 3.6 whose drinking was classified as progressive, the comparison is revealing. (The n in Figure 3.6 is 42, not 35 as in Table 3.9, because the figure includes 7 men who died.) Men who returned to asymptomatic drinking spent a much smaller portion of their adult lives "out of control" of their drinking—an average of four years as contrasted to the average of 15 years for the progressive alcoholics depicted in Figure 3.6. When the PDS and Cahalan scores were combined, the average return-to-asymptomatic drinker had experienced 11 problems and the progressive alcoholic had experienced 20 problems. In other words, the more severe, numerous, and prolonged the symptoms, the more a given patient's alcohol abuse will conform to reductionistic views of alcoholism as a progressive unitary disease. The milder and less progressive the alcohol abuse, the more the future course of a given patient can be used as ammunition against the black and white views of Alcoholics Anonymous and the National Council on Alcoholism. Thus, the concept that alcoholism is progressive is a tautology that can only be established in retrospect. If an alcoholic experiences many alcohol-related problems, the clinicians may assume that the alcoholic has lost control of his drinking, but such an assumption by no means proves that the loss of control came first. As Orford (1973) has noted empirically, the more controlled an alcoholic's past drinking the more he will wish for and be able to return to a pattern of controlled drinking in the future.

Trice and Wahl (1958) and more recently Porkorny and colleagues (1981) have obtained retrospective data that confirm the general outline of Jellinek's temporal sequencing of alcoholic symptoms in advanced alcoholics. Blackouts and frequent intoxication come first; these symptoms are followed by arrests, complaints by others, morning drinking, and attempts to go on the wagon. These symptoms are then followed by job loss and binge drinking (benders and intermittent drinking). Finally, an average of three to ten years after the start of the process, convulsions and decreased tolerance to alcohol occur and finally hospital treatment and/or involvement with Alcoholics Anonymous.

Tomasovic (1974) contrasted binge drinkers with alcoholics who drank more or less continuously. He noted that the former had been problem drinkers significantly longer (18.1 versus 14.5 years) and were twice as likely to have had delirium tremens and to have visited Alcoholics Anonymous. In a fascinating study, Park (1962) found the same general sequence in Finnish and English alcoholics that Jellinek observed in American alcoholics. Park observed roughly the same speed of progression—five to seven years from blackouts and morning drinking to voluntary hospitalizations and morning tremors. However, at each stage, he noted that the members of his English sample were five years older than those of his Finnish sample.

The 73 Core City alcohol abusers with a progressive course confirmed the general outlines of Jellinek's model, but because much of the data was gathered retrospectively, no effort was made in the Core City study to obtain precise sequencing of individual symptoms of alcohol abuse. Certainly, binge drinking and AA attendance were seen late and were most common among the abstainers who, at least in theory, had progressed the furthest. In contrast, blackouts, complaints by relatives, arrests, and alcohol-facilitated belligerence were equally common to all four groups in Table 3.9. The symptoms of alcohol abuse in the College sample occurred roughly 20 years later than those in the Core City sociopathic sample (Figures 3.3 and 3.4) but in the same general sequence. Admittedly, individual variability was enormous.

In illustrating the variability but also the reality of progression, the sequentially gathered comments of a member of the College study are particularly illustrative. Tom Braceland began drinking at age 13. Although he acknowledged no problems from alcohol use in college, he did experience blackouts. He reported that he had more fun and felt more full of energy when he did not drink. After four difficult years in the navy in World War II, Tom wrote, "I got quite drunk often in officers' clubs," and he noted for the first time occasional morning drinking and tremors after heavy drinking the night before. (It was only 30 years later that he admitted to the study that it was at this point that he secretly recognized that he might have a drinking problem.)

At age 29 Tom wrote, "Alcohol is very nice to me . . . it convinces me that the world is better than it seems. I never have hangovers." Four years later, he wrote, "I don't think I am an alcoholic, but I drink maybe a quart a week, I am unhappy with less." At age 35, he wrote hopefully, "Now things are going so well, I am changing from a heavy to a moderate drinker." But two years later he admitted, "I drink much too much; a major worry. Maybe a pint of whiskey a day on average." (In four years, he had advanced from a steady three to four drinks a day to a steady ten drinks a day.) By age 44 he wrote, "I drink all day and half the night . . . I go to a psychiatrist three times a week to bring the drinking problem under control." And three years later he began formally to go on the wagon: "I quit drinking three months ago, hopefully for life."

Tom began attending alcohol clinics as an outpatient, and by age 50 his drinking had become increasingly intermittent. He wrote, "I feel I have alcohol barely under control. I really do quit for a period of weeks or months." Four to five years later Tom admitted increasing loss of control, fear, and hopelessness. "I really don't want to stop drinking . . . never hospitalized . . . I hope I can cut down on the booze before it kills me . . . I have been an alcoholic for at least ten years . . . If I start drinking I overdo it grotesquely." Tom's sense of self-worth became increasingly undermined. "I don't like the idea of AA," he wrote. "I don't think I could be helpful to anyone else."

At age 57 Tom began to notice decreased tolerance of alcohol: "I can drink for about a month before starting to consume lethal quantities of the stuff. After a month, I have to go back on the wagon . . . at my peak, I guess, I consume 12–15 ounces of vodka. This goes on only two or three days before my stomach rebels and I have to quit." Ten years earlier, he had been able to drink 16 ounces of whiskey a day for weeks at a stretch.

At age 59 Tom again went on the wagon, joined Alcoholics Anonymous, and concurrently joined the ranks of the stably abstinent. After two years of sobriety, he wrote, "I am an alcoholic and I don't drink alcohol . . . I wish I had sought help from AA 20 years earlier . . . Booze problem licked. I feel I am beginning to grow." What is clear from Tom Braceland's history is that the progressive nature of his alcohol abuse would have been invisible within the time frame of a four-year follow-up study.

❧ Progression Revisited

Unlike abstinence for many of the underprivileged, alcohol-dependent Core City men, for Tom Braceland abstinence was not very stable. At age 61, after two years of doing well in AA, he tried to return to "social" drinking. For a few months he confined himself to two or three drinks a day; then he would start to lose control. He would then become abstinent for several months only to return to his unsuccessful experiment to drink in a controlled fashion. His only boast was that he did not "get drunk." At 64 he again became abstinent for almost two years; and then at age 66 he returned to trying to drink two or three drinks a day. The next year he required hospitalization for detoxification. For the last four years, until age 71, he has maintained abstinence.

Fifteen years later, not only were there additions to the story of Tom Braceland, but there were also additions to my understanding of the natural history of alcohol abuse. The course of alcohol abusers in the College sample contradicted my previous assertions that sustained alcohol abuse without abstinence is a progressive disorder. As mentioned earlier, Edwards (1984) has emphasized that in understanding the course of alcoholism we need to separate the concept of natural history from that of career. Natural history is the development of the individual's reactivity to alcohol abuse; career pertains to the evolution of the individual's style of abusing alcohol. Natural history is an idea borrowed from medicine and underlies Jellinek's phases of alcoholism. The term implies a biological condition with a tendency, once established, toward an inexorable progression of symptoms. In such a model environmental factors and an individual's characteristics only determine the pace of progression. Career is a concept borrowed from sociology and draws attention both to the individual and to the individual's culture and social milieu, which shape and encourage certain behaviors and constrain others. Social scientists have shown how drinking careers are influenced by "the individuality of the drinker, by the perceptions and reactions around him, by

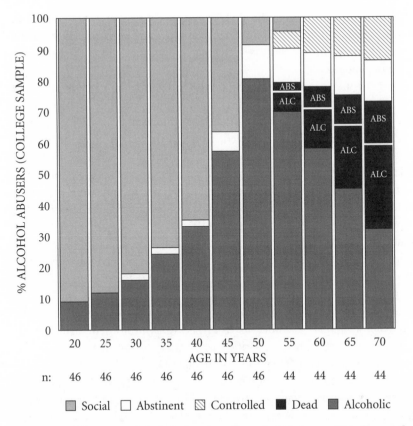

Figure 3.5A Life course of alcohol abuse by college alcohol abusers. This figure reflects the quinquennial alcohol-use status of the 46 College men who met the DSM III criteria for alcohol abuse. The 6 alcohol abusers reclassified as "social drinkers" have been excluded. The proportion of deaths among men classified as alcohol abusers is indicated by the label ALC; the proportion among those classified as stably abstinent, by ABS.

society's definition of the drinker's condition, and by individual and social processes of the most diverse kinds" (Lindström 1992, p. 52).

Figure 3.5A presents a very different model of the course of alcohol abuse from either Figure 3.2 or Figure 3.4A. It suggests that "social processes of the most diverse kinds" have done much to make alcohol abuse among the College sample follow a very different pattern from that suggested by Jellinek's model of alcoholism as a progressive disease. From age 45 to age 70 the alcohol abuse of most men in the College sample got neither better nor worse. The alcohol abusers in the College sample had more in common with the Core City men in the alcohol use category V than they did with those who became dependent.

Because of the richness of the longitudinal data for the College sample it seemed useful to increase the sample size in every way possible. In contrasting Figure 3.3 to Figure 3.5A, it can be noted that the number of College alcohol abusers depicted has almost doubled, from 26 to 46. The reasons for this increase in sample size were threefold. First, 15 alcohol abusers were identified by adding the identically studied 64 College men from the classes of 1939–1941 to the 204 from the classes of 1942–1944 whose data were originally included. Second, the change in the diagnostic criteria for alcohol abuse (from four problems on the PDS to the DSM III criteria for alcohol abuse) added another 10 alcohol abusers among the original 204 men in the College sample. Third, 1 College man did not meet criteria for alcohol abuse until age 65. However, doubling sample size did not change the pattern of College alcohol abuse up to age 47.

In keeping with the classification rules for the Core City men, 6 of the College men originally classified as "returned to asymptomatic drinking" in Figure 3.3 were arbitrarily reclassified as lifetime "social drinkers" and excluded from Figure 3.5A. They were reclassified because they abused alcohol for five years or less, their PDS scores did not exceed 4, and they spent the rest of their lives drinking in a controlled fashion. What is most striking about Figure 3.5A is that the pattern of College alcohol abuse after age 47 was different from that of the Core City sample. The College men were less likely to become stably abstinent than were the Core City men (Figure 3.4A). Only 6 College alcohol abusers were alive and abstinent during their 70th year; only 2 of these men had been abstinent for several years. Seven other stably abstinent College men had died prematurely. These 9 College men who ever achieved stable abstinence made up 45 percent of the 20 College men who ever met the criteria for alcohol dependence. No College men who did not develop the dependence syndrome ever stopped drinking for more than two years.

If the 20 alcohol-dependent men *and* the 4 long-term College alcohol abusers who successfully returned to asymptomatic drinking are excluded from the 46 men depicted in Figure 3.5A, then 22 men remain. Of these 22 alcohol abusers, all of whom met the criteria for DSM III alcohol abuse, at least 20 continued abusing alcohol until death or the present time without progression after age 50. In other words, these 20 chronic alcohol abusers spent the quarter-century between age 47 and 72 alternating between controlled drinking and a pattern of alcohol abuse that usually caused problems only to their self-esteem and to their family.

In this College cohort this pattern of alcohol abuse was much more analogous to the pattern of obesity in individuals 50–70 years old than to that of a progressive illness like multiple sclerosis or alcohol dependence. Just as some individuals with obesity always claim to eat modestly or to be on a diet, on questionnaires the College alcohol abusers often claimed to be consuming only one to three drinks a day. At the end of each two-year period, however, they would also report that they had made efforts to cut down, and that their wife and/or doctor had complained, and that they themselves felt guilty about their drinking. They rarely achieved even a year of significant abstinence, but often it took observation over several years to determine that such men should not be reclassified as simply heavy social drinkers. Rarely did their employers or physicians complain about their use of alcohol. Nevertheless, as already noted, their death rate was very high. Thus, as Figure 3.5A illustrates, at age 70, because of their high mortality, only 30 percent (14) of the 46 College alcohol abusers were still abusing alcohol.

The case of Francis Lowell, an effective and highly paid Philadelphia trial lawyer, serves as a contrapuntal case history to that of Tom Braceland. If Tom Braceland's misuse of alcohol underscored the fact that alcohol abuse sometimes has a natural history, Francis Lowell's use of alcohol illustrates that given enough education, willpower, social supports, and an undemanding lifestyle, the abuse of alcohol can simply be a lifelong career.

Without any noticeable decline in his physical health or serious damage to his legal career, Francis Lowell abused alcohol from age 30 to age 70. In college he was a heavy social user of alcohol and was very guarded about answering Grant Study questions related to his alcohol use. By age 25 he had established a pattern of very heavy weekend drinking, Friday through Sunday, and not drinking during the week. This was a pattern that he continued over the next 30 years. His heavy weekend drinking sometimes expanded into five-day binges with a loss of one or two days of work.

From age 30 on, Francis was aware that he had a problem with his drinking. He felt guilty about how much he drank; his friends criticized his drinking; he failed to keep his promises to cut down; and he avoided his relatives when drinking. At age 39 he had his first drunk-driving arrest. He had a second such arrest at age 47, but his liver chemistries remained entirely normal. He

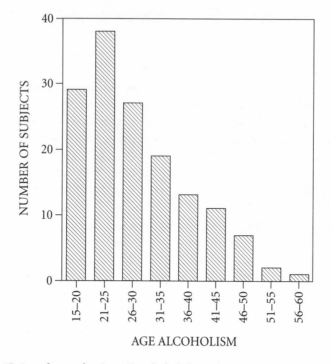

40

30

20

NUMBER OF SUBJECTS

10

0

15–20 21–25 26–30 31–35 36–40 41–45 46–50 51–55 56–60

AGE ALCOHOLISM

Figure 3.5B Age of onset for Core City alcohol abusers. Approximate age at which the 150 Core City men first met the DSM III criteria for alcohol abuse. Age of onset before age 45 based in part on retrospective data.

had his only detoxification at age 52; but his physical exam and liver chemistries remained normal. At age 56 Francis Lowell could say, "No doubt about it, I do drink heavily at times"; but he had never stopped drinking for more than six weeks. Many weeks he drank within social limits, and often he did not drink except on weekends. He attributed his successful steady pattern of alcohol abuse to the fact that his stomach would not tolerate his drinking for more than five days. And he added, "I don't want to sound pompous, but a sense of duty drilled into me from family and from St. Mark's School contributes to my control . . . you just can't let everything go."

Although after age 60 his career did not advance, by age 59 Francis Lowell was making $200,000 a year as a lawyer. Although his alcohol abuse had contributed to his losing the woman who had most touched his heart, Lowell's heavy alcohol intake did not interfere with his work and only barely with his other relationships. After age 62 his doctor began encouraging him to cut

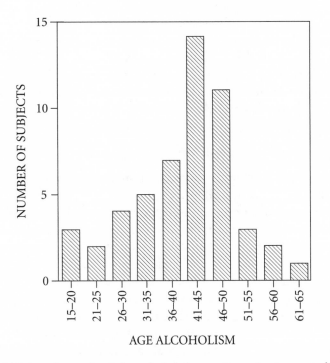

Figure 3.5C Age of onset for College alcohol abusers. Approximate age at which the 52 College men first met the DSM III criteria for alcohol abuse. Age of onset before age 45 based in part on retrospective data.

down on his use of alcohol, and at age 66 he had a seizure "possibly related to alcohol." Nevertheless, at age 70 Francis Lowell is still working 40 hours a week and making his handsome salary. Compared to his college classmates he is still very physically active and his liver chemistries are still normal. At no time in his life has he described a wish to become abstinent, and he continues to drink ten drinks a day on the weekend. In short, Francis Lowell has had a lifelong problem with alcohol, but not a "progressive disease."

While for most of the men in the Study of Adult Development alcohol *use* began in late adolescence, the transition from alcohol use to *abuse* occurred at very different ages. The most important correlates of early age of onset were the relative social instability of family of origin and the development of alcohol dependence. Contrary to expectations, for neither the Core City nor the College sample was age of onset associated with number of alcoholic relatives.

Age of onset clearly distinguished the 150 alcohol abusers in the Core City sample from the 52 alcohol abusers in the College sample. Only 9 (5 percent) of the Core City alcohol abusers appeared to lose control between age 47 and age 60. In contrast, of the 52 College men classified by age 70 as alcohol abusers by DSM III criteria, 13 (25 percent) had developed alcohol abuse after age 47. Only 1 man, however, has so far lost control after age 60. Figures 3.5B and 3.5C depict this contrast graphically.

The Problem of the Atypical Alcoholic

In Chapter 4 I will discuss the currently abstinent men in detail, and in Chapter 5 the men who returned to asymptomatic drinking. It seems appropriate at this point to discuss in detail the men in Table 3.9 classified as atypical. Young men, especially in northern European and American cultures, abuse alcohol during young adulthood without either becoming dependent or losing control. At around age 30, family responsibilities, a stable job, the breakup of the old drinking crowd all serve to allow them to return to less symptomatic drinking. However, most of the Core City men in this group tended to be from the group of erstwhile heavy drinkers who received scores of two or three on the PDS and were never categorized as alcohol abusers.

Less well understood are the atypical alcohol-dependent individuals who spend a lifetime abusing alcohol, but who never progress. In follow-up reports of clinical samples of alcoholics, these men usually fall in the group called "improved." These are the individuals who continue occasionally to abuse alcohol, but whose alcoholism seems to get slowly better instead of inexorably more severe. In short-term cross-sectional studies, this group of drinkers can seem very large. In the present study, with its longer time frame, such men were less frequently identified.

Out of the 110 Core City men who showed four or more symptoms of alcohol abuse, there were 19 individuals classified as atypical. Some achieved abstinence for as long as a year, but these men never really became stably abstinent, nor did they really return to asymptomatic drinking. Unlike progressive alcoholics, the 19 atypical alcoholics were far less likely to have experienced trouble with jobs, money, or employment, and their marriages were more stable. However, they were just as likely to perceive alcohol as a problem.

The atypical alcohol abusers by no means were individuals who were not "really alcoholic." As the second section of Table 3.9 reveals, in terms of etiological risk factors, the atypical alcoholics differed very little from those who experienced a chronic course. The atypical men were as likely to have alcoholic relatives, to be of other than Mediterranean ethnicity, and to have manifested disciplinary problems in school. Unlike the men who were able to return to asymptomatic drinking, the atypical alcoholics were more often morning drinkers, and 42 percent had abused alcohol for most of their adult lives.

Rather, the atypical alcohol abusers had almost "mastered the art" of alcohol abuse. Like their two-liter-of-wine-a-day counterparts in France, 8 of the atypical alcohol abusers drank low-proof liquor, usually between 3 and 5 quarts of beer (10–15 drinks) a day, without occupational or severe social damage. At 47, most of these men continued to view alcohol as a friend, not a foe; and there was no evidence of progression. By the DSM III criteria, only 3 of these 8 men would be called alcohol-dependent.

Patrick Reilly epitomized this subgroup. He had drunk heavily in his 20s, beaten up his wife, and had multiple alcohol-related arrests. As a young man, he had multiple alcohol-related medical problems; he was a morning drinker and frequently went on the wagon. At one point he had visited an alcohol clinic and his physician had told him to cut down.

However, with the passage of time his use of alcohol became progressively more manageable. He now sets aside one or at most two nights a week to get drunk (10 drinks) and remains abstinent for five to six days a week. By virtue of his capacity for sustained drinking, there is no evidence of dependence or "progression." However, he acknowledges that sometimes when he wakes up after his planned weekly drunk "I feel like a shitbum."

Henry Smith was one of 3 men who met the DSM III criteria for alcohol dependence but not the PDS criteria for alcohol abuse. He developed a pattern of drinking five shots of whiskey and ten beers every day at his job in the presence of an understanding boss who retained him at his job for ten years and "sends me home when I drink too much." He denied difficulties with his girlfriend of eight years. When he was a young man, his use of alcohol had led to at least 12 alcohol-related arrests. He had frequently gone on binges and experienced early morning shakes relieved by morning drinking. For the past ten years, he reported no legal, financial, or health problems. He himself felt that he had no problem: "I can stop any time I want." In no sense had he met the Jellinek criteria for alcoholic progression.

There were 3 atypical alcoholics who had achieved patterns of controlled alcohol abuse—after marital or medical confrontations—that were stable over many years. One of these 3 men drank 8 to 12 ounces of spirits three days a week for ten years. Another was abstinent except for getting drunk for 24 hours each week; his body could tolerate no more than that. The third man was abstinent except for one binge a month. In 5 of the 19 atypical alcoholics, although progression was not clear, alcohol abuse appeared to be growing more severe. With time, they may well fall into the group of progressive alcoholics.

Finally, in the three remaining cases of atypical alcoholism, there was a pattern of slow tapering off of alcohol use over several years. A reverse progression, if you will, leading from alcohol dependence toward asymptomatic drinking. While such a course contradicts the Jellinek model of progression, the fact that it occurred in only 3 out of 110 cases justifies suggestions by most alcohol clinics that abstinence remains the prescription of choice for alcohol-dependent individuals.

An example of such an atypical alcoholic was George Comeau, who began to drink at the age of 9 and was drinking heavily in his 20s. In his 30s he was drinking "two quarts of whiskey" a day and experienced multiple blackouts, arrests for alcohol abuse, and episodes of violent behavior. In his early 30s George developed seizures, joined Alcoholics Anonymous, and became abstinent for two years, only to relapse into an intermittent pattern of two months of abstinence interspersed with "a beer once in a while." When pressed, he redefined "a beer once in a while" to represent a "six-pack a month." When pressed further, he acknowledged continuing alcohol-related problems. He had been unemployed for 20 years and had been dependent on his family. His drunk arrests had continued until the present, and in the previous year he had been treated at a clinic for alcoholism. George Comeau lived entirely in the past and was in social contact with no one. His lifestyle was closer to skid row than to recovery; but with each passing year, he probably consumed less alcohol. Of all the Core City men, he was the closest to a "burned out case."*

The Natural History of Treated Alcoholism

In recent years, follow-ups of untreated alcoholics have placed the course of alcoholism per se into clearer perspective. As a result, the efficacy of our existing treatment methods has come under increasingly critical scrutiny. Previous reviews of the treatment literature by Emrick (1974; 1975) have underscored the fact that inadequate controls have invalidated many positive studies of treatment outcome. Indeed, like the small boy who declared that the emperor was naked, Orford and Edwards (1977) come close to saying

---

*Over the next 13 years Comeau's pattern of declining use of alcohol and reclusive lifestyle continued. At age 60 he remained unemployed, crippled with emphysema and cirrhosis. According to both him and his sister, Comeau had not abused alcohol for the past five years. At age 60 he drank moderately about three times a month and was in extremely poor health.

that, if proper controls are employed, the course of treated alcoholism will be found to be virtually the same as the course of untreated alcoholism. Many long-term studies of the course of alcoholism concur that treatment has little if any lasting effect (Bruun 1963; Kendell and Staton 1966; Ojesjo 1981; Vaillant 1980b).

Even when short-term treatment studies have been well controlled and have shown positive results (McLellan et al. 1982; Neuberger et al. 1981), failure to control for compliance and the law of initial values have cast the significance of such studies into doubt. The hazards of failing to control for compliance are well known to investigators in the field of obesity. During the period of acute intervention, individuals who comply with obesity treatment regimens invariably lose weight—only to regain it all by the end of one or two years. In similar fashion, Moos and co-workers (Bromet et al. 1977) and Costello (1975) have demonstrated that much of short-term success in alcohol treatment is a function of premorbid variables that influence compliance. For short periods, middle-class individuals respond well to treatment in the medical model, but that response may be short-lived and reflect premorbid variables rather than the efficacy of specific treatment. Costello (1980) has demonstrated that merely controlling for marriage and employment is enough to explain most of the outcome variance that has been attributed to treatment.

Similarly, the law of initial values (that is, the tendency of extreme physiological or psychological values to regress toward the mean over time) distorts assessment of alcohol treatment over the short term. Alcoholics, like individuals with any acute relapsing illness, will tend to present themselves for medical attention at their clinical nadir and the time of their most extreme exacerbation of symptoms. Thus, if the follow-up consists of a brief and rigid time frame, alcoholic patients will seem to improve regardless of the treatment employed. For example, the initial finding of the Rand Report (Armor et al. 1978) that 67 percent of all alcoholic patients were improved at 18 months seemed too good to be true. The men's alcohol consumption and symptoms for one month prior to their presentation at an alcohol treatment center were contrasted with their symptoms and alcohol consumption during an arbitrary month, 18 months later. Not until the Rand investigators carried their follow-up out to four years (Polich et al. 1980) and began substituting a time frame of six months for that of one month could they appreciate how evanescent had been much of the improvement that they had reported earlier.

Paradoxically, if in order to control for both compliance and the law of initial values the individual is followed for long periods of time, then the effects of specific treatment cannot be experimentally controlled. After all, investigators cannot forbid their subjects to seek treatment elsewhere. As Kendell and Staton (1966) first noted, if followed for more than a year or two alcoholics will get multiple treatments from multiple sources. Proof of therapeutic efficacy is not easy.

Thus, it is well to set forth some minimal ground rules that must be observed before we can regard treatment efficacy proven beyond a shadow of a doubt. First, since alcoholism is a chronic relapsing disease, follow-up must be prolonged—at least 5–15 years. Second, observations must occur at multiple different times. (To my knowledge, in the world literature there is no previously published study that has both followed an alcoholic clinic population for more than four years and also assessed their outcome at more than one time.) Third, in order to assess the effect of favorable admission variables upon outcome, the study must be prospective. Fourth, attrition must be minimal. Failure to observe this requirement has called several otherwise well-designed studies into question. Fifth, at outcome presence or absence of alcohol abuse must be correlated with multiple facets of social functioning. The goal of alcohol treatment is not to reduce an individual's annual alcohol consumption, but to improve the quality of his life. Sixth, posttreatment environmental variables should be controlled. To my knowledge, this has been carried out well only by Finney and colleagues (1980). Failure to observe this last requirement is a methodological defect in the Clinic study to be reported below.

In Table 3.8, the best outcomes were from untreated community samples of Goodwin, Ojesjo, and the Core City; the worst outcomes, if one includes deaths, were experienced by alcoholics who received inpatient treatment. Such alcoholics represented a more severely ill population with a poorer prognosis. It is useful to contrast, but unfair to equate, the natural histories of older alcoholics who attend alcohol clinics with younger alcoholics drawn from community samples. In this section I shall present a description of an eight-year follow-up of 100 alcoholics (the Clinic sample in Table 3.8) who sought hospital treatment for their illness, and I shall contrast their course with that of the Core City sample.

The Clinic sample comprised 110 consecutive admissions admitted for detoxification to an urban, municipal hospital (Cambridge Hospital) during the winter of 1971–72. Four patients who did not stay for 24 hours were excluded from the study, leaving 106 patients; 91 men and 15 women. At the time of admission, in anticipation of prospective follow-up, systematic data were gathered for all patients on previous employment, living arrangements, use of Alcoholics Anonymous, prison history, and so on. The criteria for diagnosing physiological dependence upon alcohol were that the patients had either required 750 mg or more chlordiazepoxide (Librium) during detoxification or manifested severe withdrawal symptoms during previous detoxifications. Hospital stay ranged from 1 to 11 days with a mean of five days.

All patients received individual counseling and two to three hours of films and group discussions a day. An internist educated patients about medical issues on alcohol use and abuse. Alcoholics Anonymous meetings were required twice weekly. After discharge, all patients knew that they could return to the program as outpatients at no cost and without appointment. All patients were encouraged to attend the twice-weekly outpatient group meetings, which were designed to guide patients toward Alcoholics Anonymous.

The Cambridge and Somerville Program for Alcohol Rehabilitation (CASPAR) program blankets the entire cities of Cambridge and Somerville and includes halfway houses, drop-in centers, freestanding detoxification units, and integrated mental health facilities. Therefore, a majority of our sample, when they relapsed, continued to have multiple therapeutic contacts with our program. In addition, over the next eight years a special effort was made every 18 months to monitor the course of these 106 patients. If abstinent, the patient was personally interviewed; if the patient was abusing alcohol and not available for interview, a relative of the patient was interviewed or recent clinical charts were reviewed. The number of days in detoxification units and in halfway houses and the estimated number of AA visits were specifically recorded. Multiple informants were used, and the records of five halfway houses, four detoxification centers, and four alcohol counseling programs were reviewed. Over eight years, we could identify, for the average subject, 15 admissions for detoxification and at least as many visits to emergency rooms or counseling centers. At each interview an effort was made to assess not only the individual's use or abuse of alcohol but also the quality of the individual's social, medical, and occupational adjustment.

The last effort to contact these men and women was during the spring of 1980; and on the average, the course of each patient was reassessed at five different times. Over the eight-year period of follow-up, 6 Clinic patients were lost, but even these patients were followed for an average of three years each. At last contact, 1 of these lost patients had been abstinent for six months, 2 were using alcohol intermittently, and 3 were still experiencing severe, sustained alcoholism.

The following list shows the characteristics (at time of admission) of the 100 patients in the Clinic sample who were successfully followed for eight years.

Age	45±10
Male	87 percent
10+ years of alcohol abuse	87
Ever previously detoxified	80
Ever in jail	71
Straus-Bacon score 0 or 1	64
Lives alone or in street	50
Lives with spouse	35
Regular employment	27
Attended college	19
Stable psychosocial adjustment (1970–1971)	17

Premorbidly, all subjects were rated on the Straus-Bacon scale for social stability. The Straus-Bacon scale is a four-point scale that gives a point for each of the following: if the subject had a steady job for the past three years, had a stable residence for the past two years, is currently not living alone, and is currently married or living with a spouse. Compared to the population of alcoholics attending private hospitals or industrial alcohol counseling programs, the Clinic sample was socially very unstable. For example, 64 percent of our sample received Straus-Bacon scores of 0 or 1; this was true of only 18 percent of the original sample from New Haven Alcohol Clinic on whom the scale was developed (Straus and Bacon 1951).

Premorbidly (1970–71) and at follow-up (1978–79) the men in the Clinic sample were also assessed for psychosocial adjustment, employment, marital stability, and number of detoxifications. The time frame was the preceding two years.

Psychosocial adjustment was assessed on a four-point scale. A score of one indicated a "skid row" adjustment—unemployed more than 80 percent of the time and living in a single room or institutionalized because of alcohol abuse. A score of two indicated a "marginal" existence—the individual might have *either* a regular job *or* a stable home situation but still manifested clear social instability attributable to alcohol. A score of three indicated a "fair" social adjustment that could not be directly blamed on alcohol abuse: such individuals might be chronically physically ill, socially isolated, or psychiatrically disabled. A score of four reflected "stable" social adjustment: the individual held a regular job or functioned effectively as a homemaker *and* enjoyed a regular residence *and* remained in contact with relevant family members *and* experienced no serious emotional or physical disability.

Half of the Clinic sample were living alone or in the streets; only a third lived with a spouse and only a quarter were regularly employed. Four-fifths of the Clinic sample were between 30 and 60; and four-fifths had begun abusing alcohol before age 30. Virtually all had experienced alcohol-related problems for more than a decade. Seventy-one percent had spent time in jail for public drunkenness, but only 5 had spent more than a month in jail. Although the average Clinic subject had experienced greater social damage from alcohol abuse than had the average Core City alcohol abuser, originally they had represented a less socially disadvantaged group. Of the Clinic sample, 61 percent had graduated from high school, and 28 percent of the Clinic patients currently classified as leading a skid-row existence had attended college.

Outcome measures for the Clinic sample were deliberately global and based on a time frame of years, not months. As dichotomously as possible, clinical outcomes were separated into categories of stable remission and chronic alcoholism. The category *stable remission* included the 29 individuals who for the past 36 months or for the three years preceding death (3 cases), had remained in the community without experiencing alcohol-related problems of any kind. Five such individuals had resumed asymptomatic drinking and 24 had been abstinent (no use of alcohol for 51+ weeks/year) for three or more years.

The category *chronic alcoholism* encompassed 47 individuals who for the last three years (or until death) had spent at least six months of the year symptomatically abusing alcohol, had manifested physiological dependence, and had required at least 1 detoxification. Over the eight-year period, all but 4 of the 47 chronic alcoholics had required at least four detoxifications, and two-thirds had been detoxified ten or more times.

The category *intermittent alcoholism* encompassed those 24 individuals who for the previous three years did not fit easily into either of the dichotomous categories described above. Many members of this category correspond to the "atypical" alcoholics described in Table 3.9. Intermittent alcoholics also included individuals who were institutionalized, who were currently abstinent for less than three years, or who managed to remain abstinent for long periods between binges.

Table 3.10 documents that not only were the categories of stable remission and chronic alcoholism dichotomous for alcohol abuse, they were nearly dichotomous for social adjustment. As a group, the chronic alcoholics were psychosocial cripples and the stable remissions were employed and were living in gratifying social environments.

Had a briefer time frame been employed, however, the course of most of

TABLE 3.10.   Association between presence of alcoholism and social adjustment at outcome.

	Clinical status (1979)		
Psychosocial adjustment (1980)	Stable remission (n = 29)	Intermittent alcoholism (n = 23)[a]	Chronic alcoholism (n = 46)[a]
Stable	66%	35%	9%
Fair	31	26	9
Marginal	3	26	30
Skid row	0	13	52

a. Social adjustment of 2 cases could not be rated.

the Clinic patients could have been described as intermittent alcoholism. By this I mean that at some time after discharge from their first admission to the Cambridge Hospital detoxification unit, 95 of the 100 Clinic patients relapsed to alcohol dependence—a criterion often used to indicate clear failure of treatment. However, within the same eight-year period, 59 percent of the clinic sample achieved at least six months of abstinence—a criterion often used to indicate stable recovery. On the one hand, 6 of the 29 men eventually categorized as stable remissions required ten or more detoxifications. On the other hand, 15 of the 27 chronic alcoholics who survived the full eight years achieved at least four consecutive months of community abstinence. Under high magnification most blacks and whites appear gray.

Figure 3.7 depicts the clinical course of the Clinic sample alcoholics over eight years. The figure illustrates that once alcoholism is severe enough to require hospital detoxification it represents—in a cybernetic sense—a very unstable state. After one year, 81 percent of the Clinic patients continued to abuse alcohol; after eight years, the proportion had shrunk to 26 percent. Figure 3.7 corroborates both the pessimism of Lemere and the optimism of Drew. Stable remissions gradually rose to 34 percent, but 29 percent of the patients died. The data from the Core City sample in Figure 3.2 and for the Clinic sample in Figure 3.7 graphically reflect the point made in Table 3.8 that stable remission from alcoholism occurs in roughly 2–3 percent of active alcoholics per year. Perhaps 10 percent of alcoholics will achieve stable remission the first time they seek clinical intervention.

The death rate depicted in Figure 3.7 was roughly three times what would have been expected for nonalcoholic men and women of comparable age.

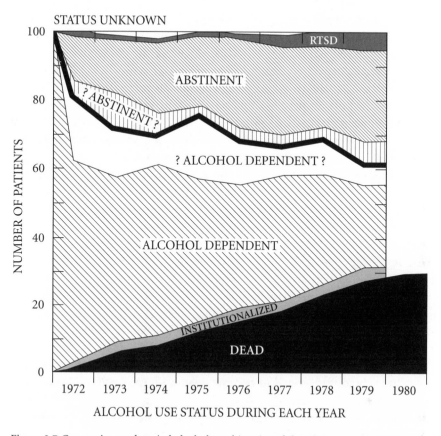

Figure 3.7 Composite posthospital alcohol use histories of the Clinic sample. Abstinent = no alcohol use for more than 51 weeks during a year (corroborated by more than one source). ?Abstinent = evidence for abstinence unreliable, or abstinent for 44–51 weeks. RTSD (return to asymptomatic drinking) = individual drank more frequently than once a month and longer than 12 months but with no discernible alcohol-related problems. ?Alcoholic = alcohol abuse for more than 2 but less than 6 months in a given year, or ambiguous evidence suggesting alcohol abuse, or no evidence of alcohol abuse but the individual exhibited clear alcohol dependence in the preceding or the following year. Alcohol dependent = unambiguous alcohol abuse for more than 6 months leading to hospitalization for detoxification. Institutionalized = in a nursing home, prison, or chronic disease hospital for more than 11 months of the year. Deaths were verified by death certificates.

One-tenth of the patients aged less than 40 years on admission were dead eight years later; and one-quarter of those aged 40–50 and almost half of those aged 50 on admission were dead. Eight of the 29 deaths were from homicide, suicide, or accident; and 9 or more were alcohol-related (for example, hepatic failure, aspiration pneumonia, or exposure). Five Clinic alcoholics died of coronary thrombosis. Mortality was highly associated with poor premorbid psychosocial adjustment. Half of the 29 alcoholics who later died had manifested a "skid row" social adjustment at first admission; and half had received a Straus-Bacon score of 0. During the eight years of follow-up, half of the men who spent ten months or more in halfway houses died.

At the eight-year mark, 5 men and women had returned to asymptomatic drinking. Such drinking ranged from an occasional glass of wine by one man to one man who regularly drank four to six cans of beer a night. These 5 individuals, however, were premorbidly very different from the other 95. At first admission, they had enjoyed far greater social stability; they had experienced far shorter periods of active alcoholic drinking; and three of them had never required previous detoxification.

Although the numbers were too small to be conclusive, no important differences were observed between the 87 men and the 13 women alcoholics. Although the men were more likely to live in the streets, to be sent to jail, and to have lost control of their drinking in adolescence, both sexes were equally likely to recover and to become involved in Alcoholics Anonymous.

At this point three questions must be asked. First, do social variables on admission predict both clinical course and future social adjustment or is it recovery from alcoholism per se that is primarily responsible for the increased social stability observed for the stable remissions in Table 3.10? Second, what is the effect of treatment, if any? Third, if treatment affects outcome, are treatment effects independent of the favorable prognostic factors on admission?

The left-hand columns of Table 3.11 confirm the previous findings of many investigators. Over the short term, social stability is an important predictor of alcoholism outcome. Premorbid marital status, employment, residential stability, first-admission status, and the absence of previous drunk arrests all significantly predicted who would become a stable remission by 1979.

Many other factors often cited in short-term studies (Gibbs and Flanagan 1977) were not important at the end of eight years. These factors included length of education, presence or absence of physiological dependence on

TABLE 3.11. Association of premorbid and outcome social-adjustment variables with alcohol abuse and AA membership.

Variable	Clinical status (1979)		Use of AA (1972–1979)	
	Stable remission (n = 29)[a]	Chronic alcoholism (n = 47)[a]	0–99 visits (n = 68)	100+ visits (n = 32)
Admission variables (1971)				
Prognosis scale items				
Stable psychosocial adjustment	28%	9%*	22%	6%*
Married	45	28	41	22*
Employed	31	13*	29	22
Never before detoxified	21	11	25	3*
2+ prognosis scale items present	31	13*	32	9*
3 or 4 on Straus-Bacon scale	31	13*	26	16
Never in jail	41	13*	29	28
Outcome variables (1979)				
Skid row adjustment	0	52*	30	22
Stable psychosocial adjustment	66	9*	24	47*
Living with spouse	60	27*	51	32
Employed	79	18*	35	58
Dead	10	40*	37	13*
300+ visits to AA	48	2*	0	60*

a. The 24 patients manifesting "intermittent alcoholism" have been omitted from this table.
*Significance $p < .05$ (chi-square test).

alcohol, a year or more of previous abstinence, previous exposure to Alcoholics Anonymous, age on admission, and adolescent alcohol abuse. As we have already seen in the contrast between the College sample and the Core City sociopaths in Figures 3.3 and 3.4, even social stability is not such an important predictor of alcoholism outcome over the very long term.

It can also be appreciated from Table 3.11, however, that when premorbid psychosocial adjustment was controlled, freedom from alcohol abuse was powerfully associated with improved future social adjustment. In 1972, 6 of the 29 stable remissions had been living a "skid row" psychosocial adjustment; none were in 1979. Similarly, only 8 of the stable remissions enjoyed a "stable" psychosocial adjustment in 1972, but 20 did in 1979. Twice as many of the stable remissions were employed in 1979 as had been employed in 1972. Compared to Clinic subjects with stable remissions, chronic alcoholics were four times as likely to die, four times as likely to be unemployed, and far more likely to be living in single rooms, halfway houses, or the streets. Age was not an explanatory variable.

Table 3.11 shows a striking finding that requires amplification. Half of the stable remissions, but only two of the chronic alcoholics, had made 300 or more visits to Alcoholics Anonymous. Once again, the question that prospective study must address becomes one of causality. Is AA attendance merely a manifestation of good premorbid social adjustment or a result of sobriety? Or does frequent AA attendance actually alter the course of the disease? The right-hand columns of Table 3.11 relate the premorbid and outcome social-adjustment variables to attendance at AA meetings. Whereas social stability in 1972 predicted stable remission, social *instability* in 1972 predicted heavy use of AA. Put differently, premorbidly socially stable alcoholics tended to become abstinent without Alcoholics Anonymous, but if socially unstable alcoholics were to recover, AA attendance seemed very important. Thus, 32 patients attended AA meetings 100 or more times (mean 600 visits) between 1972 and 1980; the number of these individuals with stable psychosocial adjustment went from 2 in 1972 to 15 in 1980.

Multiple regression analysis revealed that both the number of favorable preadmission prognostic items *and* the number of postadmission AA visits explained large and independent amounts of the outcome variance. The first four prognostic items in Table 3.11 explained 25 percent of the variance of current social adjustment and 7 percent of the variance in the categorization of clinical outcome; number of AA visits explained an additional 19 percent of the variance in current social adjustment and an additional 28 percent of the variance in the clinical outcome of alcohol abuse. If both the prognostic items and AA visits were controlled, then the Straus-Bacon scale and other premorbid variables explained little further variance.

Table 3.12 puts the relationship between Alcoholics Anonymous visits and premorbid prognostic factors into still sharper relief. There were 66 men who made fewer than 300 visits to AA *and* on admission had manifested fewer than three of the four favorable prognostic items: only 7 (11 percent) of these men achieved stable remission. There were 34 men who had more than 300 visits to AA *or* who had manifested three or four favorable prognostic items

TABLE 3.12.   Interrelationship among good prognosis, Alcoholics Anonymous attendance, and stable remission.

| | Clinical status (1979) | | |
| | | | |
Prognosis and AA attendance	Stable remission (n = 29)	Intermittent alcoholism (n = 24)	Chronic alcoholism (n = 47)
Two subgroups			
> 300 AA visits (n = 19)	48%	17%	2%
Prognosis score 3–4 (n = 15)	28	17	6
Total sample			
< 300 AA visits *and*			
prognosis score 0–2 (n = 66)	24	67	91
> 300 AA visits *or*			
prognosis score 3–4 (n = 34)	76	33	9

on admission: 22 (65 percent) of these men achieved stable remission. No clinic patient had three or four favorable prognostic items and subsequently made 300 or more visits to AA. In other words, social stability on admission and AA utilization seem clearly additive.

Four illusions obscure our view of the natural history of clinic treatment. One illusion is that early, intensive treatment of alcoholism is usually effective. The second illusion is that the chronic relapsing alcoholic is untreatable. The third illusion is that alcoholism must inevitably end in abstinence or death, and the fourth is that the course of alcoholism is so intermittent as to defy classification. Let me reconcile these illusions one by one with the Clinic results; in so doing, I hope to reconcile the black and white outcome of the Clinic study with contradicting studies in the literature.

On the one hand, the apparently high recovery rates reported in intensively treated alcoholics are often an illusion produced by studying a selected subsample of previously untreated samples of employed men who retain their jobs. For example, the outcome results from industrial alcohol programs are outstanding (Clyne 1965; Asma et al. 1971); but the design of such studies tends to emphasize successes and lose track of failures. The illusion can also result from a brief time frame. For example, Moos and colleagues (1978) reported that during the sixth month of follow-up, 46 percent of Salvation

Army clients were abstinent compared to only 6 percent who were abstinent the month before entrance. However, the rate of rehospitalization for alcoholism over the entire six months was unchanged from prior rates and the overall social functioning of these men over the six-month period was unchanged. Similarly, Ludwig and his colleagues (1969) closely monitored the course of 178 alcoholics and reported that in any given month 45 percent of them were abstinent, but that by the end of six months 8 percent had relapsed. Orford and Edwards (1977) noted that after two months 55 percent of their sample met their criteria for treatment success (fewer than ten unacceptable drinking days in the two months); by six months this figure had shrunk to 35 percent and by two years to 20 percent. At the end of their study, the drinking pattern of their untreated sample was identical to that of their treated sample. After two years, also, the outcome of the Clinic sample was not appreciably different from the natural history of an untreated sample (see Chapter 8).

On the other hand, the apparent hopelessness of treating alcoholics who make multiple visits to public clinics and emergency rooms is also an illusion—an illusion based upon sampling procedures that tend to count relapses but not remissions. For example, an unpublished review of admissions to the Springfield Free Standing Detoxification Center over six and a half years (M. Carlson, personal communication, 1980) illustrates this point. During the 78-month interval, roughly 5,000 clients received over 19,000 detoxifications. One-eighth of these 19,000 admissions encompassed the easily forgotten 2500 clients who *never* returned. One-eighth of these admissions, however, encompassed the 25 indelibly remembered subjects who returned 60 times or more—a mere 0.5 percent of the total. In other words, in the trenches of clinical warfare against alcoholism, the 25 most incurable alcoholics were admitted as often—and became far more deeply etched in the clinicians' consciousness—as were the 2500 patients who never came back yet who must have included the best outcomes.

In Table 3.8 there was a suggestion that the Clinic sample's treatment results were better than those of other studies. Instead of the usual 2–3 percent rate of improvement per year, the rate was almost 6 percent per year. If real, this difference in therapeutic outcome may be attributed to the fact that therapeutic efforts toward the Clinic sample were exerted over a much longer time. As Figure 3.7 suggests, the Clinic treatment outcomes were certainly not impressive at the one-year mark. But the CASPAR program continued to regard the relapsing alcoholic in the same way that a hospital might regard a patient with brittle diabetes. Gentle pressure for patients to unite themselves with Alcoholics Anonymous never abated. The price of this program policy, however, was not inconsequential. The average number of detoxifications among the stable Clinic remissions was four. Only 5 alcoholics never relapsed again; as a group the other 24 accounted for at least 98 subsequent detoxifications. Had follow-up not persisted for eight years, repeated detoxification might have seemed hopeless.

Among the less favorable outcomes were 14 men who required 50 detoxifications or more, but these patients did not represent 14 percent of all the alcoholics that CASPAR treats. The CASPAR alcohol program has now seen more than 8,000 different clients, and yet many of the most chronic repeaters in the system were included in our initial sample of 100 consecutive admissions. Recall that 0.5 percent of the patients made 12 percent of the visits to the Springfield Detoxification Center.

The third illusion is that alcoholism is a progressive disease that ends in abstinence or death. Unfortunately, this is an illusion that the study of the Clinic patients threatens to perpetuate. The data in Table 3.12 make alcoholism seem deceptively black and white. Three favorable prognostic items on admission or 300 visits to Alcoholics Anonymous and the patient recovers. If both variables are absent, the patient either dies or is condemned to skid row. Yet we know that alcoholism is made up of grays; in Figures 3.2 and 3.7, only the deaths and the losts are colored black or white. In each of the other categories, individuals could move back and forth from one category to another and the month-by-month course of alcoholism is nothing if not dynamic. In a careful month-by-month study of the life charts of alcohol abusers, no two of the 50 patients studied by Davies, Shepherd, and Myers (1956) had an identical course; patients oscillated from being abstinent to being desperately ill.

But to examine the course of an alcoholic's life under too high magnification is to perpetuate the fourth illusion—that clinical course cannot be categorized. In their month-by-month study of 100 alcoholics, Orford and Edwards (1977) called into question the validity of any black and white outcomes. They interviewed the wives of their subjects every month. On the average, wives felt that their husbands engaged in drinking in only 31±3 out of the 52 weeks; for only 23±3 of those weeks was their husbands' drinking unacceptable, and for 8±2 weeks their husbands engaged in perfectly acceptable drinking behavior. Admittedly, these figures are averages, but the standard errors are small. On a day-by-day basis, most alcoholics do not have trouble with their drinking. What is equally important, however, is that if the alcoholic's behavior is looked at over years, instead of weeks, this apparent instability becomes diminished. At the year's end, 20 of Orford and Edwards's men were clear clinical successes and 55 percent of their men could be unambiguously classified as problem drinkers. Only 25 percent were left in the intermediate group, a proportion similar to that of the intermittent alcoholics in the Clinic sample and the atypical alcoholics in the Core City sample.

The Clinic study, with its clear-cut results, employed methodology that differed from other studies of treatment outcomes in three important ways: eight years of repeated follow-up allowed a clarity of vision not possible in other studies; discussion of the results of the Clinic study focused upon only the 75 percent most stable outcomes; and patients who died were reclassified in terms of their adjustment in the three years prior to death.

Alcoholism and Morbidity

In Western industrialized countries alcohol is not only an important social custom but a major source of employment. To abolish the production and sale of alcohol in France and England would deprive 5–10 percent of the work force of their jobs (Jellinek 1960; Smith 1981). At the same time, the cost of alcohol abuse and its morbidity is enormous. In 1975 in the United States the estimated cost of alcohol abuse ($43 billion) was greater than the cost of all cancer and respiratory disease combined (Institute of Medicine 1980).

Recently, Zook and Moore (1980) have demonstrated that alcoholic patients tend to experience unusually long hospital stays and that they consume a disproportionate amount of hospital costs. By way of illustration, the average Core City man with eight or more problems on the PDS had spent an average of six weeks in the hospital *excluding* admissions for alcoholism; the average man with one or zero problems had been hospitalized an average of only two weeks. In addition, the greatest, if incalculable, costs of alcoholism occur through its destruction of family integrity (divorce, child abuse, delinquency, and unemployment). The resulting costs of social welfare, school failure, aid to dependent children, and criminal justice can only be imagined and are not adequately factored into the $43 billion figure.

However, society tends to deny the morbidity of alcoholism. Thus, American research expenditure is currently 40 times greater for research on cancer and respiratory disease than for research on alcoholism; much of the existing research is based upon the effect of alcoholism on the liver—the merest tip of the iceberg. Even the mortality due to alcoholism is not what it appears. Looked at in cross-section, as viewed by emergency room and medical unit staffs, chronic alcoholism appears to kill its victims at an early age through cirrhosis, violence, suicide, and nutritionally based neurological degeneration. Such a view of the morbidity of alcoholism is reflected in the work of Wilkinson and co-workers (Schmidt and Popham 1975) which suggests that 26 percent of male alcoholics have problems with liver disease and 20 percent have neurological complications. However, if alcoholism is looked at from the perspective of life-span study of community populations, the disorder appears to kill its victims at a rather late age through heart disease and through generally increased morbidity from all causes, especially those associated with heavy smoking.

Let me cite another set of examples. Goodwin (1973) and Kessel and Grossman (1961) have suggested that 10–30 percent of all suicides are alcoholics and that 21 percent of alcoholics may die by suicide. It is a fact that the four major causes of death in American males between the ages of 20 and 40—cirrhosis, homicide, suicide, and accidents—are alcohol-related. In New York City, 90 percent of cirrhosis deaths are alcohol-related (Haberman and Baden 1974) and cirrhosis deaths have long been used as a crude estimate of the extent of alcoholism in the general population. It is true that roughly 50 percent of all murders (Goodwin 1973), suicides (James 1964), and motor vehicle accident deaths (Waller and Turkel 1966; Haberman and Baden 1974) are associated with alcohol. However, such statistics are misleading. As Goodwin (1973) and James and colleagues (1963) have suggested, perhaps the majority of those intoxicated at death are not alcoholic. There are important differences between intoxication (drunkenness) and alcoholism. Lastly, it is important to keep in mind that only 2.5 percent of male deaths occur between ages 20 and 40.

Table 3.13 contrasts five major prospective longitudinal studies of mortality in alcoholics with mortality in the Clinic, College, and Core City samples. Between the ages of 40 and 70, the death rate among alcoholics is approximately three times that of age-matched controls. Before age 40, and especially among young women, the excess mortality of alcoholics may be four to six times the expected rates (Room and Day 1974). What is surprising in Table 3.13, however, is that roughly one-third of deaths are caused by cardiovascular disease alone and that in older patients the number of cardiovascular deaths equals the number of deaths caused by cirrhosis, accidents, and suicide combined. In the studies displayed, severe neurological complications were

TABLE 3.13. Mortality in the Clinic, Core City, and College samples and in large studies of alcoholic mortality.

Sample	Deaths in total sample	fo/fe[a]	% of total deaths from selected causes							
			Cardio-vascular	fo/fe	Cirrhosis	fo/fe	Suicide	fo/fe	Other violence	fo/fe
Sundby 1967	1061	2	11%[b]	1.6	2%	10	5%	8	9%	3
Schmidt and deLint 1972	738	2	35	2	9	12	7	6	12	3
Pell and D'Alonzo 1973	102	3	41	3	11	c	2	c	2	1.5
Nicholls, Edwards, and Kyle 1974	309	2.7	23	2	3	23	15[d]	25	12	11
Polich, Armor, and Braiker 1981	111	3	21	1.2	8	8	12	20	21	5
Clinic sample	29	3	17	—	14	—	3	—	32	11
Core City and College samples	20	2	35	2	20	c	15	2	10	<1

a. fo/fe indicates the ratio of observed deaths to expected age-adjusted deaths or to deaths in controls.
b. In addition 9 percent died from "apoplexy" and 40 percent of deaths were not accounted for.
c. No controls died from this cause.
d. Psychiatric hospital sample.

too rare to merit separate mention. It is true that among young alcoholics the death rates for suicide, accidents, and cirrhosis are roughly ten times as high as expected and the death rate for heart disease is only about twice the expected rate; but over the life span, the total *excess* mortality from heart disease may exceed that from cirrhosis or suicide.

The study by D'Alonzo and Pell (1968; Pell and D'Alonzo 1973) deserves special mention. By following a community sample of employed alcoholics with a mean age of 51, they found interesting differences from the other studies in Table 3.13 that were derived from younger clinic populations. They conducted a careful, well-controlled five-year prospective study of the health of 899 alcohol abusers employed at Dupont and contrasted them with 921 controls matched for age, sex, and payroll class. At the start of their follow-up, their sample of alcoholics did not differ from the controls in terms of electrocardiogram abnormalities, angina, or obesity. Nevertheless, 21 of the 68 excess deaths that occurred among the alcoholics were from cardiovascular disease and 19 more were from cancer. During the same period of observation, there were only 14 excess deaths from suicide, accidents, and cirrhosis combined. It should also be underscored that the Pell and D'Alonzo study was the only one that estimated excess mortality from comparison with a matched control group rather than by comparison with the general population.

Although the studies in Table 3.13 provide the best picture of alcohol-related mortality that we have, none gives us an undistorted picture. Since the sample of Nicholls and colleagues (1974) was drawn from four British psychiatric hospitals, that sample manifested the highest proportion of suicides. Since Polich and colleagues (1981) followed a relatively young clinic sample, their sample manifested the highest proportion of accidents. All of the studies but the one by Sundby (1967) reflect mortality of that minority of alcoholics who die before age 55. Sundby managed to follow a cohort of alcoholics until two-thirds had died. Unfortunately, the causes of 40 percent of the deaths in his sample were unknown to him, but what was most significant about Sundby's study was that only 16 percent of his observed mortality was due to cirrhosis and unnatural causes. The study by Schmidt and deLint (1972) was perhaps the best executed and may provide the fairest overall picture.

The death rate of the Clinic sample is congruent with previous studies. The death rate from accidents in this relatively indigent urban population was higher than that observed in other studies and the cardiac death rate was lower. But the most distressing aspect of the Clinic study was the fact that in a sample of alcoholics granted virtually unlimited access to detoxification and medical care, the mortality was not lower than in less intensively treated samples. Tragically, abstinence does little to reduce the increased mortality of alcoholics. In the study by Pell and D'Alonzo, currently abstinent alcoholics experienced almost as high an excess death rate (2.9 times the expected) as did the active alcoholics (3.6 times the expected).

The death rates of this book's two community samples—the Core City and the College samples—differ from the death rate of its Clinic sample in the same way that the mortality of other community samples (such as Pell and D'Alonzo 1973) in Table 3.13 differed from the other clinic samples. The high proportion of suicides in the Core City and College samples can most likely be ascribed to their relative youth. In the community samples, cardiac deaths exceed those from unnatural causes. Indeed, in the study by Ojesjo (1981) of a community cohort of alcoholics, cited in Table 3.8, 21 of the 25 observed deaths occurred after age 65; 52 percent were cardiovascular in origin; and only 1 death was from violence.

Obviously, the etiology of the excess cardiac mortality observed in alcoholics is multiply determined and can only partly be attributed to alcohol abuse. Among the many factors that add to the apparent association between alcohol abuse and increased cardiac mortality, six will be discussed here. First, alcoholics with poor physical health receive preferential admission to detoxification units (Schmidt and deLint 1972); this sampling bias will exaggerate the observed mortality rates among such alcoholics. For example, the mortality in the Clinic sample was certainly enhanced by the fact that the detoxification unit was an integral part of a general municipal hospital whose usual clientele were the chronically ill. Second, alcoholic beverages contain many ingredients, and ethanol is not the only health offender. Thus, morbidity is affected by the kind of alcoholic beverage ingested. Beer may be selectively associated with cardiomyopathy, wine with cirrhosis, and spirits with certain cancers (Schmidt and Popham 1975). Binge drinkers appear to have greater morbidity than alcohol abusers who consume a similar volume of alcohol spread out more evenly over time. Third, the mean age of the sample studied, of course, makes an enormous difference in both the cause and the frequency of death. Cardiac deaths become increasingly frequent among older samples. Fourth, the general lifestyle of the alcoholic is often characterized by personal neglect, imbalanced diet, and lack of exercise. Thiamine deficiency contributes to alcohol-related illnesses of the central nervous system, and vitamin C deficiency, especially, is associated with cardiovascular disease. Fifth, just as the combination of alcohol abuse and frequent driving is synergistic with regard to accidental death, just so the combination of alcohol abuse and smoking may be synergistic with regard to increased mortality from both heart disease and cancer. Finally, D'Alonzo and Pell point out that a significant amount of the excess cardiac mortality among the alcoholics they studied occurred among those with hypertension.

Ashley and Rankin (1980) have provided an excellent in-depth review of the multifactorial etiology that links cardiac deaths with alcoholism. Their review suggests that alcoholics do not exhibit more atherosclerosis at autopsy. Rather, alcohol-induced cardiomyopathy (Burch and Giles 1974), the facilitation by alcohol of both heavy smoking and hypertension, and the direct effects of alcohol upon myocardial contractility appear most important in explaining the increased risk of cardiovascular morbidity among alcoholics.

∼ Mortality Revisited

The last 15 years have seen an increasing recognition of the contribution of alcohol abuse to excess mortality both in the general literature and in the Study of Adult Development. Nevertheless, the fact that in recent years the *American Journal of Public Health* has five to ten articles on the dangers of smoking for every one on the hazards of drinking suggests that there may still be too little awareness of alcohol abuse as a cause of premature mortality. Between 70,000 (Harwood et al. 1984) and 110,000 (Stinson and DeBakey 1992) deaths in the United States each year can be attributed to alcoholism. Put differently, by accounting for 5 percent of all deaths in the United States each year, alcohol abuse vies with strokes and accidents for third place as a cause of death (McGinnis and Foege 1993). If heavy smoking shortens an individual's life span by an estimated 8 years (Fielding 1988) sustained alcohol abuse, albeit a less common disorder, shortens it by 15 years (McDonnell and Maynard 1985).

About a quarter of the excess deaths are directly related to alcohol abuse—for example, alcoholic cardiomyopathy, alcohol poisoning, and alcoholic cirrhosis. About a fifth of deaths are secondary to alcohol abuse. For example, 50 percent of pancreatic, upper gastrointestinal, and laryngeal cancers can be attributed to alcohol abuse. Half of the deaths are indirectly related to alcohol abuse. For example, careful studies of excess mortality by Stinson and De-Bakey (1992) suggest that alcohol abuse accounts for perhaps 40 percent of most accidental deaths, especially vehicular and fire-related deaths, and for a quarter of all suicides.

In addition, research over the last 15 years has increased recognition of the contribution of alcohol abuse to mortality in other common disorders. Thus, the above estimates of mortality due to alcohol abuse may still be too low. McGregor (1986) has reviewed extensive evidence that alcohol abuse suppresses the immune system. Such evidence helps to explain the well-known indirect contribution of alcohol abuse to deaths from pneumonia and tuberculosis. Gill and colleagues (1986) have linked alcohol abuse to an increased incidence of strokes, and Longnecker and colleagues (1988) to an increased incidence of breast cancer. Lithell and colleagues (1987) have shown that binge drinking is strongly associated with an increased risk of sudden death after myocardial infarction. Ashley (1984), Pell and Fayerweather (1985), and Regan (1990) have all documented the contribution of alcohol abuse to left ventricular cardiac dysfunction, arrhythmias, and heart failure. Likely mechanisms of action for independent effects of alcohol abuse upon heart disease also include the previously mentioned increased risk of hypertension. Finally, owing to the contribution *(vide infra)* that alcohol abuse makes to sustained cigarette smoking, the indirect excess mortality attributed to alcohol abuse for cancer and heart disease may be an underestimate.

As Tables 3.13 and 3.13A underscore, shorter studies and studies of younger cohorts emphasize alcohol-related deaths from violent causes and accidents. Longer studies and studies of older cohorts emphasize excess alcohol-related deaths from cancer and heart disease. For example, only 44 (20 percent) of the 217 deaths in Brenner's follow-up and only 149 (14 percent) of 1,061 deaths in Sundby's follow-up were from violent causes and accidents. In contrast, a 20-year follow-up of 49,464 Swedish military conscripts (Andreasson et al. 1991) found that of the 893 premature deaths in this young sample, 635 (71 percent) were from violent deaths, including 320 suicides and 203 traffic accidents. High consumers of alcohol were at 4 times the risk of suicide and 2.3 times the risk of death from traffic accidents as compared with low consumers.

In Andreasson's study of 893 deaths before age 40, only 52 (6 percent) were from heart disease and only 109 (12 percent) were from cancer. In contrast, 204 (19 percent) of Sundby's 1,061 alcohol-abuse-associated deaths were from cancer, and 186 (18 percent) were from cardiovascular disease. Sundby observed that 6 percent of his deaths were from cancer of the larynx and upper digestive tract, 12 times the expected rate.

Recent evidence suggests that two of the main health hazards of alcohol abuse are reversible with abstinence. First, Saunders (1987) reviewed controlled

TABLE 3.13A. Sources of premature mortality in five prospective studies of alcohol abuse.

Sample	Deaths in total sample	fo/fe	Cardiovascular	fo/fe	Cancer	fo/fe	Cirrhosis	fo/fe	Suicide/ accident/ murder	fo/fe
						Number of deaths from selected causes				
Marshall, Edwards, Taylor (1994)	46	3.6	13	—	12[a]	—	4	—	6	—
Core City	41	2	10	1.2	13	1.8	7	6	4	7
College	20	3	9	5	5	1.7	0	—	4	7
Brenner (1967)[b]	217	3	52	1.8	NA	—	37	10	44	6
Berglund (1985)	497	2.5	144	1.5[c]	87	1.9	21	4	171	8.5

a. All but one of the deaths due to lung cancer.
b. A prospective 4–7 year study inadvertently omitted from Table 3.13.
c. Heart disease twice as common in deaths before age 60.

and experimental studies and showed that if 80+ grams of ethanol a day experimentally increased blood pressure, abstinence resulted in a significant decrease in diastolic blood pressure. Second, it has been shown that up to 72 percent (Muuronen et al. 1989) of hospitalized alcoholics with no history of head injury show brain atrophy and half show intellectual impairment. After years of abstinence, however, they show significant improvement, especially in reduced incidence of brain atrophy. Animal research has also indicated that after cessation of chronic alcohol administration neuronal dendritic rearborization occurs (Grant 1987).

The last 15 years have also illustrated the effects of alcohol abuse upon premature mortality in the continued follow-up of the members of the Study of Adult Development. The College alcohol abusers were three times as likely and the Core City alcohol abusers twice as likely as their nonalcoholic counterparts to die prematurely.

About half of the Study of Adult Development excess deaths among alcoholics were from heart disease and cancer. This almost twofold increase in cancer and cardiac deaths among alcoholics is congruent with other large community studies of mortality from cancer and hypertension that examined the effects of alcohol abuse while controlling for other risk factors such as obesity and cigarette smoking (Klatsky et al. 1986; Brugere et al. 1986). If in Tables 3.13 and 3.13A the three large studies by Sundby (1967), Brenner (1967), and Berglund (1984) are combined, out of perhaps 900 excess deaths in alcoholics, 30 percent were from heart disease and cancer, 30 percent were from violence, and only 7 percent were from cirrhosis.

Indeed, a study by Ewusi-Mensah and colleagues (1983) made the interesting point that alcoholic liver disease appears to be twice as common in alcoholics comorbid for major depressive disorder or antisocial personality as in alcoholics in the general population. This may account for the fact that cirrhosis seems more important as a cause of alcohol-related deaths in hospital-based studies than in community-based studies like the one by Andreasson and colleagues (1991), who observed that only 2 percent of their alcohol-related deaths were from cirrhosis.

Severity of alcohol abuse made a clear difference in mortality. If the 106 College and Core City men who met only the criteria for alcohol abuse were 1.5 times more likely to die than those without alcohol abuse, the 96 men with alcohol dependence were 3 times as likely to die prematurely. (As noted earlier, the 78 Core City men who were lifelong teetotalers were also 1.5 times as likely to die as social drinkers. A disproportionate number of these teetotalers died from cancers other than lung cancer.)

The difficulty in interpreting these results is that heavy use of cigarettes and alcohol abuse were highly correlated. When the effect of alcohol abuse was controlled, heavy smoking was associated with elevated mortality risk in both samples. For example, 9 of the 13 Core City cancer deaths were from lung cancer, and 11 of the 12 cancer deaths in Edwards's 20-year follow-up of 100 alcohol abusers were from lung cancer (Marshall et al. 1990). When cigarette smoking was controlled, however, the odds ratio for mortality from alcohol abuse was still significantly elevated in both samples (Vaillant et al. 1991).

Evidence that many of the excess lung cancer and coronary heart disease deaths associated with smoking can be partially attributed to alcohol abuse is indirect and comes from a variety of sources. First, alcohol abuse greatly increases premature death among heavy smokers. This can be demonstrated by examining the interrelationship of both alcoholism and smoking to premature mortality in the two cohorts of the Study of Adult Development. Of the 297 men who abused neither cigarettes nor alcohol, 32 (11 percent) were dead by 1992. Of the 148 men who abused just cigarettes, 30 (20 percent) were dead. However, of the 128 men who abused *both* alcohol and cigarettes, 48 (38 percent) were dead, and of the 46 men who were both alcohol-*dependent* and heavy smokers (50+ pack/years), 22 (48 percent) were dead.

On the one hand, the temptation to put sole blame for the increased alcohol/smoking mortality on smoking is supported by two observations. First, the excess mortality of the 47 Core City men who achieved stable abstinence from alcohol was the same as that for the 103 alcohol-abusing men who did not achieve abstinence—twice the expected number. A major reason for this elevated mortality of the abstinent Core City men was their history of heavy smoking. Second, only 3 of the 57 Study of Adult Development men who abused alcohol *but not cigarettes* died prematurely. Very few of the nonsmoking alcohol abusers, however, were alcohol-dependent.

On the other hand, alcohol abuse exacerbates the deleterious effects of smoking. In summarizing the literature, both DiFranza and Guerrera (1990) and Vaillant and colleagues (1991) found evidence that alcohol abuse increases pack/years of smoking, but that smoking does not contribute to sustained alcohol abuse. Significantly, only 10 percent of the College non-alcohol abusers were heavy (40+ pack/years) smokers; 33 percent of the College alcohol abusers were heavy smokers; and 68 percent of the 19 College alcoholics who met criteria for dependence were heavy smokers. Ten of these 13 men were abusing alcohol *before* they became two-pack-a-day smokers. In other words, heavy smoking probably did not cause their alcohol abuse. The same association between heavy smoking and alcohol dependence held true for the Core City sample: 15 percent of the 257 men who were not alcohol abusers were 50+ pack/year smokers; 54 percent of the 68 alcohol-dependent men whose smoking histories were known were 50+ pack/year smokers.

Although most of the College heavy smokers abused alcohol before their smoking reached two packs a day, alcohol abuse in itself did not seem to cause heavy smoking. For example, the mean age of becoming a two-pack-a-day smoker was 34.8 years for the nonalcoholics compared to 33.6 years for the alcohol abusers. Rather, alcohol abuse seems to increase pack/years of smoking, because in contrast to nonalcoholics, alcoholics do not stop smoking. DiFranza and Guerrera noted that equal numbers of alcohol abusers and nonabusers tried to quit smoking but that only 7 percent of the alcoholic smokers were successful in contrast to 49 percent of the nonalcoholic smokers. The net result was that at the end of their follow-up 51 (66 percent) of their 77 alcoholic subjects were still smoking in contrast to only 31 (28 percent) of their 109 nonalcoholics. Among the College sample, by age 65, 84 percent of those who did not abuse alcohol, 62 percent of the 29 alcohol abusers, but only 24 percent of the 17 alcohol-dependent men had stopped smoking.

But if alcohol abuse prolonged the chronicity of heavy smoking, heavy smoking did not affect the chronicity of alcohol abuse. For example, among the College sample, heavy smoking was present in 67 percent of the best outcomes and in only 43 percent of the 28 most chronic alcohol abusers. The reason for this paradox was probably that in the College sample alcohol dependence was positively associated with sustained abstinence, and alcohol dependence was also associated with sustained heavy smoking. Among the Core City men nonsmokers and light smokers enjoyed the same prognosis for remission from alcohol abuse as very heavy smokers.

Not only does alcohol abuse interfere with smoking cessation, but most smokers smoke more while drinking alcohol (Schacter et al. 1977; Mello et al. 1980; Henningfield et al. 1984). A possible mechanism for this phenomenon, besides the poor self-care associated with alcohol abuse, is that the acidic urine associated with heavy alcohol intake enhances urinary excretion of nicotine (Smith 1955; Eiser 1987). Thus, a heavy drinker must smoke more to maintain a given blood nicotine level. Moreover, in chronic ethanol and nicotine treatment in mice there is evidence of cross-tolerance (Burch et al. 1988). In a recent controlled laboratory study in humans, history of past or present alcohol abuse was strongly associated with both number and potency (nicotine, carbon monoxide, and tar yields) of cigarettes smoked and daily puff duration (Keenan et al. 1990).

Since alcoholism is so much more common among smokers than among nonsmokers, the question may be asked, Is there not some common factor in both habits? As with the question of whether there is a common etiology for sociopathy and alcoholism, the answer is "yes, but. . . " Both multiproblem families and painful childhoods can enhance the susceptibility of some individuals to addictive drugs in general, and preexisting antisocial personality increases the susceptibility to behaving irresponsibly. In addition, certain social networks and occupations can serve as a common etiology for both increased tobacco and alcohol use. For example, Jessor and many other investigators have found that peer-group influence is very strong in both smoking and drinking and that the two go together. Similarly, DiFranza and Guerrera (1990) noted that alcoholics were more likely to have childhood friends who were smokers. Also, it seems clear that antisocial individuals are more likely to smoke *and* to drink heavily. Among the Core City alcoholics, heavy smokers were five times more likely to have been in jail or to have met criteria for sociopathy than were alcoholics who used tobacco only sparingly.

There does not, however, seem to be a common genetic basis for the two disorders. Kaprio and colleagues (1987) found that smoking in one twin was associated with smoking in the other twin and that alcoholism in one twin was associated with alcoholism in the other twin. But there did not seem to be any genetic predisposition for twins to abuse both substances. Similarly, if one controlled for smoking, alcoholism in Core City men was associated with alcoholic heredity with an r of .26 ($p < .001$), whereas if one controlled for alcoholism, smoking was associated with alcoholic heredity with an r of $-.04$. None of the major variables in the Core City study that predicted alcohol abuse predicted heavy smoking.

Like smoking and alcohol abuse, depression is associated with premature mortality (Vaillant 1992); and if alcoholics were three times as likely to be dead, they were also three times as likely to be depressed. Thus, it is tempting to blame depression—highly correlated with both heavy smoking and alcoholism—as a common factor and a possible cause for the high mortality seen in alcoholics. Once again, the data from the College cohort suggest that alcohol abuse is a cause rather than a result of depression and heavy smoking.

In the College sample, there were several ways by which the roles of alcoholism and depression in mortality could be distinguished. First, the association of depression with increased mortality appeared to be mediated in large part by alcohol abuse and smoking. When smoking and alcohol abuse were statistically controlled, depression was not significantly correlated with mortality. Second, only 2 (14 percent) of the 14 depressed alcoholics stopped smoking, whereas 9 (24 percent) of the 38 not-depressed alcoholics stopped smoking, at least suggestive evidence that depression made alcoholics smoke more. Conversely, 8 (57 percent) of the 14 depressed alcoholics stopped drinking, whereas only 7 (18 percent) of the 38 not-depressed alcoholics stopped drinking. In other words, depression actually increased the likelihood of alcoholics stopping drinking. While the sample is too small to be statistically significant, the pharmacology makes sense. Nicotine is a mild stimulant and may serve as an antidepressant; conversely, alcohol ingestion makes depression worse.

Third, as indicated in Table 3.13B, whether or not a smoker abused alcohol made a twofold difference in whether he was depressed (comparison B), and whether a depressed person abused alcohol made a twofold difference in how much the person smoked (comparison A). In contrast, among alcoholics, heavy smoking was not associated with being depressed and depression was not associated with being a heavy smoker. In nonalcoholics, however, depression and heavy smoking each increased the risk of the other.

Expressed still differently, smoking, depression, and alcohol abuse are all significantly ($p < .01$) correlated with one another. When smoking is controlled, depression correlates with alcohol abuse at $r = .23$ ($p < .001$). When depression is controlled, smoking correlates with alcohol abuse at $r = .37$ ($p < .001$). But with alcohol abuse controlled, depression was not significantly correlated with smoking. The numbers are small and the conclusions are inferential. However, the data all point to the conclusion that alcohol abuse, past or present, is a contributing cause of deaths attributed to excess smoking.

Hypertension and Alcohol Abuse

The medical complications of alcoholism have been well reviewed elsewhere (for example, in Kissen and Begleiter 1974), and with the single exception of hypertension, macroscopic community studies like those in this book have little additional information to offer. Until ten years ago, the relationship between alcohol abuse and hypertension was not appreciated. One reason was that, inexplicably, at the time of discharge from detoxification centers alcoholics did not appear to manifest elevated blood pressure (Schnall and Weiner 1958). It was only as investigators examined the correlation of blood pressure with drinking habits in the community that the association between hypertension and alcohol abuse became clear (Dyer et al. 1977). In assessing 300 employees referred for alcoholism to an industrial medical department, Kamner and Dupong (1969) observed that 33 percent had hypertension. In

TABLE 3.13B. Interrelationships of smoking, depression, and alcohol abuse in the College sample.

	N^a	Condition		Risk	
Comparison A		*Distribution of the 41 40+ pack/year smokers*			
	170	No alcohol abuse, no depression	16	Heavy smokers =	9%
	17	Depression, no alcohol abuse	3	Heavy smokers =	18%
	36	Alcohol abuse, no depression	15	Heavy smokers =	42%
	14	Alcohol abuse *and* depression	7	Heavy smokers =	50%
Comparison B		*Distribution of the 31 depressed men*			
	168	No alcohol abuse, no smoking	14	Depressed =	8%
	19	Heavy smoking, no alcohol abuse	3	Depressed =	16%
	28	Alcohol abuse, no smoking	7	Depressed =	25%
	22	Alcohol abuse *and* heavy smoking	7	Depressed =	32%
Comparison C		*Distribution of the 50 alcohol abusers*			
	175	No smoking, no depression	21	Alcohol abuse =	12%
	31	Heavy smoking, no depression	15	Alcohol abuse =	48%
	21	Depression, no smoking	7	Alcohol abuse =	33%
	10	Depression *and* heavy smoking	7	Alcohol abuse =	70%

a. Total n = 237, not 240, because of 3 men with incomplete data sets.

their careful comparison of alcohol abusers at the Dupont company with controls matched for age, sex, and payroll class, Pell and D'Alonzo (1973) found that hypertension (two successive readings of diastolic 95 mm Hg or above or systolic 160 mm Hg or above) occurred twice as frequently among the alcoholics. Twenty-two of the 37 cardiac deaths experienced by alcoholics in Pell and D'Alonzo's study occurred among hypertensives. The authors note that hypertensives of normal and below-normal body weight were especially likely to be alcohol abusers. By using a sample of 83,947 members of the Kaiser Permanente Medical Plan, Klatsky and colleagues (1977) document that the association between hypertension and alcoholism is independent of coffee and tobacco use.

In the Core City and College samples, rates of hypertension (a systolic of 145 mm Hg or above or a diastolic of 90 mm Hg or above) were seen twice as frequently among alcohol abusers (see Table 3.14) as among subjects without symptoms of alcoholism. Such a finding suggests, but by no means proves, a causal connection. It is perfectly conceivable that individuals with preclinical hypertension might become, for some common underlying reason, prone to alcohol abuse. For example, in some individuals blood pressure is increased during periods of heightened anxiety and anger (Whitehead et al. 1977). It is also true, however, that alcohol abuse increases anxiety and aggression and that alcohol may produce changes in peripheral blood flow that could induce elevated blood pressure.

Thus, the question must be asked: are prehypertensive individuals also predisposed to alcoholism? If so, then alcoholism might be viewed as a symptom of hypertension rather than as a cause. To address this question, the blood pressure recorded in their sophomore year of college for the 250 College men who remained in the study until age 40 was correlated both with adult hypertension and with alcohol abuse. Elevated blood pressure in college was significantly associated with hypertension in midlife. Twenty-seven sophomores had a standing or sitting diastolic blood pressure of over 94 mm Hg and/or a lying diastolic pressure over 84 mm Hg; of these, 14 (52 percent) were classified as at least borderline hypertensives at age 58 by an internist blind to college blood pressure. Of the 233 surviving men who had not had an elevated diastolic blood pressure in college, only 16 percent were classified as hypertensive at age 58. This association between college and midlife hypertension is significant at $p < .001$. The work of Thomas and Greenstreet (1973) and Paffenbarger and colleagues (1968) confirms the relationship of elevated blood pressure in college to later hypertension.

In contrast, only 4 (15 percent) of the 27 College men with elevated

TABLE 3.14. Hypertension and alcohol abuse.

Sample	Asymptomatic drinkers		Alcohol abusers	
	n	Hypertensive	n	Hypertensive
Pell and D'Alonzo 1973	921	16%	899	37%**
Core City	115[a]	10	110	25**
College	217	18	33	36*

a. 115 Core City men were selected by chance from the larger sample of 290 adequately studied Core City men without alcohol abuse.

$*p < .05$; $**p < .01$ (chi-square test).

diastolic blood pressure in their sophomore year were later classified as alcohol abusers; 29 (13 percent) of the 233 men without elevated blood pressure in college also became alcohol abusers. Thus, blood pressure in college did not predict future alcoholism, only hypertension.

Prognosis

Once heavy social drinking has begun to evolve into alcohol abuse, it is difficult to predict how far the process will continue or whether it will reverse itself. Undoubtedly, a major reason for this prognostic uncertainty is the multifactorial nature of the etiology of alcoholism. If the cause of any process is highly multidetermined, it is difficult to point to any single factor that will consistently predict the course of that process.

Nevertheless, this chapter has already addressed several factors that predict short-term, if not long-term, course. At the time when an alcoholic first seeks treatment, clinical course over the next year may be predicted with some accuracy. Many premorbid factors associated with social stability, especially occupational stability, and marriage (Bromet et al. 1977; Costello 1980) predict favorable short-term response to treatment. Conversely, the exhaustive reviews by Gibbs and Flanagan (1977) and Baekeland and colleagues (1975) of the outcome literature reveal that early age of onset, low social class, social alienation, broken marriage, many arrests, and sociopathy militate against a favorable response to treatment. For the Clinic sample, Table 3.11 pointed out that residential stability, regular employment, marriage, absence of previous arrests, and absence of previous detoxifications all correlated with a good short-term outcome. Of equal importance, however, is the observation that when such favorable premorbid psychosocial predictors are controlled

TABLE 3.15.   Comparison of securely abstinent and progressive alcoholics on premorbid variables.

Premorbid variables	Asymptomatic drinkers (n = 250±10)	Securely abstinent[a] (n = 21)	Progressively alcoholic[a] (n = 35)
Adequate maternal supervision (top third)	30%	38%	34%
Best boyhood competence (top quartile)	28	29	20
Worst boyhood competence (bottom quartile)	15	24	14
Many weaknesses in childhood (multiproblem family)	11	14	11
I.Q. < 90	28	29	29
Few strengths in childhood	23	33	37
Not a high school graduate	44	62	66
Clear family history of alcoholism	32	62	57

a. When the means of each variable for these two groups were compared by Student's T-test, no significant differences were detected.

then neither the severity of alcoholism before treatment nor the intensity of aftercare markedly affects prognosis (Costello 1975; Orford and Edwards 1977).

Most of what has been written about prognosis and alcoholism, however, is based upon clinical populations followed for brief periods, and short-term response to clinical intervention may not reflect recovery as much as treatment compliance. Social stability and compliance with conventional clinical intervention go hand in hand. Clinical populations also contain a disproportionate number of skid-row residents. Such individuals often have severe social deficits predating their alcoholism, such as schizophrenia, mental retardation, or childhood foster care. The fact that such socially deprived patients make many more repeat visits exaggerates the relationship between social incompetence and intractable alcoholism. In general population studies, skid-row residents are the exception, not the rule. Of 110 Core City alcohol abusers, only 5 men could be categorized as residents of skid row.

Over the longer term, premorbid adjustment seems less important to abstinence. Thus, the findings from the Core City study presented in Table 3.15 contradict those from studies of shorter duration. Premorbidly, the 21 "securely abstinent" alcohol abusers—men abstinent for a minimum of three years—could not be distinguished from the 35 men whose alcoholism had become relentlessly more symptomatic until the present. The blindly assessed childhoods of these two very different alcoholic outcome groups seem roughly comparable. Certainly, in terms of the childhood variables that were most important in predicting mental health (see Table 2.3), Table 3.15 reveals little difference between the securely abstinent and the progressive alcoholics. Maternal supervision, boyhood competence, childhood weaknesses, and I.Q. did not even differentiate the 21 securely abstinent alcoholics from the 21 men among the progressive alcoholics who showed the greatest social incapacitation secondary to their drinking. Early termination of education and a heredity positive for alcoholism (and its correlate, the absence of childhood strengths) were variables that predicted who would develop alcoholism, but these variables did not predict who would then recover. In Figures 3.3 and 3.4 the College men with all their "advantages" achieved stable abstinence no more frequently than the Core City sociopaths. Among the Core City sample, of these 25 men classified as both sociopaths and alcoholics, 48 percent were currently abstinent; in contrast, of the 40 Core City alcohol abusers with no antisocial symptoms except heavy drinking, only 28 percent were currently abstinent. Admittedly, there are dangers as well as benefits to hitting bottom; fewer nonsociopaths have become institutionalized or died. Nevertheless, psychological soundness may not facilitate ultimate recovery in alcoholism. This is a difference from psychiatric conditions like sociopathy, schizophrenia, and reactive depression, where clinical course is powerfully affected by premorbid adjustment.

The findings in Table 3.15 are consistent with the concepts developed in Chapter 2 that once it occurs alcoholism has a life of its own and that alcoholism is best thought of as a cause, not a consequence, of personality disorder. Premorbid childhood factors should be expected to have the greatest prognostic importance in psychiatric conditions that are symptoms of psychosocial trauma and that are not disorders in their own right. Premorbid childhood environment should be relatively unimportant in the prognosis of conditions primarily caused by culture or by adult onset of "disease."*

Several factors appear to reconcile the findings in Table 3.15 with those of

---

*After 15 more years of follow-up the categorization of excellent and very poor outcome became more certain. The number of securely abstinent men increased to 48 and their average length of abstinence was between 10 and 20 years. The number of men who were categorized as chronically alcoholic also increased to 48, and their average length of alcohol abuse was a quarter-century. There was, however, no significant change in the figures in Table 3.15. Premorbid strengths and weaknesses were equally distributed among the men with stable abstinence and those with chronic alcoholism.

previous investigators. First, the Core City findings do not indicate that premorbid variables have *no* importance in outcome. As we have seen in Table 3.9, alcohol abusers who were able to return to social drinking or whose symptomatology did not progress, as in the case of the atypical alcoholics, reflect somewhat different populations from those diagnosed as alcohol-dependent. Alcohol abusers who in response to treatment, confrontation, or insight resume asymptomatic drinking very early reflect premorbid traits usually associated with good prognosis: social stability, absence of sociopathy, late onset of alcoholism, and little evidence of alcohol dependence.

The reasons why advanced alcoholism should be relatively immune to the premorbid variables that affect the course of other psychiatric illnesses may be explained by two important ways in which alcoholism differs from most other psychiatric illness. Alcoholism destroys the very factors that facilitate recovery from illness—latent psychological (ego) strengths and social supports. First, through the ability of alcohol to damage the integrity of the central nervous system, alcoholism is a great leveler of human differences. Organic brain damage renders kings and geniuses no different from paupers and imbeciles. There is evidence that some alcohol-induced alterations in brain physiology may persist for the first year of abstinence (Williams and Rundell 1981). Second, all chronic illnesses are affected by the integrity of the patient's social network (Berkman and Syme 1979); but whereas many chronic illnesses actually draw individuals toward a sustaining network of social supports, alcohol abuse, through its facilitation of unprovoked anger, irresponsibility, and "selfish" behaviors, systematically destroys the individual's relationships and leads him or her toward social isolation and demoralization.

In most short-term studies, early onset of alcoholism is found to correlate with a poor prognosis. Indeed, investigators like Goodwin (1979) have suggested that early onset of alcohol dependence identifies genetically determined ("primary") alcoholics. This hypothesis was not substantiated among the Core City men. For example, neither of the major alcohol risk factors (ethnicity and family history of alcoholism) correlated with age of onset of alcohol abuse. Nor did major predictors of mental health—boyhood competence and childhood emotional problems—predict early alcoholism.

Rather, early age of alcohol abuse appeared to be a function of family breakdown. Among the Core City men, early onset of alcohol dependence was positively and significantly correlated with low I.Q. ($r = .34$), a variable closely linked with maternal neglect, with delinquent parents ($r = .21$), with alcoholism of the father (rather than of other relatives ($r = .18$), with early onset of a broken home ($r = .32$), and with premorbid truancy and school problems ($r = .22$). In other words, the same variables that predicted sociopathy (Table 2.14) also predicted early onset of alcoholism.

Paradoxically, as we have already seen in Figures 3.5 and 3.6, early onset of alcoholism was correlated positively with early abstinence. On the average, progressive alcoholics did not manifest their fourth symptom on the PDS until the age of 32 ± 10 years, but the men who were currently abstinent manifested their fourth symptom on the PDS at an average age of 25. Thus, the percentage of an alcohol abuser's adult life spent abstinent correlated inversely ($r = .34$) with the age of onset of his alcoholism. The younger he was when he began to abuse alcohol, the more likely he was to spend a significant percentage of his subsequent life abstinent.

Consistent with a model that views alcoholism as a disease that evolves in a predictable fashion, advanced signs of alcoholism were seen more often among men whose alcoholism had an early onset. Binge drinking ($r = .37$), multiple job losses ($r = .22$), and multiple arrests ($r = .34$) all correlated significantly and negatively with age of onset. Such observations have been interpreted by many (Goodwin 1979; Tarter 1981) as indicating that early-onset alcoholism is a different illness, but such theories ignore the temporal dimension. The longer an individual remains alcoholic, the more chronic may be his symptoms of dependence.

In their exhaustive review of prognostic studies, Gibbs and Flanagan (1977) noted that neither the age of first drink nor the number of years spent drinking heavily *without* problems affected long-term outcome. Data from Core City men did not contradict these findings.

A final set of variables that affect prognosis but are more difficult to study operationally are those psychosocial variables which support the alcoholic's denial of his own condition. How ill must an alcoholic become before he stops drinking? What first allows an alcoholic to realize that his drinking is self-detrimental? What is it in an individual's makeup or in his community that makes him recognize that he is losing control of alcohol after just a few symptoms? For example, a relative of mine at age 25 found himself reaching under his camp bed for his bottle of rum before getting up in the morning. Suddenly he had an "aha" experience: "I am becoming an alcoholic." After that he no longer kept his rum under the bed; he watched his intake; and he spent the next six decades as a social drinker. Again, a Core City man at age 24 found himself drunk and on a window ledge debating suicide. Terrified, he went back inside and never used alcohol again. In contrast, despite experiencing the most appalling consequences of alcohol abuse, other Core City alcoholics continued to deny until death that their use of alcohol was self-detrimental.

There are many factors that affect denial. First, individuals who have had alcoholic parents often experience exceptionally severe symptoms before acknowledging their own alcohol abuse. The reason does not appear to be identification with parental drinking, but may result from cognitive dissonance between their childhood hatred and condemnation of their parent's drunkenness and increasing evidence of their own alcohol abuse. The offspring of alcoholic parents experience greater than average guilt and cognitive dissonance, and both guilt and cognitive dissonance strengthen denial mechanisms. Core City men with alcoholic fathers were statistically more likely to experience multiple medical complaints than men without alcoholic fathers.

Second, the degree to which an individual's social environment accepts or denies alcohol abuse is important. If an individual's spouse or boss is an alcoholic, or is unusually tolerant of alcoholism, the individual may seek treatment late and relapse often. If one's larger community fails to distinguish between "drinking" and "alcohol abuse" (as is the case in France and in some American black urban neighborhoods; Kane 1981) denial of alcohol abuse will be enhanced. In contrast, providing nonjudgmental information about alcohol abuse, alleviating guilt about alcoholism by labeling it an illness (as in successful industrial alcohol programs), facilitating identification with culturally accepted role models who have recovered from alcoholism (such as Alcoholics Anonymous), and sharply differentiating drinking from alcohol abuse (as is the case in Italy) all reduce denial and enable the individual to recognize early that his drinking is out of control.

The recognition that alcohol abuse puts one not into but out of control is important to recovery. Within the Core City sample, the importance of such self-recognition was illustrated by the fact that 28 percent of the currently abstinent alcoholics, but only one (3 percent) of the progressive alcoholics saw alcohol as the antithesis of a tranquilizer and disavowed psychological dependence, a term defined by statements like "I drink because it makes me feel less anxious and depressed" or "I drink to help me forget my worries and to cheer myself up."

Similarly, failure to recognize early alcohol-related physical distress may have negative prognostic implications. On the one hand, among both College and Core City men, early recognition of alcohol-engendered physical distress was associated with return to asymptomatic drinking. On the other hand, it is common for alcoholics hospitalized on medical and surgical wards with multiple physical complications of alcoholism to manifest unusually resistant denial and a poor prognosis.

Habit, Addiction, and Relapse

A number of factors affect prognosis by affecting likelihood of relapse. It is just as important to consider the reasons people relapse to alcohol abuse as to consider the reasons they may be prone to develop alcohol abuse. Although in some respects this section belongs in the previous chapter on the etiology of alcoholism, it is included here to complete the canvas of the natural history of alcoholism.

It is tempting to try to focus on the risk of relapse by calculating the intensity of "craving." However, our only reliable measure of craving is the likelihood of relapse; and craving is to relapse what willpower is to abstinence—a tautology. It is better to focus on independent behavioral phenomena.

Mello has marshaled an extensive literature arguing that many of the most obvious reasons for relapse are in fact relatively unimportant (Mello 1972; Mello and Mendelson 1978). It is simplistic to think of alcoholics relapsing solely because having once been pharmacologically addicted to alcohol they "crave" the drug for the rest of their lives (Mello 1975). In the stable, unfamiliar setting of the laboratory, so-called loss of control disappears and moderate drinking by even the well-established alcoholic is a common observation (Paredes et al. 1973). But it is equally simplistic to suggest that abstinent alcoholics relapse purely to relieve tension, anxiety, or depression, or from conscious desire. "Addiction" involves more than pharmacological and emotional dependence. Work by behavioral psychologists (Conger 1956; Mello and Mendelson 1970, 1972; Ludwig and Wikler 1974; Morse and Kelleher 1970, 1977; Nathan et al. 1970; and others too numerous to mention here) provides us with the best clues to the complex learning processes underlying seemingly incomprehensible relapse to alcohol.

How can involuntary craving for alcohol be understood? Why under certain circumstances can an inveterate binge drinker drink socially in a laboratory (Merry 1966; Gottheil et al. 1973) or remain abstinent for several months in the community only to go on a self-destructive bender, losing all control over his behavior apparently following a "first drink"?

It appears that an alcoholic's craving is best understood as a verbal *ex post facto* rationalization of conditioned behavior. Thus, so-called craving identifies unconsciously learned behavior in the same way that the epiphenomenon of a visible flame draws our attention to the invisible process of combustion. At best, craving represents the cognitive correlate of a subclinical conditioned withdrawal syndrome and is likely to be evoked subsequent to any state of physiological arousal resembling this syndrome (Ludwig and Wikler 1974). At worst, craving exists mainly in the minds of alcohologists (Merry 1966; Mello 1975).

Physiological addiction plays a major role in making alcohol ingestion an even more powerful conditioned reinforcer. There is never certainty that ingesting alcohol will relieve guilt, anxiety, sadness, or loneliness, but there is certainty that it will relieve symptoms of pharmacological dependence upon alcohol—a process of dependence that begins long before it attracts medical attention. Drinking alcohol instantly relieves the anxiety, even terror, of withdrawal symptoms; and immediate consequences are far more reinforcing than delayed consequences. As Bandura points out, "it is precisely for this reason that persons may persistently engage in immediately reinforcing but potentially self-destructive behavior" (1969, p. 530).

The fact that alcohol *nonspecifically* alters an individual's feeling state also makes it a powerful reinforcer. Consider for example compulsive shoplifting, gambling, Russian roulette, and indecent exposure. None of these behaviors depends upon physical addiction; they are all under very limited conscious control; they all have a life of their own; and all undoubtedly would disappear in a laboratory setting. All, however, involve a dramatic change of affective state. We know that a change of mental state is more important when an individual is unhappy than when an individual is happy. The excitement of Russian roulette, of painful tattoos, of joining the Foreign Legion, occurs among people who are demoralized and who possess impaired social networks. It is not that Russian roulette or exposing oneself or getting drunk necessarily makes one feel *good*, but what all three share is that they make one feel *different*—analogous to the "trip abroad" that nineteenth-century physicians once prescribed to relieve depression in rich patients.

Mello and Mendelson (1972) have demonstrated that many alcoholics do not maintain stable concentrations of blood alcohol when drinking, but instead tolerate or even seek considerable variation in blood alcohol levels. This suggests that continued changes in one's state of consciousness may be as reinforcing as the relief of physiological withdrawal. Again, Morse and

Kelleher (1977) have shown that monkeys can be placed in operant situations where they will work when the only consequence of working is a painful electrical shock. It is difficult to understand the reinforcing properties of such shock except in terms of the production of a sudden change in state.

Bandura perceived alcoholism as reflecting a social learning process rather than either deviant behavior or pharmacological addiction: "Although drinking behavior is most often acquired during non-stress conditions, the habitual social drinker will experience stress reduction on many occasions. Once alcohol consumption is thus intermittently reinforced, it will be readily elicited under frustration or adverse conditions. Therefore, alcoholism typically results from habituation after prolonged heavy social drinking" (1969, p. 535). Anyone who has ever compulsively eaten too many peanuts or potato chips can appreciate the dilemma that loss of control of consumption magnifies and does not reduce distress. Learning theory per se cannot fully explain why alcohol abuse leads to loss of control, but a learning theory of alcoholism must be complementary to a theory of pharmacological addiction.

Also, chronic alcohol ingestion alters the central nervous system in ways that are not fully understood. Gordis (1976) has pointed out that in terms of physiology, the detoxified, currently abstinent patient really is different from a lifelong moderate drinker. After months of abstinence the former alcoholic's sleep electroencephalogram may remain abnormal (Williams and Rundell 1981); and after months of abstinence, alcoholics may experience brief withdrawal-like symptoms Anecdotal reports by anesthesiologists suggest that pharmacological tolerance to sedatives may persist even after a year of abstinence from alcohol or barbiturates.

Perhaps more important than physiological dependence, alcoholism reflects in its intensity a psychologically conditioned habit somewhere between fingernail biting and a proscribed sexual appetite. In fingernail biting, if conditioned cues can be overcome, and if a conscious desire to stop biting the fingernails is established, willpower may overcome the once intractable habit. There is no inner biological urge to chew one's nails. In the case of a forbidden sexual appetite, as with alcohol abuse, for a day willpower can seem omnipotent and yet after a year, willpower may be almost for naught. In the laboratory or after a New Year's resolution, forbidden sexual desire may seem utterly absent. Then, through a series of linked or "chained" conditioned cues, and often in the absence of alternative forms of sexual release, an individual may forget the strongest resolutions and become more and more focused, consciously or unconsciously, toward a specific—if detrimental—goal. At a certain point in any courtship process an individual goes on "automatic pilot." Despite its biological base, intense sexual desire can be quenched in one setting only to be suddenly rekindled in another. In similar fashion, conditioned alcoholic craving vanishes in treatment units and in behavioral laboratories only to return unexpectedly at some unforeseen point in the alcoholic's future.

Keller has fancifully described the conditioning paradigm that underlies this phenomenon: "For any alcoholic there may be several or a whole battery of critical cues or signals. By rule of generalization, any critical cue can spread like the tentacles of a vine over a whole range of analogs, and this may account for the growing frequency of bouts or for the development of a pattern of continuous inebriation" (1972, p. 161). Thus, the process of initiation of binge drinking is analogous to bulimia, compulsive gambling, wanderlust, or sexual indiscretions. In one sense, we all are addicted to food, to vacations, and to sexual activity. But detrimental addictions put an otherwise reasonable individual on automatic pilot, as it were, and seem to give the addictive behavior a life of its own that is more difficult to understand. The study of chained or linked conditioned reinforcers and of the importance of schedules of reinforcement upon drug effects (Morse and Kelleher 1977) points us in the correct direction. It has been experimentally documented that in humans (Nathan et al. 1970; Hunt and Azrin 1973; Mello 1972) and in animals (for example Falk and Tang 1980) relapse to alcoholic drinking reflects conditioned behavior, not a capricious desire or a simple response to psychological conflict.

It is possible to go even further and show that the pharmacological effects of alcohol are in large part conditioned. Marlatt and colleagues (1973) have demonstrated that in an experimental setting how much of a vodka mixture an alcoholic will drink is determined by how much vodka he thinks he is drinking rather than by the amount of alcohol actually consumed.

The qualities of a reinforcer are also tremendously affected by social and historical set. In other words, cognitive set can take precedence over pharmacology. An animal will work for a given reinforcer in a pattern that is more dependent upon the operant schedule of reinforcement than upon his "motivation." The tendency for a given drug to affect that animal's behavior will depend on the effect of the drug upon the schedule of behavior, not on the drug's effect upon the specific "motivational" properties of the reinforcer (Morse and Kelleher 1977). For example, although amphetamine decreases appetite ("motivation" to eat), it will consistently increase an animal's rate of responding on a fixed-ratio schedule of food reinforcement. In similar fashion, alcohol may produce belligerence in a barroom, frivolity at a wedding, somnolence in a library, and sexual abandon in a parked car.

Cigarettes exerted a very different sort of control over behavior in Berlin in 1946 than at the Surgeon General's office in Washington, D.C., in 1980. Craving for heroin diminishes or disappears in settings where heroin is unavailable, and increases in conditions previously associated with drug procurement (Meyer and Mirin 1979). All the physiological effects of heroin withdrawal can be reproduced through hypnosis (Ludwig and Lyle 1964). Similarly, craving for alcohol is often induced by unrecognized environmental or internal cues (Ludwig et al. 1974). The problem, of course, is that the alcoholic's impulse to drink is assumed by the alcoholic to represent character flaws or weaknesses rather than conditioned symptoms of addiction. Like the College subject James O'Neill, once conscious of craving, the alcoholic views his symptoms as a moral problem, not as a disease.

In their persuasive review of the importance of attribution and expectancy to the effects of alcohol, Marlatt and Rohsenow (1980) carry the theory of the importance of attribution and expectancy one step further. They review a large number of studies illustrating that the belief that one is drinking alcohol, even when one is not, may have much more effect upon aggression, relief of anxiety, sexual arousal, and reported craving than the pharmacological effect of alcohol per se. Thus, the individual's culturally conditioned expectancies about what alcohol is supposed to do may be far more specific than the actual pharmacological effects of alcohol.

For example, normal male subjects showed greater sexual arousal (measured physiologically) when exposed to deviant sexual scenes (such as forcible rape) than when exposed to nondeviant erotic scenes only when they believed they had consumed alcohol, regardless of whether they actually had consumed alcohol or not (Wilson and Lawson 1976). Again, experimental subjects administered significantly more intense electric shocks to the experimenter's confederate, if they received tonic water which they believed to contain alcohol than if they received alcohol and tonic which they believed to be just tonic (Lang et al. 1975).

Of course, such observations must be tempered by the fact that if the culture *believes* that the conscience is soluble in ethanol, there is also pharmacological justification for this belief. Sedative drugs do truly pharmacologically disinhibit behaviors suppressed by punishment in experimental animals (Morse and Kelleher 1977). In other words, expectancy and pharmacology interact to determine the effects of alcohol. Nonetheless, the summary statement by Marlatt and Rohsenow has clinical as well as theoretical implications: "If the individual firmly believes that a drink or two will trigger a bout of uncontrolled drinking, a single slip will quickly snowball into a full-blown relapse in accordance with the individual's expectations of losing control" (1980, p. 194).

In acknowledging the complexity of relapse, therefore, we must refrain from attributing psychodynamic motives to conditioned or unconscious learned behaviors. Consider the individual who has been hypnotized to open a window when the clock strikes three. At three o'clock, with great persistence, he will open the window. When asked why he opened it, he attempts to explain his motivation; although his explanation is confabulated, it may appear perfectly plausible to the listener. In other words, in his irrational behavior, the alcoholic resembles Pavlov's dog or Skinner's pigeons far more than he does Freud's Dora, or Breuer's Anna O., those two prototypes of the dynamic unconscious.

An early suggestion that the cure of alcoholism lay in recognizing that it reflected unconscious conditioned behavior was from a wise backwoods doctor, John Kain, in Shelbyville, Tennessee. In the early nineteenth century, Kain wrote, "In every intemperate man, there is an immutable association in his mind between stimulating liquors and the relief they afford to all unpleasant sensation which I have described as forming his disease. To him, the bottle is a catholicon, it relieves anorexia, gastrodynia, flatulence, nausea, vomiting, colic and those gloomy feelings which are worse than all. It produces an instant change from pain to pleasure, from despair to hope and transforms this thorny, rugged wilderness of a world into paradise . . . To cure him, we must break up this association and convince him, by actual sensations that his remedy has lost its effect" (1828, p. 293).

A century and a half later, John Mack, a wise urban psychoanalyst, wrote much of the same message to a young patient. Although Mack's language is tempered by advances in alcohol treatment, and by the self-psychology of Heinz Kohut, the message, like Kain's, runs counter to a motivational or psychodynamic model of alcoholism:

> The drinking becomes a vicious cycle; hence your feeling of self disgust. You feel you are not living up to what you want to be, which brings much pain and guilt. But only drink can anesthetize these awful feelings, which in turn bring a further violation of one's sense of self. You fear the boredom,

depression and loneliness that will come in the wake of giving up the drinking. Yet, strange as it may seem, I am persuaded that these feelings are the *result* of the drink, that is, they are brought about by drinking itself. Thus, the drink is more the cause of the isolation and the feelings of boredom . . . after all, you were not such a lonely adolescent once.

You like to think you can control the drinking, that you can make a decision when to drink and when not to and how much. Every rational man likes to think that he is in control of his decision-making. But once you are addicted to alcohol—and make no mistake about it, you have a true addiction—it is not within your powers to make this decision. The alcohol has an uncanny capacity to stimulate all sorts of rationalizations, but all of these rationalizations are in the service of not giving it up. It is as if the alcohol had a life of its own and took over the personality and brought about attitudes and reactions which will foster further drinking.

To sum up, during relapse there are at least five factors at work. There is a genetic predisposition, the biological factor that permits the ingestion of large amounts of alcoholic beverages without notable ill effects. Second, there is a psychological predisposition, which appears to have more to do with how a person is socialized in drinking than with specific personality vulnerabilities. Third, there is the physiological change that takes place in an individual's central nervous system as the individual becomes dependent on alcohol. Fourth, there is the learning that results from both operant and Pavlovian conditioning and which depends not only upon the pharmacological properties of the drug but upon the schedule and the environment in which it is consumed. Fifth, there is often the absence of "protective" factors such as a stable social network and adequate morale and self-esteem to promote self-care. The next two chapters will be devoted to illuminating how a largely untreated cohort of men found ways of preventing relapse.

II ~ *Patterns of Recovery*

4 ～ *Paths into Abstinence*

In a much cited paper written in 1962, Gerard and colleagues questioned whether abstinence was a sufficient or even a desirable goal of treatment for alcoholics. Since then, using more broadly based evidence, many other researchers have pointed out that abstinence per se may be a very limited criterion for recovery in alcoholism (Pattison 1968; Blane 1978). Indeed, Pattison and colleagues have asked that we entertain the proposition "that abstinence bears no necessary relation to rehabilitation" (1977, p. 192). In this chapter I shall compare the alcohol abusers in the Core City sample who became abstinent with those who did not. The major questions asked will be: How does one achieve abstinence? and What are the costs and the benefits?

Definition of Abstinence

Like the definition of alcoholism, the definition of abstinence is relative. Since alcoholism is a continuum, not an off-on phenomenon, and since remissions and relapses are common, the parameters of abstinence must be carefully defined—especially in a longitudinal study. Always it must be kept in mind that classification of a subject as abstinent is a labeling process carried out by the researcher. It is a judgment process in which the available evidence, often incomplete and occasionally conflicting, is used to place each subject in a defined category.

On the one hand, the chronic alcoholic resembles the man in the Mark Twain story who found stopping smoking so easy he had done it more than 20 times. Thus, after many years virtually every alcohol abuser in the sample, no matter how chronic, had been abstinent for at least a month. Indeed, one

231

of the criteria for the diagnosis of alcoholism is a history of having "gone on the wagon." The more physiologically dependent and the more symptomatic the alcoholic, the more likely that he has experienced multiple brief episodes of abstinence.

On the other hand, relatively few men with long periods of abstinence had never taken another drink. Ceremonial drinks at weddings or carefully controlled and planned one-day binges were not uncommon among men who had been essentially abstinent for many years. For example, one man had been abstinent for most of 15 years. He sustained his sobriety by taking Antabuse regularly and by passionately pursuing his hobby of fishing. About once a year, he alleged, he experienced a build-up of tension and increased irritability. At these times, instead of taking the Antabuse that his wife administered to him each morning, he would secrete it under his tongue. He would then engage in a compulsive and pleasureless two-week binge. The binge would stop because he was arrested or became too ill to drink further. Although he had become sufficiently involved in Alcoholics Anonymous to have spoken at meetings, he preferred his fishing buddies. Despite his 50 weeks a year of abstinence, he was categorized in this study as an atypical drinker; not as currently abstinent.

For the purpose of this book, abstinence will be defined in terms of three categories: ever abstinent, currently abstinent, and securely abstinent. Of the 110 men who manifested four or more symptoms of problem drinking and for whom adequate data were available, 49 were classed as *ever abstinent*. After abusing alcohol for years, these 49 men had spent at least 12 consecutive months using alcohol less often than once a month. During each year in which they were categorized as abstinent they had engaged in not more than one episode of intoxication and that of *less than* a week in duration. The majority of men fitting this definition were totally abstinent; and during most years for which men were classified as abstinent they claimed that they had from zero to two drinks. The definition *ever abstinent* will be used in examining how the entire sample of 49 achieved abstinence.

These ever abstinent men could be broken down into subgroups. Of these 49 men, 11 relapsed—5 to intermittent abuse of alcohol and 6 to progressive alcohol dependence—and thus only 38 men could be classified as *currently abstinent* (abstinent for at least 12 months prior to interview). For 17 of these currently abstinent men, abstinence had been of less than three years, incomplete, or achieved only because they were too incapacitated to seek alcohol: 1 man had been abstinent for four years in a nursing home; 3 had been abstinent for more than three years but engaged in binges more than once a year or maintained periods of controlled drinking; and 13 had been abstinent in the community for less than three years. The definition currently abstinent will be used when contrasting abstinent men with the 35 progressive alcohol abusers and with men classified as having returned to social drinking.

The third subgroup of abstinent men, the 21 classified as *securely abstinent,* were so defined by having stayed abstinent in the community for at least three years and remaining abstinent at follow-up. However, with the passage of time, the number of securely abstinent men will undoubtedly increase; some of the men abstinent for less than three years will remain abstinent and other alcohol abusers who are currently actively drinking will become abstinent. As will become apparent in Chapter 5, return to asymptomatic drinking was not an option for the securely abstinent because such men did not opt for abstinence until their alcohol abuse was very severe and until they had tried and repeatedly failed to return to successful social drinking. Only one of the securely abstinent men ever resumed asymptomatic drinking for a significant period of time.

Many follow-up studies of less than three years' duration assert that if an individual is stably abstinent for six months he can be presumed to be immune from future relapse. This assumption, based on relatively short-term follow-up, is not supported by the findings of this or other long-term investigations. In this study, at least 20 of the 110 Core City men had been abstinent for from six months to two years and then relapsed once more to alcohol abuse.

∿ "Abstinence" Revisited

As predicted, after 15 years of additional follow-up, the number of Core City men with secure (> 3 years) abstinence had grown from 21 men to 47 (Table 3.9A). In 1977, 12 of the 47 now stably abstinent men had been classified as only currently abstinent, 4 as returned to asymptomatic drinking, 3 as having progressive alcoholism and 2 as atypical. The remaining 8 men who were categorized in 1992 as having stable abstinence had been unclassified in 1977: 3 had begun to abuse alcohol after the age 47 cutoff for the original publication of this book, and 5 had been classified as alcohol abusers using the DSM III criteria but not the PDS criteria. The length of abstinence for the 47 securely abstinent men varied from 3 to 37 years. Thirty of the men had been abstinent for 10 years or more, with a mean length of abstinence of 19 years. By 1992, 14 of the 47 men with stable abstinence had died, many of them from causes associated with cigarette abuse.

In 1992 the 47 Core City men with stable abstinence included 18 of the original 21 men identified in 1977 as securely abstinent. Of the remaining 3 men rated securely abstinent in 1977, 1 had withdrawn from the study, 1 had relapsed to alcohol abuse, and 1 had returned to controlled drinking.

Heredity, ethnicity, quality of childhood, and sociopathy did not distinguish the securely abstinent men from the other alcoholics. Indeed, the only characteristic that distinguished the abstinent men was that 28 (60 percent) of the 47 Core City alcohol abusers with stable abstinence—and 10 out of 10 (100 percent) of College alcohol abusers with stable abstinence—had been alcohol-dependent. In contrast, only 49 (48 percent) of the 103 Core City and only 9 (21 percent) of the College men without stable abstinence were alcohol-dependent.

Fifteen years of additional follow-up allowed the study to address the stability of abstinence. By this I mean how long abstinence must persist before an individual's recovery can be considered truly secure. In cancer, remission must often last for five years before relapse is considered unlikely. In alcoholism treatment studies, however, investigators often speak of recovery after the abuser has been symptom-free for six months or one year. Two years of abstinence from alcohol abuse is considered an adequate criterion for candidacy for a liver transplant. In the earlier version of this book, without empirical evidence, I suggested that three years was adequate to define secure abstinence—but is that long enough?

Table 4.1A illustrates the association between length of abstinence and stability of remission. All of the 10 College men and 46 of the Core City men who reported at least two years of abstinence *and* who subsequently survived for at least eight years were included. Eventual relapse to alcohol abuse occurred for 41 percent of these 56 men. With each passing year, however, the likelihood of long-term abstinence became greater. After six years of abstinence, subsequent relapse to abuse of alcohol seemed quite unlikely. Thus, the mean length of recorded abstinence among the 37 men *not* reporting relapse after 6 years was 18 years (range 9–33 years).

Admittedly, without corroboration from relatives, the assertion of abstinence on a single questionnaire can be unreliable. However, the assertion of abstinence over 10 to 30 years on multiple returned questionnaires and supported by quinquennial physical exams and stable social adjustments makes such self-report more credible. For example, the one abstinent man

TABLE 4.1A.   Association between length of abstinence and the likelihood of subsequent relapse in 56 Core City and College men abstinent for two years.

	Number still abstinent	Number relapsing that year	% eventually relapsing
After 2 years	56	9	41%
After 3 years	47	5	25%
After 4 years	42	0	25%
After 5 years	42	5	16%
After 6 years	37	1	7%[a]

a. These 3 men eventually relapsed after abstinences of 8, 10, and 13 years.

who relapsed returned no questionnaires; knowledge of his relapse came from his relatives, from physical exam data, and from personal interview.

Since systematic follow-ups of abstinent alcohol abusers are seldom undertaken, I know of data from only two other follow-up studies that address the question asked by Table 4.1A: Is two years of abstinence from alcohol too short a time to provide a basis for long-term prognosis? Reanalysis of data from the previously reported eight-year follow-up of the Clinic sample (Vaillant et al. 1983) revealed that when followed from 4 to 14 years (mean 8 years), 45 percent of 33 alcohol-dependent men and women relapsed after two years of abstinence. After five years of abstinence, however, only 9 percent relapsed; and none relapsed after six years. In another two-year follow-up of 29 alcohol abusers already abstinent for two years, 6 men (21 percent) relapsed within the two years of follow-up (Loosen et al. 1990). As shown in Table 4.1A, a comparable number, 14 (25 percent) of the 56 men abstinent for two years relapsed during the next two years.

Etiology of Abstinence

A question of great interest is the relation of clinic treatment to abstinence. In recovery from alcoholism, how important is access to treatment? As can be seen in Table 4.1, the men who achieved successful abstinence did not differ from severe alcoholics in general. The treatment encounters experienced by the currently abstinent men were no more frequent, nor was the severity of their alcoholism any less.

TABLE 4.1. Severity of alcoholism among currently abstinent men and men diagnosed as alcohol-dependent.

Characteristic	Currently abstinent (n = 38)	Alcohol-dependent (DSM III) diagnosis (n = 69)
Diagnosis of alcoholism by clinician	51%	56%
At least one visit for alcoholism	54	59
Multiple clinic visits for alcoholism	38	37
Gone on the wagon	100	79
Acknowledges inability to control drinking	89	90
5+ symptoms of sociopathy (Robins scale)	32	30

Table 4.1 makes another interesting point. In short-term follow-up studies of clinic patients, sociopathy is a negative prognostic finding (Gibbs and Flanagan 1977), but, as Table 4.1 points out, by the time the Core City men reached the age of 47, symptoms of sociopathy did not appear to be a negative prognostic factor. If sociopaths make up only a fifth of the alcohol abusers but a third of the alcohol-dependent group, they also made up a third of the currently abstinent.

Twenty years ago, Gerard and Saenger succinctly described the paradox of recovery from alcoholism: "What seemed to have made a difference was a change in the alcoholic's attitude toward the use of alcohol based on the person's own experiences which in the vast majority of cases took place outside of any clinical interactions" (1962, p. 94). Of the 55 abstinent men that Gerard and Saenger studied, only 16 actually began their abstinence during clinic treatment. And as Table 4.2 illustrates, 70 percent of the year-long abstinence experiences among the Core City men were independent of clinical intervention. If the majority of recoveries from alcoholism occur outside the ken of the alcohol professional, this may help to explain why members of Alcoholics Anonymous take a different view of alcoholism from many professionals: they may have encountered a different group of remitting problem drinkers.

Table 4.2 reports the kinds of treatment that the ever abstinent men reported during their first year of abstinence. Although about half of all the alcohol-dependent men in the study were seen at least once in an alcohol clinic, clinic visits played a significant role for only a third of the abstinent. Disulfiram and halfway houses were rarely used by the Core City men and did not play a major role in abstinence. The point to be made is not that the

TABLE 4.2. Treatment experiences associated with abstinence.

Treatment experience	*Ever abstinent* *(n = 49)*		*Securely abstinent* *(n = 21)*
	Important to abstinence	*Tried but failed*	*Important to abstinence*
Psychotherapy	8%	8%	5%
Disulfiram (Antabuse)	4	8	5
Halfway house	6	8	0
Alcohol clinic or hospital	30	22	20
Alcoholics Anonymous	37	8	38
Willpower	49	?100	43

interventions were ineffective, but only that most remissions from alcoholism took place without them.

Table 4.2 also reports unsuccessful treatment experiences, but what the table obscures is the number of repeat clinic visits made by the treatment failures. Each Core City man was counted only once. However, alcohol clinics usually serve a disproportionate number of patients with poor prognosis because the small minority of chronic alcoholics who have multiple admissions are overrepresented during any given period.

The treatment experience of the College alcohol abusers was different in one significant respect. Only 31 percent of the 26 College problem drinkers were ever hospitalized or treated specifically for alcoholism; but 62 percent of the College alcohol abusers compared to 8 percent of the Core City counterparts received psychotherapy. (For the Core City men in Table 4.2, psychotherapy referred to any form of counseling with a professionally trained person that continued for several visits; for the College sample, psychotherapy was defined as ten or more visits to a psychiatrist.) Among the 26 alcohol abusers in the College sample at least 10 men received over 100 hours of individual psychotherapy, and collectively the 26 men received approximately 5000 hours. However, for only 2 College men was such therapy significantly associated with abstinence or a return to asymptomatic drinking. One of these 2 men relapsed and is now a member of AA.

To put the findings in Table 4.2 in perspective, the study that Gerard and Saenger conducted is useful. They, too, found that dynamic psychotherapy did not seem to be a useful treatment method for alcoholism. They contrasted the efficacy of several different alcohol clinics, and concluded: "The less the clinic became involved in the intricacies of the determinants of the patient's symptoms, relationships, or defenses, the more likely was the clinic to succeed in supporting change in drinking behavior" (1966, p. 192).

Gerard and Saenger observed that socially unstable alcoholics needed to be treated among peers rather than to become social outcasts in a middle-class treatment program. They also suggested that the socially least deviant patients are the most likely to respond to the medical model and therefore most likely to respond to "treatment" from an alcohol clinic. In contrast, the socially alienated patient will respond poorly to short hospital or outpatient treatment and will require a sustained effort to resocialize him into a new subculture. Chapter 3 and the compelling investigations of Edwards and colleagues (1974), Finney and colleagues (1980), and Costello (1980) make the same point. Most of the outcome variance in alcohol treatment can be explained by variation in premorbid social stability. Therefore, we should not be surprised that the treatment variables in Table 4.2 did not explain outcome in often socially unstable Core City men.

Although half of the abstinent Core City men believed that will power— their own simple decision to stop drinking—played a major role, this belief may often have been illusory. However, a dramatic example of willpower *was* provided by a man who after having been hospitalized for cirrhosis of the liver achieved seven years of sobriety. After receiving 11 units of blood for hemorrhage due to esophageal varices secondary to his cirrhosis, he left the hospital and never had another drink. He said whenever he now has the urge to drink, "I think clearly and the facts are overwhelming. One drink will lead to another; I will become ill and die." If he had one drink, he said, "It would be like committing suicide." In summarizing his case the interviewer wrote: "As he began to talk about his life and the way he had changed after he stopped drinking, I was convinced he was a member of AA. He has developed self-confidence and a positive approach to life; he resorts to prayer and knows that he can never ever have another drop to drink. He seems to have gained some insight into himself, can talk about his early life without bitterness and can accept some responsibility for the course of his life." But as far as the interviewer could tell, his change was brought about by a single "aha!" experience.*

But this man who never attended an AA meeting, an alcohol clinic, or a detoxification center is the exception, not the rule. In most cases it seemed

---

*Shortly after his interview this man returned to using and probably abusing alcohol. From age 49 to 57 he drank secretly off and on in a fashion that distressed his wife and children but neither himself nor his physicians. He is the one man classified as securely abstinent in 1977 and as a chronic alcohol abuser in 1992.

likely that the explanation "willpower," like the explanation "hitting bottom," reflects a failure of the interviewer and the subject to identify important factors associated with abstinence.

Certainly, deciding what factors are relevant to recovery from any intractable habit is at best an imprecise process. One approach is to ask ex-alcoholics what they thought made a difference. Using this approach, Orford and Edwards (1977) reported that improved working and housing conditions made a difference in 40 percent of good outcomes, intrapsychic change in 32 percent, improved marriage in 32 percent, and a single 3-hour session of advice and education about drinking at the start of treatment in 35 percent. A difficulty is that cause and effect may be confused. Abstinence may be the reason for employment and for marital reconciliation as often as it is the result of them.

An alternative approach is to disregard what the patient says and to study temporarily related contingencies. The argument for this approach is that since addiction is largely maintained by conditioning and linked reinforcers of which the patient is not conscious, just so recovery will depend on factors of which the alcoholic may or may not be aware. A key to recovery will be the alcoholic's recognition that his use of alcohol is no longer under his voluntary control. This self-discovery appears to be a highly personal process but one affected by external circumstances.

How any individual becomes "converted" or abruptly "decides" to alter his life course is a riddle that has puzzled many observers of human nature. The sudden transformation of the drunkard to a teetotaler is analogous to the sudden change of heart, the abrupt religious conversion, and the scientist's experience of Eureka. Such transformations often have long subterranean pasts. When a young bird suddenly hatches from an egg, we are not dealing with spontaneous generation. Rather, in the words of William James, we are dealing with "the process, gradual or sudden, by which a self hitherto divided and consciously wrong, inferior and unhappy becomes happy" (1902, p. 189). This hatching, as it were, reflects "subconsciously maturing processes eventuating in results of which we suddenly grow conscious" (p. 204). James suggests that the process evolves because of "the subconscious incubation and maturing of motives deposited by the experiences of life. When ripe, the results hatch out" (p. 230). It is no accident that James illustrates this whole process with the case of a "homeless, friendless, dying drunkard . . . Mr. S. H. Hadley, who after his conversion became an active and useful rescuer of drunkards in New York" (p. 201).

In the past, when I interviewed heroin addicts who had achieved stable abstinence, only 2 ex-addicts consciously linked the experience of parole with abstinence; but of 30 addicts who were on parole for more than a year, 20 became abstinent (Vaillant 1966). Initially, ex-addicts with stable abstinence had assured me, "I just got tired of the life," but as the circumstances of their abstinence were explored, it became apparent that during their first year of abstinence many of them not only had been on parole but also had formed a fresh, unambivalent relationship, had become members of fundamentalist religious groups, or had found substitute dependencies with which to replace heroin. Thus, in studying alcoholics I instructed the field interviewers to look for certain temporally related contingencies that I suspected would be important in altering drinking habits, and when questioning the ever abstinent alcohol abusers, interviewers systematically probed for likely events upon which abstinence might be contingent (see interview schedule in Appendix).

The men's answers to these questions are depicted in Table 4.3. Admittedly, these findings still depend upon self-report, and the reader must take all first-person accounts of the paths out of abstinence with a grain of salt. Table 4.3 suggests that perhaps half of the ever abstinent men found an alternative for alcohol. Some found more than one. These substitute dependencies varied from candy binges (5 men) to benzodiazepines (Valium or Librium) (5 men), from compulsively helping others (2 men) to returning to dependence upon parents (2 men), from marijuana (2 men) to mystical belief, prayer, and meditation (5 men), from compulsive work or hobbies (9 men) to compulsive gambling (2 men), from compulsive eating (3 men) to chain smoking (7 men). In addition, the increased involvement by some of the men with religion or with Alcoholics Anonymous could be construed as a substitute dependency.

For the purpose of simplification, Table 4.3 has combined medical consequences and compulsory supervision under the heading of *behavior modification.* By that term I mean the presence of events contingent upon alcohol use that systematically altered the consequences of alcohol abuse. Admittedly, the events leading to habit change are more complex than implied by such reductionistic labels, but the point to be made is that in any intractable habit, willpower is inferior to behavior modification. If an individual is to change a habit, the individual must be continuously reminded that change is important. Once one "forgets" that alcohol use is a curse not a blessing, willpower is no longer operative—and alcoholics are expert forgetters. In contrast, behavior modification—whether through disulfiram, legal pressure, or vomiting after a second drink—allows the dangers of alcohol use to intrude

TABLE 4.3.   Nontreatment factors associated with abstinence.

Nontreatment factor	Ever abstinent (n = 49)	Securely abstinent (n = 21)
Substitute dependency	53%	67%
Behavior modification		
Compulsory supervision or sustained confrontation	24	0
Medical consequences	49	48
Enhanced hope/self-esteem		
Increased religious involvement	12	19
Alcoholics Anonymous[a]	37	38
Social rehabilitation		
New love relationship	32	38

a. Alcoholics Anonymous, if frequently attended, may also be viewed as a substitute dependency *and* a variety of behavior modification *and* a source of social rehabilitation.

themselves upon the patient's consciousness as if from an external superego. "Hitting bottom," then, is not arriving on skid row. Rather, hitting bottom signals that the message "I have truly lost control of my use of alcohol" has penetrated the alcoholic's system of denial.

Confrontation and compulsory supervision without potential consequences are usually not effective. It has been reported elsewhere (Costello 1975; Baekeland et al. 1975) that the most important single prognostic variable associated with remission among alcoholics who attend alcohol clinics is having something to lose if they continue to abuse alcohol. Not only do alcoholics with stable jobs and stable marriages have the most to lose; they also enjoy the best social supports, and thus are most closely supervised. Probation, real or metaphorical, is effective only to the degree that one's probation officer, employer, or spouse really cares. Thus, at the start of their abstinence 24 percent of the ever abstinent men were under some kind of compulsory supervision from employers or courts, or under believable threat of divorce by their wives.

Just prior to the start of the abstinence, 49 percent of the ever abstinent men developed some kind of medical problem that interfered with their drinking, or began regularly to take disulfiram. The behavior-modifying symptom must prevent the alcoholic from forgetting that he is the victim, not the master, of his wish to drink. Thus, medical complaints associated with abstinence tended to be those with immediate consequences, including re-current seizures, stomach problems, alcohol-induced insomnia, and chroni-cally painful fractures that resulted from drinking. In contrast, it was difficult for the men to make an emotional connection between painless liver disease and the ingestion of alcohol.

In one of the most careful, long-term studies of abstinent alcoholics, Gerard and Saenger (1966) found that patients cited changed life circum-stances rather than clinic intervention as most important to their abstinence. The most important of these changed circumstances were increased ill health, substitutes for dependency-need satisfactions, and increasing community or family sanctions. These variables translate into the first two nontreatment factors in Table 4.3. Indeed, the ideal program that Gerard and Saenger describe for socially alienated patients encompasses the four factors described in Table 4.3—the factors that appeared most associated with remission in the Core City men.

Undoubtedly, behavioral psychology has much to teach clinicians about the parameters of successful confrontation. Certainly, in well-run laboratories, behavior modification has been shown repeatedly to be an effective tool in the rehabilitation of alcoholics (Sobell and Sobell 1976; Lovibond and Caddy 1970). The most serious drawback to such methods is that for the present, such techniques are more academic tour de force than panacea. In the real world, severe alcoholics are as unlikely to encounter a behavior-modification laboratory as is a patient with severe coronary heart disease to receive a heart transplant.

Another limitation of more readily available forms of behavior modifica-tion can be seen by comparing the ever abstinent with the securely abstinent in Table 4.3. The securely abstinent were less likely to depend upon external controls. Let me try to explain why. Disulfiram (Antabuse) is, of course, the most widespread example of the use of behavior modification in treatment for alcoholism. But although disulfiram interferes with the metabolism of alcohol and makes individuals desperately sick after even a single drink, the drug takes alcohol away and replaces it with nothing; thus disulfiram is more effective over the short term than the long term. The importance of substitute dependencies in breaking habits may explain why disulfiram has not lived up to its early promise. It is difficult to make someone abandon a habit without offering him something else in return. This observation confirmed a similar observation among heroin addicts, for whom parole was more effective over the short term than it was over the longer term (Vaillant 1966).

In an early controlled study, Wallerstein (1956) suggested that disulfiram was a useful adjunct to treatment in two groups of patients: those who request it and those who are high on traits of compulsiveness and reaction formation. However, despite the claims of Wallerstein's and many equally hopeful but less well executed studies, literature reviews (Mottin 1973; Viamontes 1972) have suggested that the efficacy of disulfiram depends not so much upon its aversive pharmacological properties as upon the enthusiasm and hope with which it is prescribed and upon the other supports provided by the clinic prescribing the drug. In a similar vein, Ditman and his colleagues (1967) and Gallant and colleagues (1968) reviewed the evidence for court pressure as an effective component in the treatment of alcoholism and found that legal sanctions resembled disulfiram in that unless combined with other treatment they were not effective.

In the treatment of addiction, Karl Marx's aphorism "religion is the opiate of the masses" masks an enormously important therapeutic principle. Religion may actually provide a relief that drug abuse only promises. Thus, as Table 4.3 suggests, a third major source of help in changing involuntary habits comes from increased religious involvement. Only recently have investigators begun to tease out the nature of this principle (Robinson 1979; Mack 1981; Bean 1975; Meyer and Mirin 1979). Let me explain what I suspect is involved. First, alcoholics and victims of other seemingly incurable habits feel defeated, bad, and helpless. They invariably suffer from impaired morale. If they are to recover, powerful new sources of self-esteem and hope must be discovered. Religion is one such source. Religion provides fresh impetus for both hope and enhanced self-care. Second, if the established alcoholic is to become stably abstinent, enormous personality changes must take place. It is not just coincidence that we associate such dramatic change with the experience of religious conversion.

Third, religion, in ways that we appreciate but do not understand, provides forgiveness of sins and relief from guilt. Unlike many intractable habits that others find merely annoying, alcoholism inflicts enormous pain and injury on those around the alcoholic. As a result the alcoholic, already demoralized by his inability to stop drinking, experiences almost insurmountable guilt from the torture he has inflicted on others. In such an instance, absolution becomes an important part of the healing process.

Equally important is the fact that reaction formation—an abrupt reversal of what is cherished and loved into what is rejected and hated—is essential for abstinence; and reaction formations are often stabilized through religious involvement. By surrendering his commitment to one set of desires to the control of a "higher power," the addict becomes suddenly capable of commitment to quite an opposite set of desires. Thus, 6 of the ever abstinent and 4 of the securely abstinent men noted increased religious involvement during the first year of their abstinence. Eight of the 38 currently abstinent men but only 3 of the 54 men who are currently abusing alcohol reported over the past decade that their religious involvement had increased. (This observation, of course, does not separate cart from horse; remission from alcoholism may be as important to increased religious participation as increased religious participation is to abstinence.)

Less ambiguous was the fact that almost two-fifths of both the ever abstinent and the securely abstinent became involved in Alcoholics Anonymous, an organization that effectively mobilizes the poorly understood ingredients present in increased religious involvement. AA not only counters alcoholism by focused social support but also "converts" individuals from one belief system to another. It is a paradox that a major goal of AA—a strictly moral and religious system—has been to view alcohol abuse as a medical illness, not a moral failing. The Core City experience was not unique. Throughout the English-speaking world, Alcoholics Anonymous is now acknowledged to be one of the most effective therapies for alcoholism (Kish and Herman 1971; Vallance 1965; Robson et al. 1965; Beaubrun 1967; Leach and Norris 1977).

The fourth and final factor that Table 4.3 associates with abstinence is the acquisition of new love relationships. One reason that marital therapy is not more effective in the treatment of alcoholism (Orford and Edwards 1977) is that the wounds that an alcoholic inflicts on those he loves and the festering sore of guilt which he incurs for himself heal so slowly. Thus, just as a stable marriage is important for motivating abstinence and treatment, just so a new love relationship—unscarred by the mixture of guilt and multiple psychic wounds that alcoholics inflict upon those whom they love—becomes valuable in maintaining abstinence. For many, this relationship was a new wife or a special relationship with a nonprofessional, helping person or mentor; for others it was learning to help others who were as troubled as themselves. For still others, this new relationship was paradoxically acquired through the death of a loved person. The explanation that I would tentatively venture for this last phenomenon is that sudden death sometimes allows the deceased to become internalized and, thus, to provide a source of fresh strength or comfort. An everyday example would be the sudden inspirational meaning that John Kennedy, after his death, acquired for people who had not been consciously affected by him when he was alive.

All of the factors in Table 4.3 are interrelated, and all are embodied in many self-help recovery programs organized along similar lines to Alcoholics Anonymous. Of the 21 securely abstinent men all but four either used Alcoholics Anonymous or used at least *two* of the four factors outlined in Table 4.3. Among those four men who had achieved secure abstinence by what appeared, at least in retrospect, to be largely willpower, all were somewhat atypical alcoholics. Three did not meet the criteria for DSM III alcohol dependence and three did not meet Cahalan's criteria for problem drinking.

In achieving abstinence, it was definitely possible to employ all the factors in Table 4.3 without reliance upon Alcoholics Anonymous. For example, the most severe sociopath in the study, a man who scored 15 on the Robins scale, has been sober for two years on Antabuse. He himself attributes change in his drinking to "hitting bottom." However, he had been a binge drinker for ten years, and why he should suddenly have realized that he was powerless over his drinking when he did requires close scrutiny. He had often been exposed to AA and insisted that he had no faith in the organization and that attending AA "would drive me out the door to get a drink." Prior to his abstinence, he had received, without success, an enormous amount of clinic treatment for alcoholism. He maintained that he could have tolerated therapy sessions, "if they didn't bullshit," but he alleged that he had never attended any therapy session where that did not happen. Although in the past he had always refused disulfiram, two years ago when he finally began to take it, he turned the responsibility for his taking the drug each morning over to his wife. Not only did he consent to take disulfiram, he also returned to the church of his childhood; and he has been a faithful attender ever since.

This erstwhile sociopath endeavored to help others by becoming a scout master, and guilt-free interpersonal satisfaction was inevitable. Finally, he found an ingenious substitute dependency. Whenever he feels a craving for a drink, he ritually takes an extra Antabuse tablet. His abstinence was not just willpower; he had devised an external threefold "higher power"—wife, disulfiram, and church—to assist his own conscience.

Again, O'Briant and Lennard (1973) have described a program at Bret Harte Hospital in California that is in no way connected with AA and that treats alcoholism as if it were a problem in social networks, existing "somewhere in the complex relationships of persons and their social contexts." Nevertheless, the Bret Harte program embodies all the principles mentioned in Table 4.3. The program suggests that the medical and psychiatric models clearly do not work in definitive treatment of alcoholism and that neither detoxification per se nor psychotherapy has proven effective. Instead, alcoholics are brought together, isolated from other contexts, and engaged in a "cooperative group enterprise in which all must participate . . . interdependence is stressed continually" (p. 60). Re-entry into the community occurs with the individual accompanied by another patient. The "construction of social contexts where the message, don't drink, prevails" is really closely analogous to behavioral modification. In their program, the average successful graduate goes to 15 meetings a month. "Treatment, then, can be an ongoing process aimed at creating a new social landscape" (p. 60).

Thus, one of the most striking conclusions that results from reviewing interviews with remitted Core City alcoholics is that recovery from alcoholism is anything but "spontaneous." Rather, the profound behavioral switch from alcohol dependence to abstinence is mediated not by hitting some mysterious "bottom" but rather by forces that can be identified and understood by social scientists and harnessed by health professionals.

One thing is clear, however: abstinence is achieved through the help of others. As Table 4.4 suggests, the efficacy of willpower as a means of producing abstinence is a little like advice to control one's drinking—willpower is useful only for those who are "a little bit" alcoholic. Among the 49 abstinent men, seeking help from Alcoholics Anonymous or a clinic was correlated with the number of alcohol-related symptoms on the PDS with an r of .50 and .60 respectively. In contrast, the allegation that abstinence was a product of willpower was negatively correlated with the PDS score with an r of $-.37$ ($p. < .01$).

In the future, we need much more research into the prospective study of the attainment of stable abstinence. In the present study, critical events that occur during the first year of abstinence have been identified in retrospect. What were the events that occurred in the year preceding abstinence? Will prospective fine-grained study validate the findings in Table 4.3? Do these same variables hold for women, for other cultures, for abstinence from smoking? We need answers to these questions.

～ Stable Abstinence Revisited

Unfortunately, follow-up of the men in this study over the past 15 years has not been sufficiently fine-grained to answer these questions. Rather, the confirmation of Table 4.3 has come from recent research literature that bears directly on relapse prevention, for relapse prevention is essential to successful treatment. In the past 15 years, experimental psychologists sophisticated in

TABLE 4.4. Percentage of men with different PDS scores citing selected factors in abstinence.

	PDS score		
Factor	4–7 (n = 15)	8–11 (n = 22)	12–16 (n = 12)
Willpower	73%	45%	25%
Substitute dependency	53	45	62
New love relationship	20	18	42
Clinic treatment	0	23	83
Alcoholics Anonymous	13	41	92

skills training have contributed a fresh and important body of knowledge to the alcohol treatment field. If research over the last 30 years has convinced the treatment field that unconscious aversion techniques do not work, the more conscious cognitive-behavioral techniques have offered great promise. Two of the more important contributors to this body of knowledge are William Miller, at the University of New Mexico, and Alan Marlatt, at the University of Washington. However, the effective ingredients of AA and the principles espoused by Miller and Marlatt have much in common: stay away from that first drink, don't become too tired, avoid loneliness, remember how it was, replace old drinking buddies with new sober buddies, seek knowledgeable help, rejoice in the new manageability of your life, practice the quote "I am responsible," think positive, develop self-restraint, remember your last drunk, think the drink through before you take it.

The first task of relapse prevention is the cognitive task of changing alcohol from a friend to a foe. This means developing the patient's ambivalence toward alcohol, building his or her curiosity about alternatives to alcohol, developing an understanding of triggers for relapse, and using cognitive techniques to help the patient remember that alcoholism is enemy and not friend.

The second task is to develop a plan to stop drinking that is shared with other people, helping the individual tell others that he or she plans to stop and how. The third task is to help the individual develop cognitive ways of recognizing when relapse is imminent—or, in the language of AA, to recognize when one is "building up to the next drink." The fourth task is to encourage the individual to seek social supports, including social reinforcers for sobriety. The fifth task is to do what all behaviorists understand, and what teachers and parents often forget: to provide substitutes for bad habits. For neither forgiveness nor punishment will change deeply ingrained habits.

Marlatt and Gordon (1985) have systematically thought through a program of relapse prevention which focuses on the "maintenance phase of habit change." From this perspective, relapse is not viewed as an indicator of treatment failure. Rather, potential and actual episodes of relapse become targets for future intervention strategies. Marlatt has developed specific intervention techniques designed to allow the individual to anticipate, and then cope with, potential relapse situations. Basically, these techniques combine behavioral skills–training procedures with cognitive intervention techniques. Marlatt has identified three general categories associated with high relapse rates: negative emotional states; interpersonal conflict; and social pressure. Obviously, such high-risk situations are often simply the last link in a chain of events leading to relapse. Often, such final events are merely the final step in a covert planning process. Such a view closely parallels the attitude of AA toward a relapsing member. Relapse to alcoholic drinking can be construed as "research" and reflects a need to use more "tools" of AA next time.

Relapse prevention can also be conceptualized by using the analogy of diabetes. The task of relapse prevention is to change overall risk and not to confuse *lapse* with *relapse*. In the early stages of treatment of diabetes, a single urine positive for sugar, like a single brief drinking episode in a recovering alcohol abuser, can, if properly responded to, lead to improvement, not relapse. Meaningful behavioral change is usually the result of a process of sustained trial and error or of what behaviorists call successive approximations. Thus, for both diabetes and alcohol abuse effective treatment means sustained contact with "coaches" or in AA parlance with "winners." A relapse to a brief drinking episode should be reported to one's treatment resource and followed up by increased precautions, and the circumstances underlying the relapse should be examined and learned from. Conversely, *unreported* or untreated relapses in either alcohol abuse or diabetes lead to the breakdown of compliance that is the death knell of effective treatment.

More important, the principles of relapse prevention that have worked in experimental treatment programs (Brownell et al. 1986) are very similar to the principles I have reviewed in linking self-help programs to successful abstinence in a naturalistic setting. First, it must be recognized that the alcohol abuser uses alcohol to produce a *change in state* that, especially in stressful situations, seems desirable. In order to prevent lapses, alternative ways of changing state must be developed and made conscious. The successful programs reviewed by Brownell and colleagues have offered physical exercise and skills training as substitutes for alcohol. Self-help groups offer coffee, cigarettes, and the fellowship of AA as substitutes for alcohol.

Second, the experimental programs also offer what Brownell and his colleagues call "self talk"—a way of making conscious the risk that one would incur by picking up a drink. This is analogous to the way self-help groups make "budding" (building up to the next drink) conscious and in naturalistic settings to the way the recovering alcoholic acquires an external conscience.

Third, the experimental programs point out that self-efficacy counteracts helplessness. Demoralization, helplessness, and the ensuing risk of relapse to drinking are reduced if you have a plan. Thus, experimental programs help emphasize the need for skills training. This often consists of helping people make conscious the decisionmaking process that leads to picking up a drink and ways of saying no in social situations. In addition, simple principles of cognitive therapy to counteract faulty attributions become helpful: for example, making the alcohol abuser conscious that even small amounts of alcohol interfere with sleep and increase depression. Such coping skills also involve rehearsing alternatives to picking up a drink in order to produce a desired change of state. In self-help groups the counterpart to such alternatives would be using "belief in a higher power" to elevate morale. Self-help groups also teach that when one is tempted to pick up a drink, "picking up the phone" is a way of producing a desired change of state.

Fourth, similar to self-help groups, experimental programs realize the importance of enlisting social support to produce lasting behavioral change. They emphasize the importance of telling other people that you plan to change your behavior. They recognize that the danger of interpersonal conflict is that it withdraws social support. In short, William Miller, Alan Marlatt, and Alcoholics Anonymous all have an enormous amount in common.

Indeed, the principles that make AA effective are being continually discovered. Rational Recovery, a mirror image of AA, believes it achieves the same self-efficacy by emphasizing "choice" and reaffirming the individuals' faith in their own "rational" self-efficacy rather than in a higher power. Rational Recovery was deliberately developed as an alternative to AA, and it explicitly includes cognitive approaches. The approach is based on the principles of rational-emotive therapy (Trimpey 1989). Its membership is largely made up of individuals who have left AA because of objections to its spiritual aspects.

An extensive review of the literature on preventing relapse by facilitating discovery of competing sources of gratification has been provided by Stall and Biernacki (1986). In their thorough examination of the evidence, the authors contrast the sources of improvement in obesity, smoking, and alcohol and opiate dependence. Their conclusions are very similar to my own from my narrower examination of the parallels between sustained abstinence from heroin and from alcohol (Vaillant 1988).

Stall and Biernacki use different semantic labels for the clinical factors in relapse prevention from the ones I use in Tables 4.2 and 4.3, but their meanings are the same. Stall and Biernacki, wisely I believe, pay little attention to willpower as an explanatory variable. However, they pay close attention to substitute dependencies for those who wish to stop smoking, and they list eating, exercise, and nicotine gum as effective substitutes. They also note the importance to abstinence of telling one's story to others and of supportive new marriages and close friends; these are congruent with "new love relationships" in Table 4.3. Finally, what Table 4.3 calls behavior modification through compulsory supervision or medical consequences (that is, an external conscience) they refer to as the association of sustained remission with worsening health problems, negative social sanctions, and increasing expense.

In describing Alcoholics Anonymous Stall and Biernacki refer to "religiosity and prayer" rather than labeling AA a source of enhanced hope and self-esteem. And, in endeavoring to distinguish between treatment-related remission and spontaneous remission, they call AA a "lay treatment." I suspect that such distinctions may not be useful. Whether a diabetic receives insulin from a clinic or self-administers the hormone is really not important in understanding relapse prevention. What is important is that the diabetic is receiving insulin. Similarly, the ingredients of relapse prevention are the same regardless of who administers them.

Stall and Biernacki discuss three other important sources of relapse prevention not included in Tables 4.2 and 4.3. First, they note that abstinent alcoholics attempt to create new identities for themselves. They point out that part of this new identity is achieved by the public announcement of the intention to stop drinking. In addition, the new identity is achieved by the mysterious "conversion" process already discussed in reference to William James's discussion of religious conversion. Thus, Stall and Biernacki remind us of Knupfer's (1972) reference to the "strangely trivial" but significant "accidents" and Tuchfeld's (1981) "extraordinary events" that can trigger stable abstinence.

Second, Stall and Biernacki note the utility of conscious, cognitive strategies for relapse prevention. Such strategies include paying attention to positive feedback for successful abstinence, recalling alcohol-related negative experiences, and avoiding relapse-provoking situations. These techniques have proven helpful, particularly in the hands of experimental psychologists like Miller (Miller and Hester, 1986) and Marlatt (Marlatt and Gordon, 1985). In contrast to "willpower," these strategies, like external supervision, convert alcohol from friend to foe and make abstinence a reinforcement rather than a deprivation.

In addition, cognitive-behavioral techniques for relapse prevention such as those advocated by Miller and Marlatt depend on the fact that the effect of alcohol upon an individual's behavior depends only modestly upon its pharmacological properties (Marlatt and Rohsenow, 1980). Cognition, attribution, and expectancy play important roles. Thus, just as detoxification in itself is not a predictor of sustained remission, just so severity of prior addiction does not in itself predict repeated relapse. This observation has also been confirmed in a large study of heroin addicts (Robins 1974).

The difficulty with such cognitive strategies is that they may be evanescent once an individual leaves treatment. This is because without external reminders alcoholics have trouble keeping in mind the positive feedback from successful abstinence and the memory of alcohol-related negative experiences. Thus, external events that restructure a patient's life in the community—for example, parole, methadone maintenance, and AA—are more often associated with sustained abstinence than are briefer "treatment" experiences (Vaillant 1988). For example, disulfiram (Antabuse) works only so long as the alcoholic remembers to take it. In this regard, the analogy of treatment for alcoholism with treatment for diabetes is again helpful. Conscious awareness of possible diabetic relapse is maintained by the daily ritual of urine testing. Such a ritual can serve as an external reinforcer to control diet.

Third, Stall and Biernacki draw attention to the importance of extinguishing secondary reinforcers. One reason abstinence from opiates under parole supervision and abstinence from alcohol under AA supervision are more enduring than abstinence achieved during hospitalization or imprisonment is that the former experiences occur in the community. Thus, abstinence is achieved in the presence of many conditioned reinforcers (community bars, other addicts, community hassles, and so on). For example, AA encourages the alcohol abuser to maintain a busy schedule of social activities and the serving of beverages (coffee) in the presence of former drinkers. Many of the secondary reinforcers are present. Only alcohol is missing. Such "secondary reinforcers" lose their potency in controlling an addict's behavior most rapidly when such events occur in the absence of reinforcement. Similarly, one of the reasons AA encourages its members to continue to attend meetings is to provide continuity of behavioral modification.

In one of the classic texts on "spontaneous remission" Tuchfeld (1981) interviewed 51 individuals who had "resolved their alcohol problems" for a year or more. Their mean length of abstinence was 6.4 years. Tuchfeld agreed that few, if any, remissions in his study could be characterized as "spontaneous," in the sense of remission occurring in the absence of external influence. His interviews of abstinent alcoholics dramatically underscored the importance of a critical event often associated with a religious or an interpersonal experience. He uses the terms "heightened reflective experience" and "extraordinary events" to describe abstinence-precipitating phenomena. These events included personal humiliation, attempted suicide, personal identity crisis, and the illness of a significant person. Such phenomena, similar to those described by James in *Varieties of Religious Experience* (1902), also reflect the hard-to-quantify experience that alcoholics call "hitting bottom." The actual circumstances of hitting bottom are mysterious, ill-defined, and unique to the individual, but they reflect the sudden realization that alcohol is no longer a friend but has become a foe.

As Table 4.4A illustrates, one of the most remarkable findings from continued follow-up of the Core City men was that no clear antecedent differences were observed between men who achieved stable abstinence and those who remained chronically alcoholic. Thus, the attribution by AA members of stable abstinence to the grace of God is metaphorically not far off the mark. Table 4.4A reveals that education, I.Q., boyhood competence, membership in a multiproblem family, and hyperactivity in youth and sociopathic behavior in adulthood failed to distinguish men who achieved abstinence from those who did not. Presence of premorbid risk factors for alcoholism did not distinguish the two groups except that the men of Irish descent were somewhat more likely to be severely alcohol-dependent and thus to join AA and become stably abstinent. Men of French-Canadian and Mediterranean ancestry were somewhat more likely to continue to abuse alcohol over the life span, but they did so with relatively few symptoms.

With the exception of binge drinking (and, of course, going on the wagon) there was no symptom that differentiated the 48 Core City men with stable abstinence (30 of whom were abstinent for ten years or more) from the 48 Core City men who abused alcohol until the time of most recent contact or until they died. With the exception of AA attendance, there was no treatment experience that distinguished the two Core City outcome groups. However,

TABLE 4.4A.   Absence of predictors of stable abstinence in Core City men.

	Stable abstinence n = 48	Chronic alcoholism n = 48
Possibly significant differences		
Risk factors for alcohol abuse		
Irish ancestry	36% (n = 17)	25% (n = 12)
French Canadian–Mediterranean ancestry	8% (n = 4)	25% (n = 12)
Symptoms of alcohol abuse		
Ever a binge drinker	63%	43%
Treatment factors		
30+ AA visits by age 48	27%	6%
Not significant[a]		
Childhood antecedents		
Boyhood competence, I.Q., education, childhood environmental strengths, childhood environmental weaknesses, childhood social class, maternal relationship, paternal relationship		
Risk factors for alcohol abuse		
Hyperactivity, number of alcoholic relatives, antisocial behavior		
Symptoms of alcohol abuse		
DSM III alcohol dependence, number of Cahalan problems, problem drinking score (PDS), blackouts, clinic treatment, morning drinking, pack/years of smoking, symptoms of sociopathy		

a. Spearman correlation coefficients −.13 to +.13.

even if abstinence is correlated with AA attendance, the difficulty is establishing causality. Detractors of AA would argue that frequent attendance at AA is a consequence, rather than a cause, of abstinence, while advocates of AA would argue that AA attendance is the cause and abstinence is the result.

Stable abstinence was much less common among the College alcohol abusers. When the expanded sample of 52 alcohol-abusing (DSM III criteria) College men was examined, only 10 men by age 70 had been abstinent for three years or more. Four of these 10 had achieved their abstinence through intense involvement with AA. All but 2 of the abstinent College men were two-pack-a-day smokers for 25 years or more. Their heavy smoking contributed to the fact that 7 (70 percent) of the 10 College men with stable abstinence had died by age 70. Four died of heart disease and 2 of lung cancer.

Among these 10 men, owing to the relatively late onset of their alcoholism and their high premature death rate, only 4 achieved ten or more years of abstinence.

All of the 10 securely abstinent College men came from the subgroup of 19 College men who had been alcohol-dependent. As noted elsewhere, this association of symptom severity with abstinence confounds the search for predictors of good long-term prognosis in alcohol abuse. For example, 8 of the 10 *most* symptomatic College alcohol abusers achieved secure abstinence and 8 of the 12 *least* symptomatic College alcohol abusers returned to asymptomatic or controlled social drinking. Thus, the best outcomes came from the two extremes of severity of alcohol abuse—a pattern echoed among the Core City men.

The Relationship of Alcoholics Anonymous to Abstinence

To its detractors, Alcoholics Anonymous is unscientific, smacks of fundamentalist religion, excludes those who do not espouse its views, and is not open to other forms of help for alcoholics. To its admirers, AA is an organization made up of winners. As one Core City member put it, "If you come to an uncharted minefield and see footprints, you had better follow them—very closely."

The effectiveness of Alcoholics Anonymous reported here is at variance with the rather gloomy view contained in other recent reviews of alcohol treatment (Baekeland et al. 1975; Orford and Edwards 1977). I believe that the reason for the discrepancy is the difference between a short-term and a long-term perspective.

One reason that the scientific literature takes such a skeptical view of Alcoholics Anonymous is that AA *is* so unscientific. It asks its members to take the following 12 steps:

Step 1: We admitted we were powerless over alcohol—that our lives had become unmanageable.
Step 2: Came to believe that a Power greater than ourselves could restore us to sanity.
Step 3: Made a decision to turn our will and our lives over to the care of God as we understood Him.
Step 4: Made a searching and fearless moral inventory of ourselves.
Step 5: Admitted to God, to ourselves, and to another human being, the exact nature of our wrongs.
Step 6: Were entirely ready to have God remove all these defects of character.
Step 7: Humbly asked Him to remove our shortcomings.

Step 8: Made a list of all persons we had harmed, and became willing to make amends to them all.

Step 9: Made direct amends to such people whenever possible, except when to do so would injure them or others.

Step 10: Continued to take personal inventory and when we were wrong promptly admitted it.

Step 11: Sought through prayer and meditation to improve our conscious contact with God as we understood Him, praying only for knowledge of His will for us and the power to carry that out.

Step 12: Having had a spiritual awakening as the result of these steps, we tried to carry this message to alcoholics, and to practice these principles in all our affairs.

Any such rigid set of beliefs that are religiously adhered to but not scientifically proven (be it macrobiotics, fundamentalist Christianity, or insistence on daily jogging) tends to irritate the scientific community. The fact that Seventh Day Adventists really do live longer (Berkman and Syme 1979) by no means mitigates the mistrust that many thoughtful people have toward their dogmatic prohibition of coffee, cigarettes, and alcohol. Researchers prefer to study variables that they can experimentally manipulate and observe without bias. But like the study of political parties within one's own country, the study of AA tends to polarize its observers into believers and nonbelievers. Perhaps AA resembles the pixie dust in J. M. Barrie's *Peter Pan* that enabled Wendy to fly; for AA to work, one must be a believer. At present the actual effectiveness of AA has not been adequately assessed.

Virtually the only real follow-up study of the effects of Alcoholics Anonymous was carried out by Bill C. (1965). Over a period of several years, he tried to follow 393 members of AA who ever attended ten or more meetings of a single group during the period 1955 to 1960. Of these, 149 (38 percent) were lost to follow-up; and of the remaining 244, 50 percent had remained sober until 1964 and almost 20 percent more had been sober for more than a year but relapsed. Both selection bias and attrition leave the study so methodologically flawed, however, that it convinces no critics.

But the criticisms of the research world sometimes seem overdone. Baekeland, Lundwall, and Kissin report: "As a primary treatment method, compared to alcohol clinic treatment, AA seems to be applicable to a narrow range of patients in whom it may not be as effective" (1975, p 281). They continue: "It seems possible that the population served by AA is quite different from that which goes to hospitals and clinics and also that the general applicability of AA as a treatment method is much more limited than has been supposed in the past" (p. 306). Yet in questioning the broad effectiveness of AA, they point out that in the United States AA, by virtue of reaching an estimated 650,000 individuals in a given year, reaches twice as many alcoholics as do clinics and medical practitioners combined.

Reviewing short-term studies of clinic attenders, Armor and colleagues (1978) pointed out that only 13 percent of the clinic patients that they followed attended AA regularly. However, like Baekeland, Lundwall, and Kissin, Armor and his co-workers studied a subgroup of alcoholics who at the time they were studied had elected to attend a clinic, not AA. It is not surprising, then, that such patients did not uniformly switch to AA. Armor and his co-workers write: "If other treatment is available, the impact of AA on general remission rate is minimal" (1978, p. 120). But they immediately add: "If attention is directed to this outcome (total abstention) only, regular AA participation appears to make a substantial and consistent difference" (p. 120). Indeed, their actual figures suggest that even when alcoholics opted for alcohol treatment centers, they were *twice* as likely to be abstinent for six months if they attended AA. In their more recent four-year follow-up, Polich, Armor, and Braiker (1981) suggest that AA may be the *most* effective treatment to induce abstinence. Four years after admission, 74 or 14 percent of their total sample attended AA "regularly" (as opposed to "occasionally"). Forty-five percent of these 74 men had been abstinent for a year and another 12 percent for six months or more. This was three times the percentage of abstinence in the sample as a whole.

The Armor study, however, does not address the challenge put forth by Orford and Edwards: "Directing clinic patients toward Alcoholics Anonymous can enhance the likelihood of AA involvement, but evidence for the contribution of AA as an adjunct to clinic treatment is not easily found . . . attendance may actually cause improvement for a small subgroup, or AA attendance may be an epiphenomenon" (1977, p. 57). In other words, abstinence may facilitate AA attendance, not vice versa.

A second reason for the scientific community's skeptical view of AA is that thus far follow-ups have been too short. What most investigators ignore is that they are parochially concerned only with the subgroup of alcoholics who attend their clinics. After an alcoholic leaves a clinic, he escapes the clinic's influence. In contrast, Alcoholics Anonymous, a community grass-roots organization, remains in a position to influence the alcoholic's behavior for a much longer period of time. An individual's relationship to a community-based self-help organization is intrinsically different from his relationship to a medical model clinic. He "belongs" to the first; he only "visits" the latter. One visit to an alcohol clinic may be far more effective than a single visit to an AA meeting; but AA involvement, if it develops, is often measured in hundreds of visits spread over years, and the people who find AA early in their alcoholic careers do not come to clinics. Thus, in this book's examination of alcoholics drawn from the community, a higher percentage of Core City alcoholics became abstinent through their association with AA than with clinics, and more of the College sample became abstinent through AA than through psychotherapy. When a sample of 100 alcoholic clinic attenders (the Clinic sample) were followed for eight years, 48 percent of the 29 remitted alcoholics eventually attended 300 or more AA meetings; but such a finding would not have been observed on short-term follow-up.

In the Core City sample, the nature of involvement with AA among the currently abstinent varied enormously. For some, AA was merely a catalyst that was important only in the first weeks of abstinence. For others, AA attendance was frequent for a year or two and then declined. For still others, AA became a part of their stable life structure. The 18 men whom AA specifically helped had attended an average of 300 meetings, but a few of them had attended fewer than 75 meetings.

Certainly the way the four factors in Table 4.3 interact with and are incorporated by Alcoholics Anonymous is complex, and the process by which AA becomes effective in reversing alcohol dependence is not always sudden. Let me offer an illustration of a Philadelphia carpenter, Joe Hamilton. His childhood had been one of the worst in the study. As he put it: "My home life was full of booze, I never knew a way of life that was sober. Alcoholics Anonymous helped me to learn to live without a drink. What sustained me was seeing other people sober and that they seemed serene."

At age 33, Joe recognized that he was an alcoholic. For seven years he tried psychiatric counseling, repeated psychiatric hospitalizations, and tranquilizers without results. In 1968 when he was 40, a doctor sent him to his first AA meeting. He attended AA off and on from 1968 to 1973; during that period he abused chlordiazepoxide (Librium)—a long-acting tranquilizer that shares many pharmacological properties with alcohol. In 1973, at age 45, Joe finally gave up Librium *and* alcohol. That year his alcoholic father died, and since that event he has been completely abstinent from alcohol; he now attends about 200 AA meetings a year.

What happened in 1973 that made Alcoholics Anonymous able to catch hold? The answer may lie in three other events that occurred in the life of

Joe Hamilton that year. First, he joined the Episcopal church and through his church he became involved in social issues in a very active way. In 1973, he also lost his father, and shortly afterward he met his present wife. Each event in its own way may have contributed to his giving up drug dependence. His own perception was: "AA has to be first in my life . . . if anything else is helping me, it would be my woman and my church. They give and share a lot with me. This is different than when I was drinking . . . it's incredible the number of people I can depend on."

A North Carolina truck driver, Fred Murphy, provides a more expanded illustration of the interaction of the four natural healing factors presented in Table 4.3. Fred had spent most of his childhood in foster homes. Despite superior intelligence, he quit school after eighth grade. By 15, he was abusing alcohol, but morning drinking and frank dependence did not begin until age 28. His age-31 follow-up interview was conducted in an urban jail. Fred's score for sociopathy was as high as almost any in the study. At age 36, Fred was living a skid-row existence, covering himself with leaves to protect himself from rain, begging for drinking money, and throwing stones through windows of alcohol halfway houses for drunken sport—and perhaps also as a covert plea for help.

Eleven years later, I interviewed him in a trailer camp in the piney woods region of North Carolina. He was living among shabby furniture in a shabby trailer with a shabby lawn and three shabby rose bushes by the door. His kitchen, however, was spotless and well stocked with new appliances. An imitation damask tablecloth graced the kitchen table.

Fred Murphy could have been sent from central casting to fill the role of Tennessee Williams' Stanley Kowalski. His 200 pounds of muscle were well tattooed, and his opening line was: "I had trouble adjusting when I came out of the joint." He then described as much personal tragedy and pain as any other man in the study, but he spoke without rancor. Early in the interview he told me that a man should never cry, but it was easy to see the sadness just underneath the surface of this ex-prizefighter's face with its flattened, multiply fractured nose. As he talked, Fred revealed an extraordinary capacity to identify, to take people inside, and to love others without ambivalence. He let me know how extraordinarily appreciative he was of all the people who had touched him. This included everyone from his foster mother and his old school teacher, who had reinterviewed him during the earlier Glueck follow-ups, to his children, with whom he had stayed in touch throughout his shattered, vagrant life.

As I interviewed him at the kitchen table, his young careworn wife initially impressed me as a rather plain victim of slums, addiction, and social deprivation. When she offered me a cup of coffee, I accepted; Fred turned to her and said, "Hey, he turned it down when I offered it to him." His wife replied, "You're not nice, that's why." She said this with such humor and with such a disarming smile that her whole face became suddenly and unexpectedly beautiful. Later, when I asked him what was his greatest satisfaction in life, Fred jerked his thumb in his wife's direction and said, "Being married to her . . . we're pretty tight. I have to pinch myself every now and then to find out if it's really true."

Fred recollected the process of getting sober as follows. When he was 36, a friend called him a coward and Fred started to threaten the friend with his fist. The man said, "Wait a minute. I'm sure you can beat me up, but you can't face life. You're a yellow bastard." Fred commented to me, "It just bugged me that he could say that. It was 1964 and that was when I started to get sober." After flirting with AA for three years, at 39 (1967) he had his last drink. He had gone through the "AA 12 Steps," and he had had several AA "sponsors." He had gone on "commitments" (speaking at meetings) and had belonged to a group. He explained that AA served as both his church and his social club. In his 11 years of sobriety, he estimated that he had been to a thousand meetings. Six years ago he had given up speaking at meetings, and in recent years he had gone only once a month.

I asked him during the past decade what he did when he wanted a drink, and he said he called his sponsor. "When you walk into the phone booth and get out a dime, you know you're not going to drink."

Not every alcoholic, of course, has Fred's gift for substituting people for alcohol. Besides incorporating the natural healing factors in Table 4.3, AA may be effective for other reasons as well. As Bales (1962) suggests, willpower and self-control can be enormously enhanced if they are derived from belonging to a group. Edwards and his colleagues articulate this issue well:

> Identification is the very essence of the affiliation process. The role played by the sponsor may sometimes be important, but can be exaggerated. Identification is not with any one established member so much as with fragments of a whole series of life histories which are synthesized into identification with the group ideal. The importance of identification in group dynamics was stressed by Freud, and identification assumes particular importance in the leaderless group which must have a clear and firmly established picture of the ideal member. Although this picture may partly be based on the statistical norm, it derives also in some measure from the group's fantasy and wish fulfillment (1967, p. 203).

AA transforms conflict solution via direct expression of impulses (acting out) into reaction formation (turning instinctual wishes into their opposites); alcohol, instead of being a source of instant gratification, becomes the cause of all life's pain. Freud summed this process of reaction formation up by the quip: "A young whore becomes an old nun." Not only does AA capitalize on group identification, but also, with its unyielding insistence upon abstinence, AA capitalizes on reaction formation. But by definition, reaction formation is an unstable, fragile defense. Thus, it is far easier to maintain a regular daily pattern of pleasureless early morning jogging than to alternate such a pattern with weeks of self-indulgent sleeping in. Trying to reestablish training and self-discipline is more difficult than maintaining it in the first place. Thus, it seems self-evident to both alcohol clinics and old timers in AA that it is frequently disastrous for an alcoholic (or a smoker) to return to social drinking (or smoking) after rigid abstinence. Indeed, once relapse has occurred, once adherence to a rule of absolute abstinence is broken, previously sober alcoholics often find it enormously difficult to return effectively to a program they *know* is successful. Undoubtedly, factors like shame and concern with social acceptance by sober AA members also play a part.

The role that maturation and defensive transformation play in remission from alcohol dependence is difficult to assess. Often the evolution of an impulse-ridden life into one of temperance seems intimately associated with the same process of reaction formation by which the adolescent free spirit becomes "over 30."

Among the Core City sample, the process of maturation was epitomized by one of the few real sociopaths in the study. In spite of superior intelligence and a better-than-average family environment, he had spent much of his young life flirting with organized crime. He had experienced many arrests for violent behavior and had spent more than two years in jail. At 40, without any kind of treatment or contact with AA, he stopped drinking. As he looked back on his life, he sounded like the most brainwashed AA member: "I just quit cold. The more I thought of what I'd blown in the past, the more I didn't want to drink . . . I traced all my troubles and stupid things I did to alcohol . . . I haven't the slightest inclination to touch it now . . . I got a good look at myself and realized that I could not be a social drinker, I always had to empty the bottle. I thought I was having a ball at the time, I couldn't see the light through the trees . . . you think you're so sharp with the guys, but you're really a shitbum." After 40, he deliberately sought a new circle of friends with whom to identify, to replace his "street" drinking friends. He said he still tried to have one or two drinks at New Year's but "I couldn't drink last New Year's. I had a small whiskey and water and couldn't finish it." The development of such a shift in life course cannot be explained by such simple terms as "hitting bottom," "burning out," or "growing up." Rather, the process by which intrapsychic structures change and produce lasting changes in character and modulation of impulses is one of the most complex, if poorly understood, processes in psychology.

AA also counters the tendency of the alcoholic to project all his problems onto the outside world with a credo of assuming responsibility for *all* his problems—a position that some critics of AA regard as a gross oversimplification. But the insistence of AA on this point transforms externalization of responsibility into self-responsibility. Lastly, and perhaps most important, in AA denial of alcoholism is transformed into a public, almost exhibitionistic insistence upon the admission: "I am an alcoholic."

However, Alcoholics Anonymous was not a universal panacea for the Core City alcoholics. Some Core City men, especially under compulsion, attended AA for up to 200 meetings without real improvement in their drinking patterns over eight years. Some men in the Clinic study attended 100 AA meetings without improvement; often such attendance was the price of admission to detoxification units and halfway houses. But there was no evidence that such individuals then recovered through some other means.

An example of a man who failed to recover despite extensive contact with AA was a 47-year-old New Jersey farm worker, Tom Reardon. Tom grew up in a very disrupted home and despite adequate intelligence dropped out of school in the eighth grade. He remembers his alcoholic mother giving him alcohol from age 7 on, but he did not clearly abuse alcohol until his 30s. Since then, he had been treated on multiple occasions by clinics and prisons, with Antabuse and psychotherapy, but without any improvement. He almost boasted of his more than 200 drunk arrests. Since 1964 he had been going to AA about 50 times a year. Three times, he had achieved eight consecutive months of sobriety, but he always relapsed to alcoholic drinking. In recent years, he had been ordered by the court to attend AA meetings monthly; this order made him extremely resentful. He pointed out that he would go to AA even if nobody forced him to do so and that he attends AA principally for companionship. He attends one meeting regularly. Since he feels it is hypocritical to go when intoxicated, he only attends when he is sober. He keeps a little black book with names to contact in AA but confesses, "I have never used the list."

Although a few individuals report that their contact with AA began when they were compelled to attend, to force regular attendance does not seem generally useful. As with church or country club membership, reliance on AA has to be an individual decision. Thus, for the past ten years, Tom has lived an isolated marginal existence. His only social contacts are his employer and his AA companions. Unlike Fred Murphy, Tom Reardon never learned to pick up a telephone.*

To put individual case histories into a more systematic perspective, let me contrast the Core City men who benefited from Alcoholics Anonymous with those who did not. The large literature on this subject has been well reviewed by Leach and Norris (1977), Robinson (1979), and Bean (1975). Most studies suggest that AA users tend to come from the middle class and to be more extroverted and less sociopathic than nonmembers. However, previous studies have been handicapped by contrasting very nonrepresentative samples. Sober, cooperative volunteer informants actively involved with AA are contrasted with alcohol clinic attenders, many of whom are still actively drinking and who are usually involuntary subjects. Active alcoholism is a powerful barrier to membership in the middle class. To properly understand who does and does not attend AA one must study a single universe of alcoholics from which both the attenders and nonattenders have been drawn.

The sample of the Core City men seemed ideal for such purposes. Table 4.5 contrasts the 17 men in the Core City sample with a year of abstinence who used AA extensively (50 or more visits) with 32 abstinent men who attended AA less frequently. Some of the latter believed that AA had been helpful; and three men, including Tom Reardon, used AA extensively but relapsed and gave AA no credit for their year of sobriety.

Ethnicity appeared significant. Although alcoholics of Irish parentage did not enjoy better prognosis than other ethnic groups, they were proportionately more likely to achieve abstinence through Alcoholics Anonymous. Since Catholic Italian alcoholics were the ethnic group least likely to use AA, Catholicism or a strongly religious upbringing cannot be invoked as the major explanation. Three other explanations seem more likely. First, joining AA is like joining a social club or a church. In Boston, both the bars and liquor stores catering to alcoholics and many of the organizations treating the disorder, including Alcoholics Anonymous, have been dominated by men of

---

*At age 55, while intoxicated, he died in a fire in his home.

TABLE 4.5. Variables significantly associated with the use of Alcoholics Anonymous by the ever abstinent.

Variable	50+ meetings (n = 17)	0–49 meetings (n = 32)
Irish ethnicity	65%	13%**
8+ symptoms on PDS	88	59
Alcohol-dependent (DSM III)	94	72
Blackouts	94	69
Morning drinking	94	75
Binge drinking	82	75
Maternal neglect	29	62*
Warm childhood environment	65	34*
Verbal I.Q. < 80	4	23

*$p < .05$; **$p < .01$ (chi-square test).

Irish descent. Indeed, in Boston alcoholism has been unfairly called "the Irish Catholic disease." Second, in contrast to the case in Latin countries, in Ireland, abstinence of all kinds is a virtue. A key element in Irish Catholicism is the cycle of sin, guilt, and repentance (Bales 1962; Stivers 1976)—a cycle that is quite congruent with the 12 steps of Alcoholics Anonymous.

Third, as noted in Chapter 2, the men of Irish descent who abused alcohol tended to become more heavily alcohol-dependent than alcohol abusers of other ethnic backgrounds; and as can be appreciated in Tables 4.4 and 4.5, the more symptomatic alcoholics were more likely to seek help through Alcoholics Anonymous. The sheer number of alcohol problems, especially blackouts and being classified as alcohol-dependent rather than as an alcohol abuser, correlated significantly with the number of AA visits, $r = .26$ ($p < .05$). (Although the association of morning drinking and binge drinking with AA did not reach statistical significance in this study, both items were significantly correlated with AA in other studies: Edwards et al. 1967.) I suspect the explanation for these relationships may be the same as the reason for seeking abstinence in the first place—that all other reasonable alternatives had failed. Attendance at AA meetings is not usually a hedonistic prescription. Sitting on hard chairs in smoke-filled church basements, drinking bad coffee, and listening to poor sound systems and often poorer speakers several evenings a week can feel more like treating one's wounds with iodine or major surgery than with opiates.

Besides ethnicity and severity of alcoholism, having had a warm childhood seemed to facilitate AA membership. Although this finding may represent a chance association in a small sample, the observation is consistent with the fact that a certain amount of Eriksonian Basic Trust may be necessary to "Let go and let God," to turn one's problems over to a "higher power," and to gain strength from group membership. Baekeland, Lundwall, and Kissin (1975) found that high intelligence also correlated positively with AA. In the present study, I.Q. was also modestly but significantly ($r = .20$, $p < .05$) correlated with AA attendance. Although maternal neglect was correlated with low verbal intelligence, multiple regression suggested that both variables made significant negative contributions to the frequency of AA attendance.

None of the other significant predictors of mental health in Chapters 2 and 7 (such as childhood environmental weaknesses, childhood emotional problems, and boyhood competence) predicted AA involvement. Adult outcome measures like education, adult mental health (measured by the HSRS), sociopathy (measured by the Robins scale), adult social competence, and maturity of defensive styles as an adult were also insignificantly correlated with the use of AA. Adult social class correlated insignificantly ($r = .03$) with use of AA, as did parental social class. In the highly educated College sample all men fell in social class I or II by age 50, yet among the alcohol-dependent College men extensive use of AA was as common (4 out of 9) as among the Core City men (24 out of 71)—but these numbers, obviously, are too small to permit conclusions.

In a thoughtful study, Edwards and his colleagues (1967) speculate that AA excludes those who would threaten its cohesion. However, neither in their study nor in this one did criminal records, introversion, or sociopathy distinguish members from nonmembers. To the degree that it exists, exclusion from AA probably depends more upon issues of identification or nonidentification on the part of prospective members. An AA motto is "Identify, don't compare." As in church or fraternal order membership, alcoholics, if they are to make use of AA, must find members with whom to identify.

Perhaps the best testimonial for AA was provided by a 60-year-old socially sophisticated member of the College sample who long had scoffed at AA:

I've been in AA only about 2½ months now [At this writing, two years later, he is still in AA] and my only regret is that I didn't join the fellowship about 25 years ago. Then, it might have seemed to me to be not more than a bunch of meetings with odd people in church basements. Now those meetings, which I attend almost every day, except weekends, come to me as a revelation. Most alcoholics, I believe, grow up in a glass isolation booth which they build for themselves to separate themselves from other people. The only person I ever communicated with was my wife . . . AA shows us how to dissolve the glass walls around us and realize that there are other people out there, good loving people . . . I rarely talked to a woman without wondering whether we were going to wind up in bed and I rarely talked to a man without trying to figure out who outranked whom. I discovered friendship in AA, a word which had always sounded phoney as hell to me. This is more important to me than their help in keeping me off booze. I haven't had a drink since joining the fellowship but except for three days, booze had not been a problem for me in about two years. Those three days scared me, however, for obviously drinking was becoming compulsive again and I was on the way back to the nightmares of two years ago and before that.

I love the AA meetings and love being able to call people up when I feel tense. Occasionally, someone calls me for help and that makes me feel good.

I get much more out of this than I got from decades of psychiatry. My relationship with a psychiatrist always seemed to me to be distressingly cold. I hated the huge bills. For $50 an hour, one doctor kept assuring me that I was nutty to worry about money, and at the time I couldn't keep up my life insurance. I wish there were some form of Alcoholics Anonymous for troubled people who don't drink. We old drunks are lucky.

∿ Alcoholics Anonymous Revisited

For the last ten years the life of this now 72-year-old member of the College sample has been manageable but not without alcohol-related difficulties. After three years of abstinence he drifted away from AA. After another year he wrote, "I occasionally drink a little each day for months before overdoing it and going back to AA." A month after that writing he became abstinent again for two years. At 67 he again tried social drinking. In a few months he again lost control of alcohol and has reported stable abstinence up to 1992.

Despite this College man's less than perfect outcome, research during the last 15 years has revealed growing indirect evidence that AA is an effective treatment for alcohol abuse. Direct evidence for the efficacy of AA, however, remains as elusive as ever. One difficulty is that the subject of AA, like the subject of controlled drinking and the subject of whether alcoholism is a disease, evokes adversarial argument rather than dispassionate reflection. For example, William Miller (Miller and Hester 1986), an advocate of professional intervention, suggests that the evidence is clear that AA is ineffective. However, in an otherwise very scholarly review, he cites only four articles pertaining to AA. In contrast, in a more even-handed review of the efficacy of AA, Emrick (1989) was able to cite 56 studies that evaluated AA; 15 of these demonstrated that AA was superior to alternative treatments. Admittedly, since none of the studies he cited was without flaws, Emrick was forced to conclude that the effectiveness of AA has yet to be proved.

Ironically, one of the more interesting studies supportive of AA, reported after Emrick's review, is Miller's own follow-up study (Miller et al. 1992). During his four-to-eight-year follow-up of his own behavioral-self-control-trained clients, Miller noted how many attended AA, and stated, "A chi-square analysis revealed no overall relationship between long-term outcome and AA attendance by categories" (1992, p. 257). However, recalculation of his data revealed that 54 percent of his 13 clients who had made more than 100 visits to AA were abstinent, in contrast to only 20 percent of the 81 clients who had gone to fewer than 100 meetings—a difference that is statistically significant ($x^2 = 5.32$, $p < .03$) with the Yates correction. Since the purpose of Miller's treatment program was *not* abstinence, certainly not to involve his clients with AA, and since the majority of his good long-term outcomes *were* abstinent, the importance of AA to good outcome is probably significant.

In a balanced review, Nace (1992) has examined some of the facets of AA that attract criticism. First, because of its perhaps necessarily ideological nature, AA members are not encouraged to take a scientific and dispassionate approach to the study of its efficacy. The prevalence in AA of paraprofessional counselors and program administrators who are also recovering alcoholics further confounds dispassionate research. Personally based loyalty to the ideology of AA often comes into potential conflict with the empiricism of the research community. Second, although AA as an organization does not hold opinions, individual members, like members of any partisan group, can be extremely and erroneously opinionated. Third, AA certainly functions as a cult and systematically indoctrinates its members in ways common to cults the world over. The negative side effects of AA, however, are perhaps more benign than those of any other cult with which I am familiar. For example, in contrast to other relatively benign cults like fraternities, psychoanalytic institutes, fundamentalist Christian sects, disarmament groups, political parties, and even the Oxford Group on which AA was modeled, AA has avoided schisms. Nevertheless, in the absence of proven scientific efficacy, critics are legitimate in suggesting that mandated AA attendance may be criticized as a failure of proper separation between church and state. In response, AA as an organization has tried to redress this difficulty by emphasizing the importance to its membership of "wearing two hats" when becoming involved in the alcohol-treatment field.

On the positive side, Nace has clarified the ways in which AA captures the effective ingredients of most successful psychotherapies and most major religions. He underscores that AA allows the individual *release* (freedom from the compulsion to drink), *gratitude* ("a pigeon comes along just in time to keep his sponsor sober"), *humility* (a shift from self-centeredness to self-acceptance), *tolerance* ("live and let live"), and finally and perhaps most important, forgiveness for past sins. Nace summarizes:

> The alcoholic who comes to AA is not asked to change, only to listen, identify and keep coming back. The style of interpersonal contact is non-threatening . . . humor and friendliness abound. Nevertheless, the meeting is serious . . . relapses or "slips" do not represent a failure on the part of the alcoholic or of AA. Rather, slips are further demonstration of the power of alcohol and, therefore, of the necessity of AA as a counter-force . . . The AA program treats shame by enabling the alcoholic to accept his or her need for others by promoting the acceptance of others as they are . . . and by valuing and reinforcing traits of honesty, sharing, and caring. (p. 492)

Would that all "religions" and fraternal organizations were as benign.

There have been two lines of indirect evidence supporting the efficacy of AA. First, AA has continued to attract believers. The last 15 years have brought increasing evidence that AA is applicable to very diverse populations, and no longer is AA a self-help group serving middle-aged, middle-class, white, Protestant, English-speaking, extraverted males. Rather, Emrick (1989), in his elaborate literature review, was unable to identify clear demographic differences between alcohol abusers who did and did not use AA. No personality differences have been identified between AA attendees and nonattendees (Thurstin et al. 1986). The single exception is that severity of alcoholic symptomatology positively predicts AA membership. Race, education, gender, socioeconomic status, age, social stability, gregariousness, and mental health, however, do not differentiate AA members from nonmembers. For example, Nace (1992) reports that in the United States 22 percent of the AA membership is currently less than 31 years old, 35 percent of members are women, and 46 percent of members are comorbid for significant polydrug abuse. Minority groups of all kinds—young adults, African Americans, homosexuals, polydrug abusers—have been increasingly welcomed.

In the past 20 years the worldwide growth of AA has also been dramatic (Makela 1991). By 1986 two-thirds of the membership of AA resided outside the United States. For example, Mexico, which in 1965 reported no AA groups, in 1986 reported 8,510 groups to the AA General Service Office in New York City. There are three times as many AA groups per capita in Costa Rica and in El Salvador as in the United States. Admittedly, Islamic, communist, and very poor nations report little AA activity. In addition, national wine consumption correlates negatively and beer consumption correlates positively with the strength of AA. However, in the past 20 years AA membership has increased tenfold in Hindu poverty-stricken India, in Anglophobic wine-drinking France, in Catholic Spain, and in Buddhist Japan. There are between 2,000 and 5,000 members in each country. In addition, since the advent of *glasnost,* AA has gained a foothold in Russia. The first AA group was not formed there until after 1985; since then the number of groups has been doubling every year: by 1992 there were between 30 and 50 Russian AA groups.

Cross-cultural differences, of course, play an important role in how AA is conducted. AA meetings are run very differently in Zimbabwe, which reports 85 members, and in Brazil, which reports 77,000 members, from the way they are run in the United States. In many countries Anglo-American influence remains unduly strong. For example, only one of the 16 weekly meetings in Hong Kong is held in Chinese (Makela 1991); and if there are now ten AA groups in Saudi Arabia, they may be largely made up of Anglo-American employees of oil companies.

AA has also continued to expand within the United States, and in the past 20 years its membership has quadrupled. The General Service Office in New York City reported that in 1986 there were 585,823 members in the United States, but on the basis of a general population survey the number of individuals who have included AA in their efforts to find help is probably much higher. Room and Greenfield (1993) note that 3 percent of the adult American population—perhaps 3 to 4 million people—reported having attended AA at least once for an alcohol problem.

While controlled studies of AA have proven too difficult to carry out, naturalistic studies offer evidence that AA is effective. The study by Miller and colleagues (1992) has already been mentioned. In my discussion of the Clinic sample in Chapter 8, I offer evidence that AA attendance was associated with good outcome in patients who otherwise would have been predicted not to remit. In a ten-year follow-up Cross and colleagues (1990) found AA involvement the only statistically significant predictor of abstinence.

Mann and colleagues (1991) offer evidence that increasing AA membership may be partly responsible for the recently observed declines in cirrhosis morbidity and mortality in Canada and in the United States. Studying in contrasting American states the differential effects of rising AA membership, increases in utilization of professional treatment services, and declining cirrhosis morbidity, the investigators found no significant relationship between increase in professional treatment services and declining cirrhosis rates. However, both decreases in per capita alcohol consumption and increases in AA membership were significantly and independently associated with declining rates of cirrhosis.

Walsh and her colleagues (1991) reported a well-designed study of the treatment of 227 employee assistance program (EAP) clients referred for alcohol abuse; 56 percent were alcohol-dependent. Clients were randomly assigned to one of three treatment groups: short hospitalization followed by AA, AA alone, or choice of treatment. All clients were mandated to attend AA three times a week for a year—probably the most intensive use of AA in any well-controlled study in the literature. Very good results were obtained: 41 percent of the clients were abstinent for the last 6 months of the 24-month follow-up, and 23 percent were abstinent for the entire period. The effect on job retention was substantial and sustained for about 80 percent of their clients. The three treatment groups did not show a difference in job improvement, but during the first three months hospitalization combined with AA was significantly more effective than AA alone. The difficulty with the study is that there was no group randomized *not* to receive extensive AA treatment. Thus the detractors of AA can say hospitalization is superior to AA, and the advocates of AA can point to the fact that the entire sample did unusually well. The jury is still out.

The Consequences of Abstinence

In America, the benefits of abstinence have been so stridently set forth by both the Puritans and the zealots of temperance movements that humanists have become understandably suspicious and impatient. In their much quoted papers, Pattison (1968) and Gerard and colleagues (1962) have pointed out that although abstinence, like virginity, is officially encouraged, it may be no more pleasurable or health-promoting than indiscretion. The insistence of both Alcoholics Anonymous and the National Council on Alcoholism upon abstinence as the *only* treatment for alcoholism has caused thoughtful scientists to call the whole concept of abstinence into question (Blane 1978), especially in the absence of careful follow-up studies. Clinical vignettes are common of alcoholics who upon stopping drinking have become profoundly depressed or even psychotic; so are stories of marriages that break up when a previously jolly alcoholic spouse becomes a sober grouch. Finally, since five out of six American Nobel Prize winners in literature have been alcoholic, it is hard for clinicians entirely to dismiss the assertion by alcoholic artists that when drinking they are most in touch with their muse.

Experimental evidence is needed to put these concerns about abstinence into proper perspective; and the effect of abstinence upon the lives of the Core City men sheds light upon what hitherto has tended to be treated as a largely theoretical issue. How does the life adjustment of abstinent alcoholics compare with that of those who continue to abuse alcohol? Certainly, secure abstinence did not allow the Core City alcoholics to recover excellent physical health. Thirty-eight percent of the securely abstinent men, 31 percent of the progressively alcoholic men, and only 19 percent of the men who lacked a history of alcohol abuse are currently chronically physically ill. The literature reviews in Chapter 3 suggest that recovered alcoholics suffer an increased death rate almost equal to that of active alcoholics.

Nevertheless, Table 4.6 makes abstinence appear more than just a Puritan's hair shirt. Although the securely abstinent were once just as symptomatic and just as antisocial as those men whose alcoholism continues to progress, the securely abstinent are less likely to die and are far more able to enjoy their survival. Their responsibility as parents, their success as employees, and their marital enjoyment are comparable to men for whom alcohol has never been a problem. When drinking, the securely abstinent often received a psychiatric diagnosis, but their current psychiatric functioning did not differ appreciably from the controls for whom alcohol had never been a problem. In terms of psychiatric disability, there is now a vast difference between the securely abstinent and the progressive alcohol abusers. Given adequate time to rebuild their lives, abstinent alcoholics resemble the general population far more than they resemble actively drinking alcoholics or nonalcoholics with personality disorders. The implication is either that abstinent alcoholics "outgrow" youthful psychopathology or that many of the symptoms of alcoholism are incorrectly diagnosed as mental illness. My own interpretation (Vaillant 1980a) of the data is that most alcoholics are depressed because they drink and not vice versa. But many disagree.

Pattison presents perhaps the best available review of studies which suggest

TABLE 4.6. Comparison of securely abstinent and progressive alcoholics on current adult adjustment.

Adult adjustment	Alcohol never a problem (n = 250±10)	Securely abstinent (n = 21)	Progressive alcoholism (n = 35)
Ever alcohol-dependent (DSM III)	0%	71%	74%
Dead	3	5	14
Current object relations in top 40%	46	30	21
Enjoys his children	25	43	11
Enjoys his marriage	55	52	9
Significant psychiatric disability (1978)	24	29	72
Psychiatric diagnosis for non-alcohol-related problem (ever)	23	33	45
Annual earned income (1978)	$17,000	$15,000	$9,000[a]

a. Current income was known for only 28 of the 35 progressive alcoholics; since the less well studied men tended to be having even more trouble with their lives, the progressive alcoholics' average income may well be even lower than indicated here.

that abstinence might not be valuable; and he summarizes his argument as follows: "Enforced sobriety can be disastrous to personality integration, particularly when alcohol is the mechanism by which borderline characters, or psychiatric personality structures maintain ego integration, diminish hallucinations or delay overwhelming anxiety" (1968, p. 273). Certainly, alcohol may be a pharmacological source of relief, especially for alcoholics experiencing actual or conditioned alcohol-withdrawal symptoms.

But the real question is whether alcohol abuse is or is not a means of buffering psychiatric symptomatology that emerges in adult life. There are three long-term studies of abstinent alcoholics that shed light on this subject (Gerard et al. 1962; Kurtines et al. 1978; Pettinati 1981). Gerard and co-workers found an enormous amount of psychopathology in their follow-up of 50 abstinent clinic patients (30 of whom had been abstinent for three years). According to these authors, 54 percent of their abstinent patients were "overtly disturbed" and only 10 percent were classified as "independent successes"—a definition based upon having reached a "state of self-respecting independence, of personal growth and of self-realization." Equally important, Gerard and Saenger observed that some abstinent patients (4–24 percent) actually fared worse in some areas of adjustment than when they had been drinking.

This study, then, is the evidence on which Pattison (1968) and others base their belief that heavy alcohol intake may in fact be a means of maintaining psychological homeostasis. Belasco captured the essence of this dilemma when he wrote: "As Pattison points out, the correlation of abstinence with overall emotional adjustment cannot be assured, and the potentially adverse consequences of abstinence cannot be ignored" (1971, p. 44). In evaluating such arguments, however, it is important to keep in mind that Gerard, Saenger, and Wile were following a public clinic population; they did not have any means of ascertaining how troubled their sample had been *prior* to the onset of alcoholism. Nor did they provide comparison information for nonalcoholic controls.

The study by Pettinati observed that MMPI's obtained on patients abstinent for four years showed "profiles within normal ranges, showing no significant pathology." In contrast, MMPI's administered to the same patients when they were first admitted for detoxification four years earlier showed "significant pathology, especially on the scales of depression and psychopathy" (1981, p. 3).

The study by Kurtines and co-workers contrasted 60 newly sober (three weeks to four months) alcoholics both with 62 alcoholics who had been abstinent for more than four years (and an average of 8.9 years) and with 61 randomly chosen but unmatched controls. On virtually all scales of the California Psychological Inventory (CPI), the authors found the newly sober alcoholics significantly ($p < .001$) less "normal" than the controls. The alcoholics with much longer sobriety fell about halfway between, being "relatively non-neurotic but moderately socially maladjusted." Although statistically significant, the differences on the CPI scale between the controls and the men with stable abstinence were not very striking. The controls were more "socially mature" and "empathic" than alcoholics with stable sobriety but the latter were more "conflict free" and exhibited a more "comfortable sense of personal worth."

Table 4.7 makes a more rigorous test of Gerard and Saenger's hypothesis. In the table I have tried to equate their terminology with that of Luborsky's Health-Sickness Rating Scale (HSRS). As might be anticipated, since they were drawn from a public clinic population, the abstinent alcoholics of Gerard and Saenger appeared more psychologically disturbed than even the progressive alcoholics drawn from the Core City community sample. Nevertheless, in Table 4.7 the progressive alcoholics appeared far more psychologically disabled than the control Core City subjects for whom alcohol was never a problem. This was in spite of the fact that the HSRS raters of the Core City subjects had been instructed to regard alcoholism as if it were a physical illness rather than evidence of psychological dysfunction.

TABLE 4.7.   Relative mental health of alcoholics achieving abstinence.

HSRS score[a] Gerard and Saenger's terminology[b]	Gerard and Saenger's abstinent alcoholics (n = 50)	Core City sample			
		Asymptomatic drinker (n = 227)	Securely abstinent (> 3 yrs) (n = 20)	Currently abstinent (< 3 yrs) (n = 12)	Progressive alcoholic (n = 29)
0–60 Overtly disturbed	54%	8%	0%	25%	38%
61–70 Inconspicuous inadequacy	24	16	30	33	34
71–80 Alcoholics Anonymous	12	29	40	25	28
81–100 Independent success	10	47	30	17	0

a. Thirteen of the asymptomatic drinkers, 6 of the progressive alcoholics, and 3 of the abstinent alcoholics were less than completely interviewed and thus HSRS ratings could not be confidently ascertained.

b. My correlation of the HSRS with the terminology of Gerard and Saenger is admittedly arbitrary.

What is most instructive about Table 4.7, however, is that the 21 securely abstinent men appear to be functioning about as well as those for whom alcohol had never been a problem; whereas the 12 men who had been abstinent for 1–3 years more closely resemble the progressive alcoholics. On the one hand, such findings do not support the hypothesis that sobriety—at least for the majority of alcoholics—is deleterious; on the other hand, the findings do not suggest that once sobriety is achieved alcohol treatment clinics may consider their task accomplished. If psychotherapy does not induce abstinence in most active alcoholics, many newly abstinent alcoholics may gain much from psychotherapy.

Release from stable bondage, however painful, rarely brings instant relief. Analogous to the situation of returning prisoners of war (Hall and Malone 1976; Sledge et al. 1980), in the early stages of remission from alcoholism, depression and divorce are common and cognitive function and occupational stability are poor. Newly abstinent patients often return as virtual strangers to families and occupational responsibility from which they have been long separated both by alcoholic haze and by mutual recriminations. Reentry both into the occupational world and into family responsibilities should be made slowly. Alcoholics Anonymous is undoubtedly wise to encourage recovering alcoholics to "keep it simple" and to delay occupational ambition. In similar fashion, some family therapists advise recovering alcoholics to reassume family responsibilities and intimacies very gradually. Over the short term, abstinence, like returning from a POW camp, may indeed be painful. The more severe and prolonged the alcoholism, the longer time will be required for convalescence. If Tables 4.6 and 4.7 suggest that the return of the alcoholic to his best premorbid adjustment is possible, it is, nonetheless, worth remembering that the securely abstinent men in our sample had been abstinent for an average of ten years.

The argument may be raised that perhaps the securely abstinent resemble the controls because these men were particularly premorbidly favored by emotional stability, intelligence, and social class. However, if the premorbid variables that best predicted mental health did not predict who would become abstinent or who would continue to abuse alcohol in Chapter 3, neither did these variables predict short and long abstinence. The data in Table 4.7 cannot be explained by differences in premorbid adjustment.

Actually Tables 4.6 and 4.7 are quite in keeping with other studies that have assessed alcoholic outcome in terms of both abstinence and social adjustment. In a two-year follow-up study, van Dijk and van Dijk-Koffeman

(1973) contrasted the physical health, "mental condition," housing, social adjustment, and family, work, and financial situations of 50 patients who became abstinent or returned to asymptomatic drinking with those of 81 patients who continued to experience frequent episodic alcohol abuse. On each of these parameters the abstinent patients tended to improve and men who continued to abuse alcohol became worse. In the abstinent group, 70 percent of the alcoholics showed clear overall social improvement as contrasted with only 5 percent of the 81 patients who continued to abuse alcohol. Sixty percent of the latter but *none* of the former actually became worse on the adjustment variables studied.

Pokorny and colleagues (1968) carried out a similar study that examined the post-discharge life adjustment of 22 abstinent patients with three matched groups of patients with increasingly severe current drinking histories. In every category of life adjustment, the abstinent patients fared best and the heaviest drinkers fared worst. In the eight-year prospective study of 100 Clinic alcoholics, abstinence was associated with progressive social improvement, whereas continued alcohol abuse was associated with progressive deterioration of social, occupational, and physical well-being. Even Gerard and colleagues make the point that, however disturbed their abstinent alcoholics might have been, they were still five times as likely to be employed as the patients in their study who continued to drink.

In suggesting that abstinence is powerfully associated with social recovery, I do not wish to imply that alcoholic residents of halfway houses who have *never* been stably employed or capable of intimacy will miraculously demonstrate these skills once sober. Nor do I wish to dismiss the valuable contribution of Pattison (1968). The study of alcoholism has been plagued by oversimplification; and abstinence per se is certainly an oversimplified goal of treatment. If Table 4.7 suggests that long-term abstinence has advantages over chronic alcoholism, the table also illustrates that men could be abstinent for one to three years and yet remain psychiatrically disabled.

There is a second serious limitation of abstinence. In some ways, severe alcoholism resembles mania, for although both are profoundly disruptive to society, to families, and ultimately to the individual's physical health, both alcoholism and mania not only increase an individual's capacity to deny unpleasant reality but also can provide a genuine existential sense of comfort and omnipotence. The individual's right to continue abusing alcohol must be taken seriously.

A third drawback of abstinence is that for some alcoholics sobriety may no more be a blessing than effective antibiotics are to a long-time resident of a comfortable tuberculosis sanitorium. To give up the sick role and to be expected to function independently in a world for which they feel poorly prepared represents an enormous stress to both recovering alcoholics and consumptives. Once abstinent, the alcoholic may resemble a child who, having missed years of school due to physical illness, now returns in adulthood to the classroom. Not only are there problems of self-esteem, but there are also tangible deficits in life experience that must be made up. Both clinicians and recovering alcoholics report that emotional growth may stop or even regress during the years spent abusing alcohol. Losses have gone ungrieved; social supports have gone untended; age-appropriate advances in occupational proficiency have not taken place. Even when family structure has remained intact, the alcoholic has often evolved into a stranger to his family. It is small wonder that many alcohol clinic patients, when first sober, function poorly.

The possible relation between alcohol abuse and creativity must also be addressed. The College sample included several creative writers. At some point a majority of these men abused alcohol. A majority of these alcoholic wordsmiths also had alcoholic relatives, Scotch-Irish ethnicity, and a lifestyle conducive to drinking outside of the usual businessman's 5–7 P.M. cocktail hour. After 40 years of follow-up, I believe that, with one possible exception, all the men wrote better when sober than when drinking. Admittedly, assessment of creativity is subjective, but that perhaps is the point. Most of us believe that we dance better with a few drinks in us; our partners seldom agree.*

ᵔᵕᵔ The Consequences of Abstinence Revisited

A fourth potential drawback to abstinence from alcohol is that it is often associated with heavy smoking, which is hazardous to physical health. Certainly, on average the abstinent Core City men continued to abuse cigarettes (mean = 58 pack/years) as severely as the men who continued abusing alcohol (mean = 62 pack/years). However, long-term follow-up confirmed that one of the consequences of abstinence from alcohol was, nevertheless, better physical health. Table 4.7A reveals that at age 60 the 26 Core City men who were able to return to controlled drinking enjoyed health as good as that of

---

*When at age 65 the College men were rank ordered according to creative achievement over their entire lifetimes, there was no observed relationship, positive or negative, between creativity and alcohol abuse (Vaillant 1993).

TABLE 4.7A. Comparison of the physical health[a] of different outcome groups among the Core City men at age 60.

	Age 60 outcome			
	No alcohol abuse ever (n = 220)	Return to controlled drinking (n = 26)[b]	Stable abstinence (n = 47)[b]	Chronic alcohol abuse (n = 47)[b]
Good health	41%	46%	40%	19%
Chronically ill	43	35	32	43
Dead	16	19	28	38

a. Recent physical exams rated by an internist kept blind to other study data.
b. Numbers smaller than in Table 3.9B because of unavailability of physical exams for some men.

the sample as a whole and that the 47 Core City men who achieved stable abstinence enjoyed health roughly equal to that of the men who never abused alcohol. The health of the chronically alcoholic men appeared clearly worse. Owing to small numbers the almost twofold difference in abstinent men, as compared to alcohol-abusing men, remaining well at age 60 did not reach statistical significance ($p = .09$).

Finally, and most important, it must be remembered that abstinence is a means, not an end. It is a puritanical goal that removes but does not replace. It is justifiable as a treatment goal only if moderate drinking is not a viable alternative and only if sight is not lost of the real goal—social rehabilitation. Even in Alcoholics Anonymous, the term *sobriety* has the far broader, more platonic meaning of serenity and maturity. The pejorative term *dry* is reserved for individuals who are abstinent from alcohol but otherwise remain unchanged from their former alcohol-abusing selves. The lesson of this chapter is not that abstinence is good, but that uncontrolled, symptomatic abuse of alcohol is painful.

5 ∼ Return to Asymptomatic Drinking

Twenty years ago, D. L. Davies (1962) startled the world of alcohol treatment by reporting normal drinking in recovered alcoholics. His provocative report and others that followed it (summarized by Pattison et al. 1977) challenged the belief that alcoholism should be conceptualized as a progressive disease whose treatment was abstinence. Armor and colleagues wrote, "We have found no solid scientific evidence—only nonrigorous personal experience— for the belief that abstention is a more effective remedy than normal drinking" (1978, p. 171). Over the years, the original amazement, disbelief, and even outrage evoked by Davies's original report of return by alcoholics to asymptomatic drinking has diminished. Now at scientific conferences on alcohol treatment, return to social drinking is often presented as the preferred goal of treatment (Carroll 1978; Edwards and Grant 1980), and programs directed solely toward abstinence may sound almost apologetic.

By now those who advocate the resumption of social drinking by alcoholics have accumulated far more compelling evidence in their favor than the original seven cases presented by Davies. Epidemiologists like Cahalan (1970) have found that after four years 50 percent of their identified problem drinkers seem to be drinking normally. Students of experimental drinking behavior (Merry 1966; Paredes et al. 1973; Mello and Mendelson 1970; Gottheil et al. 1973) and many others have shown that in a laboratory setting, confirmed alcoholics can drink with moderation. Other work shows that the concept of loss of the capacity for controlled drinking is, at best, a relative concept (Marlatt and Rohsenow 1980). Hodgson and colleagues suggest that "The control of drinking, like any other behavior, is a function of cues and consequences, of set and setting, of psychological and social variables; in

278

short, control or loss of it, is a function of the way in which the alcoholic construes his situation" (1979, p. 380). Finally, building on the fact that contingencies and schedules of reinforcement have a great deal to do with what we call alcoholic drinking, learning theorists (Caddy and Lovibond 1976; Hamburg 1975; Lovibond and Caddy 1970; Sobell and Sobell 1978a) have shown that alcoholics can be successfully taught to return to social drinking in the community.

Perhaps the most dramatic case of return to asymptomatic drinking in the literature was reported by Kendell (1965). This case was an alcoholic whose uncontrolled drinking began at 24 and became increasingly severe between the ages of 30 and 40, but who at 42 developed an inexplicable nausea in response to whiskey and suddenly could not drink more than two pints a day of beer or four pints on the weekend. His "recovery" from uncontrolled drinking had persisted for five years. When reinterviewed Kendell's asymptomatic former alcoholic was quite unable to explain how his aversion arose, but his case illustrates the close relationship between involuntary behavior modification and return to "social" drinking.

By way of introduction, Kendell's case serves to make two important points. First, what such alcoholics return to is not carefree or social drinking but controlled or asymptomatic drinking. It is possible for some alcoholics to drink again in safety just as it is possible for some diabetics and some obese people to eat sweets—just so long as they observe numerous safeguards. Kendell's case developed an inexplicable aversion to whiskey and an inability to drink more than a limited quantity of beer; thus he developed the capacity for controlled, not "normal," drinking.

The second point is that the assertion that an alcoholic has returned to asymptomatic drinking demands definition and must take into account the frame of reference of the observer. Unfortunately, the laboratory is not the clinic. Thus, despite the claim of researchers that alcoholics can return to social drinking, clinicians who work in the front lines of public alcohol-treatment centers tend to continue to view abstinence as the only goal. They observe alcoholics for longer periods of time than laboratory researchers and under more naturalistic conditions. Max Glatt, a clinician who had devoted the greater part of his professional life to working with alcoholics, wrote, "The cardinal rule at the present state of knowledge still remains that the alcoholic has to refrain from taking alcoholic drinks altogether for the rest of his life" (quoted by Robinson 1974, p. 124).

In clinical settings, alcohol workers are confronted with individuals who have tried again and again to cut down and failed or who after detoxification and a period of successful abstinence have attempted social drinking. Such clinic patients report having tried one beer or a highball; having found nothing terrible happened, they then tried two drinks with equally benign results; yet a few months later, dependent on alcohol, they once again re-applied for admission to a detoxification unit.

Sheila Blume, a highly experienced clinician, betrays utter exasperation in her critique of the Rand Report (Armor et al. 1978, p. 263): "I find the authors' statement in their summary very puzzling. They state, 'In accepting normal drinking as a form of remission we are by no means advocating that alcoholics should attempt moderate drinking after treatment. Alcoholics who have repeatedly failed to moderate their drinking, or who have irreversible physical complications due to alcohol, should not drink at all.' I know of no other kind."

Similarly, to the family of the alcoholic, drinking by their alcoholic relative may be an all or nothing phenomenon. Having been repeatedly traumatized by his previous drinking bouts, the family of an alcoholic may find themselves demoralized by an episode of intoxication that seems harmless enough to an outsider. Thus, successful return to social drinking is a matter of definition. In her pioneering article charting the "spontaneous" recovery of "ex-problem drinkers," Knupfer (1972) included among her "reformed" drinkers men who still experienced a few, as contrasted to many, alcohol-related problems. In this book, such individuals would be labeled alcohol abusers.

The whole truth about the feasibility of alcoholics' resuming controlled drinking will be found neither with the advocates of abstinence who work in the trenches of public alcohol clinics nor among advocates of return to social drinking who work in the safety of the laboratory. There are many reasons why this should be so. First, clinicians tend only to encounter alcoholics during periods of relapse. Alcoholics who return to asymptomatic drinking feel too well or too guilty to recontact the clinician. Nor, like many abstinent alcoholics, will controlled drinkers be reported to the clinician via the grapevine, as is true sometimes of abstinent alcoholics attending AA meetings.

Second, since alcohol dependence is more severe among clinic populations, even clinicians who follow recovered patients will encounter alcoholics who return to social drinking less frequently than will epidemiologists who study community populations of alcoholics. Consider the findings reported in Chapter 3. On the one hand, in the Core City sample of alcohol abusers, drawn as it was from the community, 18 of the 110 identified alcohol abusers had returned to social drinking. On the other hand, in the Clinic sample, drawn as it was from a hospital detoxification unit, after eight years only 5 out of 106 patients were observed to return to asymptomatic drinking—or proportionately only a quarter as many. Indeed, the Clinic sample figure of 5 percent is remarkably similar to the proportions noted in the clinical literature. In his original report, Davies (1962) noted that 7 out of 93 alcoholics returned to social drinking. Gerard and Saenger (1966) found that 35 of their 797 clinic patients (4 percent) returned to social drinking. Other studies that have followed clinic patients have reported that between 5 and 10 percent will resume a stable pattern of asymptomatic drinking (Selzer and Holloway 1957; Norvig and Nielsen 1956; Moore and Ramseur 1960; Reinert and Bowen 1968; Kendell and Staton 1966; Bailey and Stewart 1967; Rakko-lainen and Turunen 1969; Orford and Edwards 1977).

Third, return to asymptomatic drinking will be most evident in fine-grained analyses of alcoholics' drinking like those by Orford and Edwards (1977), Sobell and Sobell (1978), and Armor and colleagues (1978) which report on drinking behavior in time frames as short as one month. Initially, Armor and his colleagues wrote, "The data give no reason to believe that normal drinking is prelude to relapse . . . at any one time about as many alcoholics are drinking normally as are abstaining for relatively long periods" (pp. 154–155). When, after four years of follow-up, their concept of "relatively long periods" was changed from one to six months to one to two years, the same group of investigators found that many of their social drinkers had relapsed (Polich et al. 1981).

Finally, what might be viewed as abstinence or alcohol abuse by the clinician may both be labeled return to social drinking by the researcher. For example, the reason why the group of alcoholics "trained" by the Sobells to drink in a "controlled" fashion achieved a greater proportion of "well-func-tioning" days at the end of two years than did the group taught to be abstinent was that the former group actually spent more time *abstinent* (Sobell and Sobell 1976). Similarly, in their eight-year follow-up of felons, Goodwin and colleagues (1971) suggested that half of the remitted alcoholics had returned to "social drinking"; however, their definition of social drinking—using al-cohol once a month for a year—is a definition that could be redefined as virtual abstinence. At the other end of the spectrum, Armor and colleagues (1978) put the upper limit of "social drinking" as drinking regularly for a

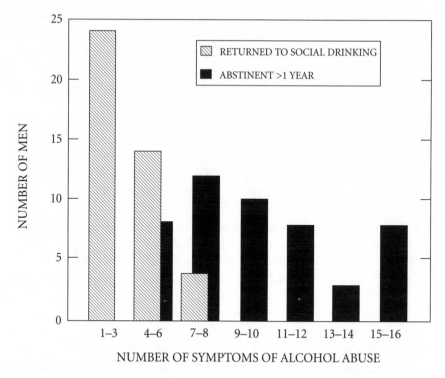

NUMBER OF SYMPTOMS OF ALCOHOL ABUSE

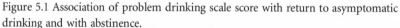

Figure 5.1 Association of problem drinking scale score with return to asymptomatic drinking and with abstinence.

month (or six months) without exceeding three ounces of absolute alcohol (the equivalent of seven martinis) in a day. A clinician or a relative might suggest that such a definition could embrace many alcohol abusers.

This chapter will first examine the differences in the severity of alcoholism among the Core City men who could and could not return to asymptomatic drinking. Next, the differences in the antecedents and in the consequences of these different outcomes will be searched for. Finally, the etiological factors that might contribute to return to asymptomatic drinking will be explored.

Return to social drinking is defined here as drinking more often than once a month for two years without experiencing any problems on the PDS. There were 42 men who were so classified who had ever had scores of two or more on the PDS.

TABLE 5.1.   Severity of alcoholism and other drug use in returned-to-social drinkers and in those whose pattern of alcohol abuse conformed to the model of a progressive illness.

	Currently abstinent or progressive alcoholism (n = 69±4)[a]	*Returned-to-social drinking (n = 42)*
Severity of alcoholism		
Alcohol dependence (DSM III)	75%	21%***
7+ Cahalan symptoms	72	19***
Abused alcohol > 80% of adult life	19	5*
Binge drinker	70	24***
Multiple alcohol-related job problems	41	2***
Multiple alcohol-related medical problems	30	0***
Morning drinking	81	17***
Ever attended clinic or AA	56	10***
Other drug use		
Heavy smoker (2+ packs/day)	55	26**
Regular use of mood-altering drugs	34	14*

a. Information was not always available for the most severe alcoholics.
*p < .05; **p < .01; ***p < .001 (chi-square test).

Figure 5.1 illustrates that for the Core City men the severity of prior alcohol abuse was the critical difference between alcohol abusers who recovered through abstinence and those who recovered by return to asymptomatic drinking. Only 11 of 38 men who at time of interview had been currently abstinent for a year or more had fewer than eight problems on the PDS; none experienced fewer than four items; their average score was 9±3 items. In contrast, only 18 of the 42 men who had ever experienced two or more problems on the PDS and who now at time of interview were drinking asymptomatically ever experienced four or more symptoms on the PDS, and none experienced more than 8. Of these 42 returned-to-social drinkers, the average PDS score was 4±2. Figure 5.1 suggests an almost complete separation of symptom severity between the currently abstinent and the returned-to-social drinkers.

Severity of alcoholism is difficult to define with precision. To strengthen their resolve, men who have chosen abstinence as a course may tend to exaggerate the pain of their alcohol abuse. Thus, Table 5.1 contrasts 73 currently abstinent or progressive alcoholics with 42 returned-to-social drinkers along as many different dimensions of severity as possible. Only one-fifth of the now asymptomatic problem drinkers had ever met either Cahalan's or the DSM III's definition of alcoholism. Reports of binge drinking and morning drinking were rare, and multiple medical problems—the hallmark of the emergency room alcoholic—were virtually never experienced. Only 4 of the men were known to have sought help from an alcohol clinic. The returned-to-social drinkers were also less likely to use other drugs heavily.

Skeptics may suggest that our interviewers were taken in by men who merely denied their alcohol abuse. In some cases, this may have been true; but wives' reports when available, absence of arrest records, and recent physical exams all supported the fact that these men were reporting their use of alcohol correctly. More convincing, perhaps, was the fact that the mean duration of reported asymptomatic drinking (after a period of alcohol abuse) was 11 years. An alcoholic can deny symptoms for a year but not for a decade.

∼ Asymptomatic Drinking Revisited

Fifteen years later, however, this last sentence betrays bravado. Alcoholics *can* deny symptoms for a decade. Unlike the case of stable abstinence, the number of men with stable return to controlled drinking did not increase with time. At age 60, only 18 Core City men manifested stable return to controlled drinking (Table 3.9A). Only 6 of these were among the 42 men classified in 1977 (Table 5.1) as having, even briefly, returned to asymptomatic drinking. By 1992 the other 36 Core City men were no longer classified as having stably returned to controlled drinking, for the following reasons: 6 had withdrawn from the study, 9 had relapsed, 6 had become stably abstinent, 8 had never met the DSM III criteria for alcohol abuse, and 7 were DSM III alcohol abusers who had been reclassified as social drinkers because of their brief history of alcohol abuse.

Table 5.1A shows that the 18 Core City men who are currently classified as experiencing sustained return to controlled drinking had experienced more severe alcohol histories than had the 42 former alcohol abusers who had appeared to be drinking in an asymptomatic fashion at age 47. As a result, Table 5.1A reveals the difficulty of predicting who among the Core City alcohol abusers would eventually maintain a pattern of returned to controlled drinking and who would not. The men who returned to controlled drinking

TABLE 5.1A. Contrast between Core City returned-to-social drinkers and abstinent or chronic alcohol abusers at age 47 and age 60.

	Return to asymptomatic drinking	*Sustained return to controlled drinking*	*Stable abstinence or continued alcohol abuse*
	Age 47 *n = 42*	*Age 60* *n = 18*	*Age 60[a]* *n = 96*
Severity of alcoholism			
Alcohol dependence (DSM III)	21%	50%	58%
7+ Cahalan symptoms	19	39	55
9+ PDS symptoms	0	28	45
Binge drinker	24	50	50
Multiple alcohol-related job problems	2	17	25
Multiple alcohol-related medical problems	0	6	20
Morning drinking	17	39	66
Ever attended alcohol clinic or AA	10	44	40
Heavy smoker	2	39	44
Presence of risk factors for alcoholism			
Two or more alcoholic relatives	31	11	35
No Mediterranean ethnicity	79	83	89
School behavior problems	2	6	10
Hyperactivity	7	0	15[b]
IQ > 99	24	11	42[b]
Dead or poor health at age 60	—	50	70

a. Range 84–96 depending on missing values.

b. $p < .01$ (significance of differences between the 18 RTCD men and the 91 men who became abstinent or remained alcoholic at age 60).

were a little more likely to have Mediterranean ancestry and somewhat less likely to have alcoholic relatives, hyperactivity, and behavior problems when in school. There were no differences in their childhood environments or in their adult mental health. Surprisingly, those who returned to controlled drinking by age 60 were less likely to manifest above-average intelligence. The fact that 6 of the 18 men had either very poor mental health or an I.Q. under 80 or both may have meant that over time they were more likely to find themselves in restricted living settings where alcohol abuse was less possible. The relatively good objective physical health of the men who reported return to controlled drinking also supports the veracity of their reports.

It is instructive to look at the 9 Core City men who had met DSM III criteria for alcohol dependence and yet in 1992 were classified as having returned to controlled drinking. Three men were on the borderline between social drinking and abstinence. The first was a very severe alcoholic with a PDS of 17 who had maintained a pattern of controlled drinking for eight years prior to his death. He reported drinking only one to two beers a month, just above the limit used to define abstinence. His control over alcohol use may have been facilitated by the fact that he was blind and thus lacked easy access to alcohol. A second man had been drinking in a controlled fashion for 20 years, but he often tested his control by abstaining from alcohol for periods of three months to a year. The third man had experienced progressive alcoholism until age 50 when he began a steady reduction in his drinking. He had been problem-free for the last eight years and had reported complete abstinence for the last three months.

Two men had maintained a stable pattern of controlled drinking for more than 20 years, but in both of these cases the original classification of alcohol dependence was in question. In 2 other men with former alcohol dependence the classification of return to controlled drinking was made on rather doubtful evidence. The control of the eighth man over alcohol was facilitated by living in a supervised group home and by his chronic schizophrenia, which left him without the social skills to obtain money to buy alcohol.

Thus, in only one case was there an unambiguous evolution from clear alcohol dependence to a pattern of controlled drinking without extenuating circumstances. This man manifested severe alcohol dependence (PDS = 9) and yet has been a daily drinker without problems for the last nine years. The shift in his pattern of alcohol abuse may have been facilitated by a new marriage in 1980.

Case Histories

Larry Green's case history illustrates both that reports of *recent* return to asymptomatic drinking were sometimes unreliable and that with time the truth emerges. Larry Green met both the Cahalan and the PDS criteria for alcohol abuse but not those for alcohol dependence. When he was 47, his interviewer rated his pattern of alcohol use for the previous four years as "probably social." Larry denied having ever been "high" or "tight" prior to that time, but for ten years he had been going nightly to barrooms, and as he put it, "who goes to a barroom and just has five drinks?" He also had been drinking in the morning "when I felt like it." Ten years earlier his doctor had warned him of severe liver disease, but at that time he could not cut down his intake of alcohol. Then, four years prior to the interview, he had been granted welfare because of "cardiomyopathy secondary to alcoholism." Un-employed, he had left the city to live with his mother in the country; since then, he maintained, he had been unable to afford to go to barrooms or to abuse alcohol. He said he now drank a couple of vodka highballs a night without problems. His classification as a returned-to-social drinker seemed dubious, but we had no good evidence to doubt his word.

Four years after the interview, Larry Green was admitted to a local hospital. His admission physical exam revealed "an emaciated man devastated by the chronic effects of alcoholism with clear evidence of ascites" (that is, severe liver disease). Seven days later Larry Green, aged 51, was dead of "cardio-myopathy due to alcoholism" and cirrhosis. Despite his own perceptions, his use of vodka over the past eight years had not been asymptomatic.

As Edwards wrote: "The fact of dependence will rob the individual's drug taking behavior of some of its plasticity; the degree will be determined by the degree to which dependence has been established" (1974, p. 190). While stages of physical and psychological dependence are difficult to define, the more the abuse of alcohol is under conscious control, the more easily it can be modulated voluntarily. The more that alcohol use reflects conditioned, habitual involuntary behavior (whether on a physiological, a psychological, or even a social basis), the more difficult it will be for the patient to return to moderate use of alcohol.

Consider, as an analogy, how easily the amount of eggs or cereal one eats for breakfast can be modulated but that the number of salted peanuts one eats at a party is less simple to control. In contrast, consider how difficult it is for a long-standing two-pack-a-day smoker, who knows that cigarettes are injurious to his health and who no longer enjoys the cigarettes he does smoke, to exert conscious control over cigarette use.

The literature is uniform in concordance with the findings depicted in Figure 5.1. The alcohol abusers who successfully return to asymptomatic drinking were previously less dependent on alcohol than alcohol abusers who achieve remission of symptoms only through abstinence. In their careful two-year follow-up of 100 clinic patients, Orford and Edwards (1977) noted

10 patients who appeared to have returned to asymptomatic drinking and 11 who were abstinent. The two samples could be almost completely dichotomized along the dimension of physiological dependence. In their four-year follow-up of alcohol clinic attenders, Polich and colleagues (1981) contrasted 117 men who had abstained for a year, 57 men who had returned to asymptomatic drinking, and 196 symptomatic drinkers. Like the heavy drinkers in the College sample, described in Chapter 3, the 57 men who resumed asymptomatic drinking represented a particularly stable group. They were more likely to be married, to be employed, and to be well paid than either the men who chose abstinence or the symptomatic drinkers. Vogler and colleagues (1977) contrasted 20 men who chose abstinence with 73 men who returned to controlled drinking. The latter reported only half as many years of heavy drinking, a third as many lost jobs and a sixth as many prior detoxifications. In short, severe alcoholics usually seek out abstinence as a goal and heavy social drinkers often seem capable of reversing their pattern of abuse.

In line with such findings, Polich and colleagues (1981) observed that young, employed alcohol abusers without physiological dependence actually did better at four years if 18 months after treatment they had achieved "controlled" drinking rather than abstinence. In contrast, alcohol-dependent men over 40 were better off at four years if at 18 months they had attempted to abstain. Alcoholics who chose abstinence were twice as likely as asymptomatic drinkers to view alcoholism as an irreversible disease that led to death and to believe they were alcoholic. The grim truth, however, was that after four years of follow-up the age-adjusted death rate of these heavy but "controlled" drinkers was one and a half times that of the abstainers.

On the one hand, the patient remanded to a clinic for the first time for driving while intoxicated or the individual whose spouse has only just insisted that he get help for a drinking problem may sometimes represent a population for whom clinical support of reduced alcohol consumption may very well be a legitimate first step of treatment. On the other hand, the more the patient's history reveals past failures at controlled drinking, the more insistently clinicians should support a goal of abstinence rather than of reduced intake.

In saying this, I do not mean that when observed for a period of weeks or even months, severe alcoholics—especially under favorable circumstances—cannot markedly cut down on their drinking. Alcohol abuse is nothing if not plastic. Nevertheless, when the lives of the men in both the Core City and the College samples were looked at in a perspective of years rather than months, the issue became increasingly black and white. There appeared to be a point of no return beyond which efforts to return to social drinking became analogous to driving a car without a spare tire. Disaster was simply a matter of time.

An attractive hypothesis is that the less emotionally stable and the more environmentally and genetically vulnerable the alcohol abuser, the more likely he is to experience such a point of no return. After all, Figure 3.1 illustrated that positive mental health was highly associated with the capacity to use alcohol in moderation for a lifetime. However, this hypothesis does not explain return to asymptomatic drinking. Statistically, the men who returned to asymptomatic drinking did not experience more childhood strengths or fewer weaknesses than did the progressive alcohol abusers. The two groups of alcohol abusers did not differ in I.Q., boyhood competence, attained education, maternal supervision, or number of alcoholic relatives. The 18 returned-to-social drinkers who ever experienced four or more symptoms on the PDS did so at just as early an age as alcoholics who continued to abuse alcohol.

Ethnicity was the one premorbid factor that perhaps was prognostically influential. Although the numbers are small, it may be significant that of the 31 alcohol abusers of Irish extraction, 36 percent are currently abstinent, while this is true for only 19 percent of the 21 alcohol abusers of Mediterranean extraction. It is consistent with Irish culture to see the use of alcohol in terms of black or white, good or evil, drunkenness or complete abstinence, while in Italian culture it is the distinction between moderate drinking and drunkenness that is most important (Jellinek 1960).

An argument might be made that although virtually all the Core City sociopaths abused alcohol, not all become dependent. Therefore, if in middle life such non-alcohol-dependent sociopaths returned to asymptomatic drinking, their poor childhoods might statistically dilute the good childhood adjustment of the other psychologically healthier men who, through strength of character, returned to social drinking. This argument is untenable. In fact, Table 5.2 documents that very few of the returned-to-social drinkers exhibited multiple problems on the Robins scale. On the one hand, when alcohol abuse began as a "symptom" of an antisocial life style, it still progressed to become indistinguishable from "real" or "primary" alcoholism. On the other hand, in both the College sample (Vaillant 1980a) and the Core City sample, whether the alcohol abuser progressed to dependence or was able to return to social drinking remained remarkably independent of premorbid adjustment.

Table 5.2 confirms the supposition that the later life adjustment of those

TABLE 5.2.   Differences in adult adjustment between the returned-to-social drinkers and those whose pattern of alcohol abuse conformed with the model of a progressive illness.

Adult adjustment variable	Currently abstinent or progressive alcoholism (n = 68±5)	Returned-to-social drinking (n = 42)	Significance[a]
Number of symptoms on Robins's scale of sociopathy	4.6±2.9	2.6±1.2	< .001
% of adult life married	54±34	71±31	< .01
HSRS score	67±16	76±10	< .001
Physical health (1 = best; 5 = dead)	2.5±1.1	2.0±1.0	< .05
Enjoyment of children (1 = clear; 3 = none)	2.2±1.1	1.6±0.8	< .01
Income (1978 dollars/year)	11,000±7,000	15,000±7,000	< .01
% of adult life unemployed	20±23	7±12	< .001

The two middle columns are headed by *Average score and standard deviation of ratings on adult adjustment*.

a. Student's T-test was the statistic used.

who successfully returned to social drinking was clearly superior to that of those whose alcoholism progressed. Although their childhoods were not different, the percentage of adult life spent married and employed, and the level of income and of physical and global mental health were very different between the progressive alcoholics and the returned-to-social drinkers.

What were the paths that led alcohol abusers to return to social drinking? Certainly, these paths were not the formal avenues of treatment described in Table 4.2. No Core City men returned to asymptomatic drinking through clinic treatment; only four reported attending Alcoholics Anonymous. One man returned to asymptomatic drinking while receiving psychotherapy, and one man credited the help he received at a halfway house.

In half of the cases, the returned-to-social drinkers reported that effective confrontation had made them recognize that a change in their drinking patterns was essential. But confrontation in alcohol abuse is common. Indeed, the more symptomatic the alcoholic, the more frequent and the more dramatic such confrontation is likely to be. Thus, confrontation alone cannot explain why some men return to asymptomatic drinking while others progress to dependence. The compelling question becomes why was the man who returned to social drinking less deaf and blind to confrontation than his more symptomatic alcohol-dependent counterpart? What is the process by which any agreeable habit creates cognitive dissonance and then becomes ego-alien? What are the forces that as a result of such dissonance lead to behavioral change?

A Core City subject who illustrated this riddle was Carl Erickson, a 48-year-old man who had abused alcohol from age 30 until his retirement from the army at age 40. During army duty, he developed a pattern of drinking a quart of whiskey and a case of beer (22 drinks a day) over the weekend. For the next three days he would suffer from gastric pain. As a result of alcohol, he experienced multiple accidents and blackouts and his marriage suffered.

When Carl was 48, his wife supported his assertion that for the previous eight years his drinking had caused no problems. But how did he come to "realize that drinking was controlling my life" and then successfully control his drinking? At age 40, a series of six linked events occurred that facilitated Carl Erickson's return to asymptomatic drinking. First, he changed to a civilian job, which meant leaving an environment of inexpensive post exchange alcohol and heavy-drinking army buddies. Second, toward the end of his army tour his wife had become increasingly angry with his coming home late. He "began to realize the drinking was controlling my life," and he stopped drinking outside his home. Third, he said that a friend in AA had been "an eye-opener" for him. He began to notice that people who drank at work got into multiple accidents and that they had difficulty performing their work when drinking. Fourth, he spoke of the films that his AA friends had showed him that made him realize the physiological effects of heavy drinking. He explained, "you have to realize yourself what it does to you, what alcohol does to your body." Fifth, it must be remembered that already his stomach complaints had kept him from drinking throughout the week. Finally, he had controlled his drinking by keeping his social life at a minimum and thereby avoiding many opportunities to drink.*

Again, in understanding remission or change of habits, it is important to ask the right questions of the right people. Serially linked questions and attention to the subjects' associations are important. For example, Knupfer

---

*The subject has been followed until 1992, and he has maintained a pattern of drinking three beers a week.

(1972) cites an alcoholic in remission who reported that he just "quit" because he thought it would be better for his health. Probing revealed that "quit" meant cutting down to one or two drinks a day, and interviewing his wife revealed that he had developed an ulcer that caused him to be sick if he exceeded two drinks.

Table 5.3 expands on this vignette. It contrasts the events that were associated with abstinence and with return to asymptomatic drinking among the Core City men. As might be expected, substitutes for alcohol were unimportant for men who never gave up drinking. Rather, it was medical consequences, dramatic confrontations, and altered contingencies associated with drinking that appeared most important for the men who returned to asymptomatic drinking. Since many progressive alcoholics manifest the most extraordinary ability to deny the consequences of their drinking, what allowed those who returned to social drinking to become and remain conscious of the need to control their drinking remains somewhat mysterious. Analogous to the behavior modification studies of experimentally induced return to social drinking, some Core City men experienced environmental cues or learned techniques that helped maintain in their consciousness the need to limit intake. These cues ranged from one man's recurrent memories of having killed a man while drunk to another man's sudden recognition that his morning shakiness meant he was alcohol-dependent. Nine men developed disturbing medical consequences that interfered with their ability to abuse alcohol. For example, a man who had abused alcohol for 20 years cut down when he began to experience alcohol-associated palpitations, nightmares, and one-sided headaches. Bailey and Steward (1967) reported six problem drinkers who had returned to social drinking for two and one-half years and whose spouses supported this assertion. In four of their cases, alcohol-related aversive medical problems facilitated their return to social drinking. Obviously, there is much further research to be done; this book offers only the most preliminary answers.

Often external control was attained more laboriously and ingeniously than just by conscious linkage of heavy drinking with distressing physical symptoms. I think of a middle-aged two-pack-a-day smoker who became a controlled smoker by timing each cigarette he smoked for the rest of his life. The point is that "control" is critical, and although such control employs cognitive processes the process is more complex than willpower. Of the 22 returned-to-social drinkers depicted in Table 5.3, 7 men manifested such a pattern of carefully controlled drinking. They would limit themselves to heavy

TABLE 5.3.   Nontreatment factors associated with abstinence and return to social drinking.

Factor	Important for	
	Return to social drinking (n = 22)[a]	Abstinence (n = 49)
Substitute	5%	53%
Behavior modification		
Compulsory supervision or sustained confrontation	41	24
Medical consequences	27	49
Enhanced hope/self-esteem		
Increased religious involvement	5	12
Alcoholics Anonymous	0	37
Social rehabilitation		
New love relationship	18	32

a. This includes the three men who met the DSM III criteria for dependence and the one man who met Cahalan's criteria for problem drinking but who did not experience 4 or more problems on the PDS.

drinking one night a week. The beverage chosen was almost always beer (one to four quarts at a sitting), and what distinguished this pattern from their prior use of alcohol was that once they ritualized their intake of alcohol it no longer interfered with their lives.

For example, one Core City man would take a cab to the bar at 10:30 every Saturday night and a cab home when the bar closed at 1:00. He knew that he could not moderate how much he drank, and so for years he had imposed these external limits on his drinking. Similarly, a College man on rare occasions would buy two two-ounce "nips" of gin, take them back to his house, and, with his wife in attendance, drink them. Such patterns have been well described by Reinert and Bowen in their valuable paper on return to asymptomatic social drinking. Such a drinker, they write, "must be on guard . . . must choose carefully and even compulsively the time, the place and the circumstances of drinking; and he must rigidly limit the amount he drinks" (1968, p. 268).

Besides the 7 Core City alcohol abusers who returned to controlled drinking, there were 12 men who returned to more spontaneous social drinking. Several of these men were successful in using the familiar strategies that repeatedly fail for many progressive alcoholics. These strategies included switching from high- to low-proof alcohol, avoiding drinking at bars, and moving to new environments. Finally, there were 2 men who had switched to beer, who continued to be heavy daily drinkers (5 quarts of beer—12 drinks—a day), but who did not admit difficulties. It appeared doubtful whether these 2 men were actually drinking asymptomatically.

∿ Return to Controlled Drinking Revisited

When the original version of this book was published in 1983, it provided support both to the advocates of abstinence and to advocates of helping alcohol abusers return to controlled drinking. In a personal communication, a prominent publicist of controlled drinking, Stanton Peele, noted that in Table 5.3 I had identified 22 alcohol abusers who had returned to a stable pattern of controlled drinking, whereas in Chapter 4 I had identified only 21 men with stable abstinence. At Peele's instigation I began tracking these two samples. The results of 15 years of further follow-up are summarized in Table 5.3A. The 21 men who had achieved three or more years of abstinence have tended to maintain that abstinence until death or until the present time. As noted in Chapter 4, one man returned to controlled drinking, 1 relapsed after 13 years, and 1 has been lost to follow-up. The mean length of abstinence of the remaining Core City men is 20 years. Such stability of abstinence manifested by the men in Table 5.3A would seem at stark variance with the Sobells' undocumented assertion that "The strength of the abstinence consensus is matched only by the lack of evidence that stable abstinence is ever achieved by very many of those individuals who had uncontestedly been considered severely dependent on alcohol" (1987, p. 245).

In contrast, of the 22 men originally classified as returned to asymptomatic drinking, only 5 are currently classified as returned to controlled drinking. Three men have been reclassified as social drinkers because of minimal symptoms; 4 have been lost to follow-up or withdrawn from the study; 7 have relapsed; and 3 have become stably abstinent. In short, prolonged follow-up of alcoholics who maintain that they are abstinent does not reveal surprises. In contrast, prolonged follow-up of individuals who claim they have returned to controlled drinking often reveals relapse, gullibility of the original interviewer, or subsequent abstinence.

Indeed, Griffith Edwards's (1985) recent follow-up of the famous seven cases of D. L. Davies with which I began this chapter is a case in point. In

TABLE 5.3A.   The long-term course of men identified in 1976 as enjoying either stable abstinence or return to controlled drinking.

	1976 Status	
1992 status	3+ years of abstinence n = 21	3+ years of controlled drinking n = 22
Abstinent	18	3
Controlled drinking	1	8[b]
Relapse	1[a]	7
Dropped out or lost	1[a]	4[c]

a. Prior to relapse or loss of contact both these men were abstinent for 13 years.

b. Three of these 8 men abused alcohol only briefly with minimal symptoms.

c. The mean length of controlled drinking prior to loss of contact was 8 years.

1962 Davies had reported sustained "normal drinking" in seven men over a follow-up period of 7–11 years. Edwards refollowed the same sample, extending the total observation period to approximately 29–34 years and whenever possible using multiple sources of information. He found convincing evidence that five of Davies's subjects had experienced significant drinking problems both during Davies's original follow-up period and subsequently. Of his two remaining subjects, one man was never severely dependent on alcohol.

In 1989 one of the Sobells' 14 allegedly successful outcomes was quoted by Maltzman (1989) as saying that "the data in the Sobells' table for the second follow-up year identified by my initials, O. L., shows me as being drunk only three days for that entire year. Similar data in the third year follow-up table . . . shows me as being drunk only six days for the entire year. Actually, I was drunk . . . approximately 92 days per year" (p. 469).

In reinterviewing the College men I have discovered that I, too, am overly trusting. I personally interviewed a long-time College alcohol abuser when he was 67 and had retired to East Hampton, Long Island. He told me that his alcohol use had come under control in the last few years because of a painful bleeding ulcer. He asserted that while their social life made abstinence for him and his wife impossible, he avoided hard liquor and kept only "small amounts of beer and wine in the house." Three years later in his questionnaire, he wrote that he consumed only two or three drinks a day. However, since, "several other illnesses had taken their toll," his doctor had told him he should "cut down his alcohol use because of other medications." He also wrote that his doctor had prescribed folic acid (a common vitamin supplement for alcohol abusers) but that "I don't know why." On the basis of his assertion of five years of apparently problem-free drinking, I classified him in Figure 3.5A as having returned to controlled drinking during the period from age 66 to 70.

His age-72 questionnaire arrived after the manuscript had been completed. He still only hinted at the clinical reality. He acknowledged that medical illnesses had continued to take their toll. He had fallen and broken his left arm; his toe had been amputated "due to arthritis"; and he had had a subtotal gastrectomy because of continued gastric hemorrhage. He did admit that he had recently gone on the wagon on his doctor's advice and that he sometimes felt guilty about his drinking.

Then his hospital reports arrived. His age-70 medical chart revealed that he had been drinking at least a bottle of wine (5–6 drinks) a day. This high alcohol consumption was the probable cause of his gastrectomy. Alcoholic neuropathy had definitely been the cause of the loss of his toe and the reason for his mysterious folic acid prescription. Examination of both his blood and his liver enzymes provided further evidence of alcohol abuse. His age-72 hospital chart revealed that the cause of his broken arm was a fall sustained after an evening of heavy drinking. On admission, his blood alcohol level had been 200mg/100ml and his liver enzymes revealed worsening damage. On discharge he became only the second of the 52 College alcohol abusers to be diagnosed with alcoholic cirrhosis.

On the one hand, I must sympathize with the gullibility of those who believe that controlled drinking is as common an outcome as their interviewees insist. On the other hand, the reader may feel more sympathetic with the intellectual intransigence of the alcohol clinic workers who seem so unduly mistrustful whenever alcohol abusers assert their resumption of "problem-free" drinking.

An example from the College sample of the instability of apparent return to controlled drinking is provided by Donald Davies. In 1970 his wife had begun complaining about his drinking. He himself reported having "many regular" drinks, and he had had repeated difficulties with drunken driving. Soon both he and his friends joined his wife in believing that he drank too much. By 1974 he was having three drinks at lunch and three drinks at cocktail time, and was consuming at least a pint of whiskey a day. He began to have blackouts, and would feel nervous the morning after a hard night's drinking. He noted that he drank like his sister who was an alcoholic but had never admitted it.

In 1975 Donald Davies tried to cut down to half a bottle of wine a day. Nevertheless, his wife continued to believe that her husband's "pattern of life revolved around the next drink." By 1977 he was drinking enough sherry that his physician recommended that he cut down. In 1979 he went on the wagon. In 1981, after a year and a half of abstinence, he again began to drink two drinks a day, writing to the study that "we shall see." On this evidence, for the age 60 quinquennial evaluation he was classified as return to controlled drinking.

By 1983 Davies had increased his intake. He felt guilty about his drinking and his wife again complained. In 1985 he challenged, "I am obviously a heavy drinker, but am I a problem one?" He was now back up to more than eight ounces of hard liquor a day; and he responded "yes" to all four questionnaire possibilities: "Some people think I drink too much"; "My wife thinks I drink too much"; "I feel guilty about my drinking"; and "My doctor has told me to cut down." In 1987 he again reported that he was drinking without problems. In 1989 he again reported drinking six to seven drinks a day. This time he chose not to answer the yes/no questions designed to identify problem drinking. Instead he wrote, "I suppose there are some people who feel I drink more than is good for me; most of them I left behind in Lake Forest." In 1991 he again did not answer the yes/no questions regarding problems. Instead he wrote, "I suppose I'd be classified as a heavy drinker, make that four to six drinks a day." On this basis at age 65 and 70 the study again classified Donald Davies as abusing alcohol.

After ten years of following a treatment cohort of 99 men, Edwards and his colleagues (1986) reported a single case of a man who after a 25-year career of alcohol abuse had achieved six to seven years of controlled drinking. In part, his control was maintained by a recurrent bleeding ulcer, which meant that "I will always feel that I need to constantly monitor my drinking behavior" (p. 131). In other words, instead of relying on willpower he had acquired a permanent external monitor to remind him to maintain control. Fortunately, six pints of beer made him feel "physically very uncomfortable . . . the whole of my stomach would just become so bloated and uncomfortable" (p. 132).

The conclusion, then, should not be that alcohol-dependent individuals never return to social drinking but only that it is a rare and often an unstable state. One often-cited longitudinal study of return to controlled drinking was carried out by Nordstrom and Berglund (1987). In a follow-up of the best outcomes among 324 alcoholics over 11–31 years, they were able to identify 15 men (5 percent) who returned to controlled drinking for 5 years or more.

In perhaps the best-designed study of clinic-treated alcohol abusers that has been done to date, Helzer and colleagues (1985) found that only 2 percent of alcoholics returned to social drinking for more than one or two years. Helzer and his colleagues took care to avoid the methodological pitfalls that often plague outcome research: they established the validity of their diagnosis of alcohol abuse; they used a minimum follow-up period of three years; they corroborated all self-reports with reports by family members; and they obtained a representative sample of alcoholics by sampling contrasting treatment facilities. Out of 1,289 men and women with a definite diagnosis of alcoholism, 66.5 percent were classified as continuing to abuse alcohol, 15 percent as having been totally abstinent, and 12 percent as heavy drinkers (having more than six drinks at a sitting for more than four days a month). Only 14 of their 1,289 subjects met their three criteria for sustained moderate drinking: being totally abstinent for no more than six of the previous 36 months, not exceeding an intake of six or more drinks four times a month, and no interview or recorded evidence of alcohol-related medical, legal, social or occupational problems over the preceding three years. Such limits, after all, would not exclude most lifelong social drinkers. Helzer could have increased the number of individuals who returned to controlled drinking to 41 if he had included those who alternated between occasional drinking and abstinence. But even 41 out of 1,289 alcohol abusers is not an encouraging proportion.

Behavioral Training

Alcohol abuse must always create dissonance in the mind of the abuser; alcohol is both ambrosia and poison. Sometimes such dissonance may be resolved in a manner analogous to sudden religious conversion or career change. A symbolic straw breaks the already heavily burdened camel's back. Thus, in a few cases, salutary change in the Core City and College men's drinking habits appeared to be derived from the effect of a traumatic event such as the death of a parent. An example was a Core City man who was a very heavy, but not alcohol-dependent, drinker: until the age of 40, he would drink a quart of whiskey each night on the weekends and during the week he would have many drinks in bars. For the previous five years he had been asymptomatic—drinking entirely at home and never exceeding six cans of beer in a day. Initially he said he had changed his drinking because of reduced finances. Then he revealed that shortly after his father had died, a close drinking friend had been stabbed to death outside the barroom where they used to drink. He said that his friend's death had frightened him: "I thought there was a message there." Somehow the death of his father magnified the importance of the death of his friend. At this point, he gave up frequenting bars and drinking hard liquor. Such a sequence of events is understandable enough to a novelist, priest, or psychoanalyst who takes for granted that internalized loved ones play an important role in our behavior. However, scientific proof of such suppositions is not easy to produce. Such temporal relationships are difficult to establish as distinct from coincidence and must remain clinical conjectures.

Both laboratory studies (Marlatt and Rohsenow 1980) and studies by social psychologists (Jessor and Jessor 1975; Plant 1979) have shown that social environment is an enormously important determinant of drinking patterns. Many men with only two or three symptoms of alcohol abuse reported resuming moderate drinking habits when they got married or changed their social network.

Whereas religious involvement appeared important to abstinence through its effect on hope, morale, and self-esteem, religious involvement appeared to facilitate return to asymptomatic drinking by altering the social network. An illustration of this was a man whose drinking from age 21 to age 37 was out of control. Beginning at breakfast, he would consume six quarts of beer (15 drinks) a day. In his mid-thirties, he married a woman who belonged to a very close-knit religious sect. Having himself been raised "a hard-headed Roman Catholic," he initially would have nothing to do with his wife's religion. At 37, while driving his wife to her religious meeting, he set out to prove her belief system wrong. Having come to scoff, he stayed to pray. His drinking pattern changed. Now, after religious meetings, he drinks one glass of beer three times a week. This is usually in the company of a friend with whom he discusses the meeting. He seldom drinks on the weekend, but on selected holidays he will still drink heavily. At such times, by ceremonial design and without complications, he will consume 10 to 15 shots of whiskey.*

---

*Unfortunately, since he was 49 years old—12 years after his return to controlled drinking—no information has been obtained from this man. At age 52 he formally withdrew from the study. He did not say why.

Although in retrospective studies reactive drinking is often invoked as a cause of progressive alcoholism, among the Core City men periods of *de novo* alcohol abuse following a painful event were seen much more often among the men who returned to asymptomatic drinking. Indeed, reactive alcohol abuse appeared most commonly in the 20 men who not only returned to asymptomatic drinking but also never manifested more than three symptoms on the PDS. In such individuals, a death or a traumatic divorce would precipitate a few months of symptomatic heavy drinking; after which time the individual would spontaneously cut down and return to his earlier pattern of drinking. In other words, truly reactive drinking—motivated by a genuine wish to drown one's sorrows—rarely produced drinking with "a life of its own." Many men, however, would date the onset of their alcoholism by a specific traumatic event and minimize the import of the alcohol-related problems that predated the event.

An illustration of reactive alcohol abuse was provided by a man who had had two or three drinks a week during his entire adult life. All his life he said he had been "afraid of drinking because of my father," who had been an alcoholic. When he was 49, his wife left him, and he found he had nothing to do after work; he spent a lot of time in cocktail lounges "floundering around." For six months, he drank about ten drinks a day until he developed an ulcer that required surgery. When informed by his physician that his high alcohol intake was the cause of his ulcer, he "had a good talk" with himself, remained abstinent for three months, and then returned to his pattern of drinking three drinks a week. He said that the increased sensitivity to alcohol that resulted from his stomach surgery helped to moderate his drinking.

These observations from the Core City men who returned to social drinking should be viewed against the actual findings of three other studies that are often cited by investigators who question the need for abstinence in the treatment of alcoholism. For one thing, although alcohol abusers who return to asymptomatic drinking have been less damaged by alcohol abuse than those who seek abstinence, their outcome is not necessarily better. Gerard and colleagues (1962) found that the 41 men "still using alcohol but no longer with a drinking problem" were not better off than the abstinent men. Indeed, when they compared their 41 asymptomatic drinkers with their 55 abstinent alcoholics, twice as many of the former were found to be "at a lower end of the scale of social participation"; at follow-up six asymptomatic drinkers, but only one abstinent drinker, were alienated from family. The former had somewhat worse relationships with their employers and spouses.

Second, the men in the Rand Report who returned to "social" drinking were not entirely asymptomatic. "Normal drinking" defined by the Rand Report was not more than an average of three ounces of absolute alcohol a day (six to seven drinks) *and* no "serious symptoms." "Serious symptoms" were regarded as absent if in the past *month* an individual had had fewer than three blackouts, fewer than three days missed from work due to alcohol, and not more than four episodes of morning drinking. By the criteria of this book, even one of these symptoms in a *year* would be considered evidence of alcohol abuse.

The third and most challenging study was the Sobells' effort to train severe alcoholics to drink in moderation (Sobell and Sobell 1976, 1978a). Between 1969 and 1971, at Patton State Hospital in California, the Sobells administered to 20 (admittedly selected) alcoholics individualized behavior therapy consisting of electric shock avoidance, practice sessions of controlled consumption of alcohol, and individual therapy sessions directed toward problem-solving skills. They also presented their subjects with videotape replays of their drinking behavior both in and out of control. The Sobells used three carefully matched control groups: one to assess a similar intensity of treatment but with abstinence instead of social drinking as the goal, and two less intensively treated groups, one of which was encouraged to return to social drinking and the other to seek abstinence. The Sobells claimed that monthly they followed 69 of their original 70 subjects; geographical dispersion was no deterrent, and they used multiple collateral sources. After two years the outcome for the 20 patients chosen for the experimental groups for return to controlled drinking was clearly better than for the other three groups. In the second year, 35 percent of their experimental sample achieved "good days" for 98 percent of the year or better ("good days" meant less than seven ounces of hard liquor a day); and 85 percent of the men were able to spend at least 85 percent of the year with "good days." As noted previously, most of these "good days" were spent abstinent. In contrast to the patients in the two groups for whom abstinence was recommended, the patients in the intensely treated returned-to-social-drinking group seemed to get progressively better over time and experienced significantly fewer arrests, hospitalizations, and alcohol-related problems. As previously noted, however, they also spent more days abstinent!

The validity of the Sobells' work has been challenged by Ewing and Rouse (1976), who found that their own early success in teaching alcoholics to return to asymptomatic drinking proved four years later to have been evanescent. Sobell and Sobell (1978b) have responded by pointing out not only that Ewing and Rouse selected alcoholics who were recalcitrant to accept traditional treatment and who had a relatively poor prognosis, but also that only 14 of their 35 subjects completed as many as six treatment sessions and that Ewing and Rouse's outcome criteria may have been too stringent.

The Sobells' findings have been more convincingly challenged by Pendery and colleagues (1982) who in a painstaking 10-year follow-up of the Sobells' 20 cases found a far more disappointing clinical outcome. They summarize: "The results of our independent follow-up of the same subjects, based on official records, affidavits, and interviews, stand in marked contrast to the favorable controlled drinking outcomes reported by the Sobells and Caddy et al. Our follow-up revealed no evidence that *gamma* alcoholics had acquired the ability to engage in controlled drinking safely after being treated in the experimental program" (p. 174). At the ten-year mark for the Sobells' original 20 subjects, 9 continued to experience, at least intermittently, damage from alcohol abuse; 4 had died from alcohol-related causes; and 6 had achieved complete abstinence for several years. Only 1 subject had continued to drink in a controlled fashion for the 10-year period, and that individual was probably never alcohol-dependent. But perhaps it is not surprising that the lives of experimentally treated alcoholics would look very different in a 10-year study by critical outsiders than they did over two years to investigators intimately involved in the alcoholics' treatment. If we are to resolve our confusion about alcoholism, objectivity and longitudinal study are essential.

Probably the most serious limitation of the Sobells' treatment does not lie in their methods or assumptions; certainly their work has played a valuable heuristic role in advancing our understanding of alcoholism. Instead, the problem with the Sobells' work is more practical then scientific. Their success proved to be a tour de force rather than a therapeutic beacon for others to follow. Thus far the Sobells have been unable to respond to their own challenge that "The foundation of validating successful treatment lies in replication" (1973, p. 617). The Sobells' work was done in 1970 and 1971 and reported in book form in 1978, and after a decade they have not yet replicated their findings.

～ Behavioral Training Revisited

Further follow-up of the Sobells' career reveals that as investigators they have been absolved of any distortion of their research data, and they have continued to be productive and respected investigators. However, although they remain based at the Addiction Research Foundation, a well-endowed Toronto research institute where replication of their original findings would be possible, after almost 25 years they have never, to my knowledge, tried to replicate their original study.

It is also instructive to review the careful follow-up of 140 alcohol abusers reported by William Miller and colleagues (1992). They had treated these patients with behavioral self-control training to facilitate their return to controlled drinking in a series of replication studies. Fifty-two percent of the sample met DSM III criteria for alcohol dependence. Miller and colleagues followed these patients for $3\frac{1}{2}$–8 years. While 10 percent of their entire sample successfully returned to controlled drinking, 16 percent preferred abstinence. In addition, the vast majority of their patients were still abusing alcohol (45 percent); or were lost to follow-up (29 percent). A patient's own goal at intake, whether to seek abstinence or return to controlled drinking, only weakly predicted who would achieve abstinence and who would successfully drink in a controlled fashion. Nor did the amount of behavioral self-control training that Miller's research subjects received predict their outcome. Rather, discriminate function analysis suggested that stable return to controlled drinking was best predicted by having few severe symptoms of alcohol abuse on admission and not having alcoholic relatives.

Conclusion

Alcoholism is a problem that affects millions of people. The development of a treatment that does not spread in exponential fashion (as have, for example, penicillin, Alcoholics Anonymous, and renal dialysis) cannot be regarded as particularly helpful. In a nation with 5 to 10 million alcoholics, alleviating the suffering of 20 patients over a two-year period is hardly a giant step forward in public health. Nor have other psychological laboratories who have reported success in returning alcoholics to asymptomatic drinking achieved this success with more than a handful of patients (Hamburg 1975).

Heart transplantation and lunar travel are of the greatest heuristic importance, but they are of little use to the millions who suffer from heart disease or an itch to visit the moon. Similarly, it is important for alcohol specialists to know that it is theoretically possible for alcohol-dependent individuals to be taught to return to asymptomatic drinking; it is equally important for them to appreciate that abstinence may be a more practical and statistically more useful therapeutic focus.

III ∼ *Methodology*

6 ~ *The Sample*

As explained in the introductory chapter, the data presented in this book come from the Harvard Medical School's Study of Adult Development, which has followed 204 men in the College sample and 456 men in the Core City sample for approximately 40 years. This study vies with the Terman Study (Terman and Oden 1959) and the Oakland Growth Study (Block 1971; Eichorn et al. 1981) as being the longest study of adult development in the United States. The Oakland sample has been more thoroughly studied, but it is smaller and has suffered more attrition. The Terman sample includes both sexes and is larger than the Study of Adult Development and of longer duration (from age 10 to age 70), but after childhood the Terman subjects have been neither studied in depth nor reinterviewed. In contrast to most studies of adult development, all these projects have the advantage of collecting information about their samples at many different times—a strategy that provides a more dynamic view of change than observing individuals at only one or two different times.

The College Sample

In 1938, thanks to a generous gift from William T. Grant, the Harvard University Health Services under the leadership of Arlie V. Bock, M.D., undertook a study of "healthy" college sophomores. The early years of the study resulted in several dozen publications, most of which are reviewed in three books, *What People Are* (Heath 1946), *Young Man, You Are Normal* (Hooton 1945), and *College Men at War* (Monks 1957). The research program was directed by Clark Heath, M.D., from 1938 until 1954; by Charles McArthur,

307

Ph.D., from 1954 to 1972; and since 1972 I have been director of the study. The study has always remained the administrative responsibility of the Harvard University Health Services.

When the Grant Study began in 1938, the average subject in the College sample was 18 years of age. Each man has been studied until the present, when the average subject has passed his 60th birthday. In all, 268 men were chosen: 64 were drawn from the Harvard classes of 1939–1941, and 204 came from a more systematically studied 7 percent sample of the classes of 1942–1944. Virtually all were initially studied in their sophomore year. One-tenth of the men were selected by chance factors (for example, 4 percent by being self-referred, and 2 percent for being younger brothers of subjects already selected for the study). The other nine-tenths of the sample were selected in the following fashion. About 40 percent of each class were excluded because of mediocre academic achievement. Known medical or psychological difficulties led to the exclusion of 30 percent more. The names of the remaining 30 percent of the class were submitted to the college deans, who selected from this group about 100 students whom they recognized as "sound." From that subgroup—now narrowed down to 10 percent of the original class—one sophomore in five was not actually accepted into the study, because of schedule conflicts or poor motivation. Once accepted into the study, the College subjects were most loyal. During their college years only 10 of the 268 subjects dropped out, and since then only 2 men have withdrawn.

After being accepted into the study, each man was seen by a psychiatrist for eight interviews. These interviews focused on the man's family, his career plans, and his values. The psychiatrist attempted to get to know the subjects as people rather than as patients. No effort was made to look for pathology or to interpret the men's lives psychoanalytically. The psychiatric interviews included a history of early sexual development, but unfortunately the psychiatrist did not inquire into the boys' friendships or dating patterns. Thus, many early questions relevant to the vicissitudes of middle life went unanswered.

The College sample subjects were also seen by a family worker, Lewise Gregory Davies, who took a careful social history from each sophomore subject and traveled the length and breadth of the United States to meet the subjects' parents. In each boy's home, she took a family history that included characterizations of the grandparents, aunts, uncles, and first cousins. She also obtained from the mother a history of the child development of each boy and a family history of mental and physical illness including alcoholism. In keeping with the research methodology of the 1930s, such histories were more anecdotal than systematic.

Each College subject received an unusually thorough two-hour physical exam, including records of his daily habits, past illnesses, and physical response to stress. Each man was studied by a physical anthropologist, Carl Seltzer, who recorded his somatotype, determined whether his physical habitus was predominantly masculine or feminine, and made exhaustive anthropometric measurements. A physiologist, Lucien Brouha, also studied each subject and measured his insulin tolerance, his respiratory functions, and the physiologic effects of running on a treadmill for five minutes or until near exhaustion. Finally, a psychologist, Frederic Wells, gave each man tests designed to reflect native intelligence (the Alpha verbal and Alpha numerical), a vocabulary test, a shortened Rorschach test, and a block assembly test designed to assess manipulative dexterity and the comprehension of spatial relationships. In 1950 the men and their wives were interviewed in their homes by a social anthropologist, Margaret Lantis. To many she administered the Thematic Apperception Test.

As measured by college board scores, the academic achievement of the chosen students fell in the top 5 percent to 10 percent of high school graduates, but their average Scholastic Achievement Test (SAT) score of 584 did not put them beyond the range of many other able college students. Because one of the criteria for selection had been successful academic achievement, 61 percent of the study subjects graduated with honors in contrast to only 26 percent of their classmates. In native ability, however, the study subjects were only slightly superior.

Socioeconomically, the College sample made up a privileged group, but not exclusively so. In 1940, one-third of their fathers made more than $15,000 a year, but one-third made less than $5,000. One-third of their fathers had had some professional training, but half of their parents had no college degree. Half of the men had had some private education, but often on scholarship. In college, 40 percent received financial aid, and half worked during the academic year to pay a significant part of their educational expenses. Eighty percent were Protestant, 10 percent Catholic, and 10 percent Jewish. The study contained no blacks.

The College sample was not selected to be representative of any group, but the net was cast in such a fashion as to have a high likelihood of retrieving a large group of men who would lead satisfactory lives—regardless of the observer's bias. The sample was not made up of volunteers who "wanted to be studied." The emphasis was on selecting men at the independent end of the independent-dependent continuum. The subjects, a majority of whom were first-born sons, had deliberately chosen to go to a difficult and competitive college. Then they had been further selected for their capacity to master this situation. Put differently, the sample had been chosen for its capacity to equal or to exceed its natural ability. The happy-go-lucky but equally stable youngster, who characteristically searched for a good time, was probably underrepresented. The Stoics outnumbered the Dionysians.

World War II forced these men into a common experience that permitted them to be compared with their fellows on grounds other than academic excellence. They performed well on the battlefield (Monks 1957). Only 11, instead of a statistically expected 77, were rejected for service because of physical defects, and only 3, instead of an expected 36, were rejected for psychiatric reasons. The proportion wounded and killed (5 men) did not differ from that experienced by the armed forces as a whole. Only 10 percent went into the army with commissions, but 71 percent were officers at discharge; 45 percent entered the navy with commissions, but 90 percent were officers at discharge.

After graduation the College sample men were followed until 1955 by annual questionnaires. Since 1955 they have been sent questionnaires every two years. These questionnaires are lengthy and designed to benefit from the men's high verbal skills. They pay special attention to employment, family, health, habits (vacation, sports, alcohol, smoking, and so on), and political views. Use of alcohol is specifically inquired about. The men were reinterviewed in 1951, and a random 50 percent sample were reinterviewed again in 1968–1970. In addition, all of the men in whom problem drinking was suspected were reinterviewed between 1971 and 1976. Complete physical exams were obtained in 1969, 1974, and 1979.

In the mid-1970s, when the men in the sample had been out of college for 25 years, 95 percent had married and 15 percent had divorced. The modal man in the College sample has the income and social standing of a successful businessman or physician, but displays the political outlook, intellectual tastes, and lifestyle of a college professor. The subjects remain healthier and occupationally more successful than their classmates. Their mortality remains 50 percent less. Four times as many have held class offices as would have been expected by chance. Although they are less intellectually gifted than the Terman sample (Terman and Oden 1959), their achievements as measured by inclusion in *Who's Who in America* and *American Men and Women of Science* are comparable to those of the Terman subjects.

A quarter of the men became lawyers or doctors; 15 percent became teachers, mostly at a college level; and 20 percent went into business. The remaining 40 percent are distributed throughout other professions like archi-tecture, accounting, advertising, banking, insurance, government, and engi-neering. The proportions in each occupational subgroup are no different for the College sample than for their classmates.

Psychologically, the College sample in adult life have fared better than the population as a whole, but it is hard to say how much better. Limitations in psychiatric epidemiology make such comparisons difficult. Under the criteria that Srole and his associates (1962) used in their epidemiologic survey of the mental health of urban America, 70 percent of the College subjects might have fallen in the 19 percent that Srole and associates considered "well." By the standards of the Health Sickness Rating Scale (Luborsky 1962), 20 percent of the men at age 47 received a score of less than 70 and so might be defined as psychiatrically ill. In college, the Grant Study psychiatrist estimated that 55 percent of the men could have benefited from psychiatric consultation. By the time the men in the College sample were 30, 10 percent had seen psychiatrists, and by age 48, the number had increased to 40 percent.

In summary, the College sample subjects were relatively psychologically healthy, but the precise differences between their health and that of any other group is impossible to ascertain. Chosen as they were for academic success and aided by ethnicity, sex, the G.I. Bill of Rights, and the economic climate of 1945–1965, the Grant Study subjects were socially upwardly mobile to a degree that may be uncommon in future historical epochs. Nonetheless, the College sample provides a vivid, if historically limited, view of how the male life cycle may progress under favorable circumstances (Vaillant 1977).

The Core City Sample

The men of the Core City sample were drawn from the 500 boys ages 11–16 selected by Sheldon and Eleanor Glueck (1950) as controls for their prospec-tive study, *Unravelling Juvenile Delinquency.* From 1940–1944 these boys were chosen from Boston inner-city schools on the basis of not being known to be seriously delinquent. Like the College subjects, the Core City men were originally studied by a multidisciplinary team of physicians, psychologists, psychiatrists, social investigators, and physical anthropologists. For reasons of financial expedience the Gluecks reduced the sample from 500 to 456 by excluding all subjects born after July 1, 1932. About five-sixths of the surviv-ing 456 Core City men were reinterviewed at ages 25, 31, and 47.

In 1970 the Gluecks deeded their case records to the Harvard Law School

Library. Since 1974, my co-workers and I have actively followed the men in this sample as part of the Study of Adult Development at Harvard Medical School. Administratively, these files remain the responsibility of the Harvard Law School.

Originally, the Core City subjects were selected as matched controls for a cohort of 500 youths who were remanded to reform school. A boy in the delinquent group was matched with a boy in the nondelinquent group by four variables: age, intelligence, neighborhood crime rate, and ethnicity. Thus, the 60 percent of Boston census tracts with the highest rates of juvenile delinquency contained 95 percent of the subjects. Thanks to the tact and preparation of the Gluecks and their staff, the refusal rate was kept to 15 percent. The subjects' average I.Q. was 95. The parents or grandparents of 70 percent of the boys had been born in Italy, Ireland, Great Britain, or Canada, and 61 percent of the parents were foreign born.

The fact that the subjects were controls for a study of urban delinquency imposed several sources of bias. The Gluecks' original sample included no blacks and no women. Besides the obvious ethnic and intellectual constraints resulting from matching the controls to reform-school residents, another major source of bias was that the sample excluded about 10 percent of schoolboys because by age 14 they had already manifested serious delinquency. Thus, just as the College sample probably excluded passive, underachieving, but otherwise perfectly healthy college students, the Core City sample probably excluded some ambitious, energetic students who manifested early delinquency but who enjoyed subsequent good outcome. Both samples probably excluded men whose abuse of alcohol began in early adolescence.

The Gluecks' original methodology involved two parallel investigations of each boy and his family. Findings obtained from interviews with the boy, his school, and his family were compared and integrated with findings obtained from public records, especially those of the Massachusetts Board of Probation and the Boston Social Service Index. For 30 years the Massachusetts Board of Probation had cross-indexed arrest records throughout the state; and for half a century the Boston Social Service Index had cross-indexed every Boston family's contact with every welfare or social agency. The Gluecks' painstaking search of probation, mental health, and social agency records allowed documentation of familial delinquency, alcoholism, mental illness, and mental retardation for three generations. Data for the Core City sample, especially for alcohol abuse, were probably more complete than the data for the College sample.

Certainly, the simultaneous use of interviews with boy, parent, and teacher and of multiple longitudinal recorded sources of public information revealed far more evidence of psychopathology than could be obtained by cross-sectional data collection alone. In the follow-ups of these men at ages 25, 31, and 47 the same technique was used. An effort was made to check interview data against public records and data from mental health agencies, hospitals, and law enforcement agencies.

Excerpts from a representative case illustrate how each item of social history was verified or alternative data presented. The example is from one of the delinquent subjects, but the controls were studied in identical detail. (See Glueck and Glueck 1968, appendix, for the description of a complete case record.)

This case illustrates the ambiguities that arose with the use of multiple data sources and longitudinal data, and the way they were resolved. In the interview, the parents remembered the "age the boy first left home" as 11 years and three months, but the field investigation revealed an age of ten years and ten months recorded by a child placing agency. For the category "mental disease of the mother" the interview datum was "seems to be quite normal," but the field investigation revealed that a child welfare agency reported that the mother had fainting spells and "neurasthenia" and that eight years earlier a child placing agency had alleged that she had "attempted suicide."

The advantages of using both personal interview data and longitudinal field work were further illustrated by the Gluecks' efforts to document this mother's household routine, her son's delinquency, and her husband's alcoholism. In many instances, ambiguity could be resolved by the use of redundant evidence. With regard to "household routine," the interviewer noted "some semblance of routine, not a well-ordered house, however." Again, such an observation would be hopelessly ambiguous had it not been for the field investigation. Two years earlier the boy's parole division had described the "mother in bed near noon with a plateful of cigarette stubs beside her." Four years before that, a social agency had recorded: "Mother in bed all hours, baby in filthy condition." And three years earlier still, a child welfare agency had noted: "Children brought to school very unkempt."

The interview with the mother revealed that the subject had been smoking since 13, hopping trucks since 12, and impulsively stealing only recently (at age 16). The field investigation revealed a report from a child welfare agency that when the boy was 8, "the mother says boy set fires in the house only once," but that he was stealing from stores, and that the "landlady says boy broke many windows in houses and autos." At 10 he had been truanting and "mother says boy unmanageable since infancy and on the street at all hours." At 11 he had run away from a foster home, and at 12 he had threatened a schoolmate with a knife. The school report at age 10 revealed truancy, stealing, and an "E" in conduct. At 15 his school research report circled the following traits: truancy, stealing, cheating, unhappiness, depression, and suspicious- ness. Such traits and many others were systematically marked present or absent on the research protocols of school reports of all subjects. Thus it was possible to compare subjects systematically on whether the school perceived such traits to be present.

The interview data were ambiguous regarding possible alcoholism in the subject's stepfather. The mother described him as a man who until recently had been "quite a heavy drinker who would drink anything," but who now "only bought a small bottle of wine every day." She alleged that alcohol never interfered with his work. On the basis of such a description, it would be difficult to describe alcoholism as present or absent as an environmental factor. In contrast, the field investigation turned up information from a social agency that the stepfather had been laid off, "probably from drunkenness," five years before; from the board of probation that he had a long arrest record for breaking and entering *and* drunkenness; from a child welfare agency that the "stepfather sometimes takes boy and half-brother to the movies but is apt to be too drunk to be a companion." Follow-up revealed that two years after the interview with his wife, the stepfather had been arrested three times for alcoholism and twice committed to a state hospital for alcohol abuse. Three years after that he died; Vital Statistics reported that the cause of his death was "cirrhosis and alcoholism." Clearly, ambiguity recedes in the face of redundant data gathered over time. In similar ways, the assessments of vague but important judgments like parental affection and supervision could be documented from several points of view and at several times.

However, dependence upon redundant evidence can distort evidence in two ways. First, an individual from a very large family would have more relatives at risk for different kinds of psychopathology. For this reason, the number of available relatives was recorded for each case as a check on this source of bias in assessing familial histories for psychopathology. Second, recent immigration of parents into the United States sharply reduced the availability of information from public records.

Originally, the Core City men were severely disadvantaged. Half of them lived in clearly blighted slum neighborhoods; half were known to five or more social agencies, a third had I.Q.'s of less than 90, and a quarter repeated two grades or more. Half of their homes had no tub or shower (by way of contrast, in 1940 only 16 percent of all Boston dwellings were without tub or shower). Indeed, in 1940 only 30 percent of the Core City subjects' homes had hot water *and* central heat *and* electricity *and* a tub and toilet. Thirty-one percent of the parents of the Core City men were in Social Class V by the criteria of Hollingshead and Redlich (1958), and more than two-thirds had recently been on welfare.

Like the College sample, these Core City men were helped in upward mobility by being white, by the educational opportunities of the G.I. Bill, and by the economic prosperity of the United States between 1945 and 1965. Under other historical circumstances, they might have experienced more limited advancement.

Comparison of the Two Samples

Table 6.1 depicts the attrition from the Core City and the College samples. No member of either sample has been permanently lost. The credit for the low attrition must go to Sheldon and Eleanor Glueck and to the original staff of the Grant Study, who from the beginning created trusting relationships with these men. Most of the men in both samples were reinterviewed at age 31; and 87 percent of the surviving Core City sample and a randomly selected 50 percent of all the participating College subjects were reinterviewed at age 47. However, almost none of the men has an absolutely complete data set. This is especially true of the College subjects, who were contacted 24 different times.

The general characteristics of men lost to follow-up was determined in the following manner. By 1978, 51 men in the two samples had died; almost all had been active participants in the study until their deaths, and in all but a few cases death certificates documented probable cause of death. The 27 Core City subjects who had asked to withdraw from the study were known to be living after 1975, and most of them were interviewed at the age of 31. In almost all cases public records (and alumni reports for the 6 dropouts from the College sample) have allowed characterization of the dropouts' occupational success, marital status, arrest records, and general adjustment over the past decade.

Table 6.2 contrasts the demographic characteristics of the two samples. Outcome variables that depend upon parental social class and conventional

TABLE 6.1. Attrition in the College and Core City samples between 1940 and 1980.

	College sample	Core City sample
Number in original cohort[a]	204	456
Lost to follow-up	0	0
Dead before 1979	22	39
Living but withdrew from study	6	27
Living but data very incomplete	0	7
Living, good current data (1979)	176	383
Interviewed at age 31	90%	82%
Interviewed at age 47[b]	50%	87%

a. Actually 268 men were in the original College sample, but 64 men in the classes of 1939–1941 were excluded because the methodology of the study was still under development and there were inconsistencies in their original data base. Only the 204 men in the classes of 1942–1944 have been consistently studied. Originally 500 Core City youths were selected, but the decision was made to follow up only those 456 men born before July 1, 1932. Neither decision should have introduced significant bias.

b. The 50 percent figure for the College men actually represents 100 percent of a randomly chosen subsample. The remaining 50 percent are being reinterviewed as close to their 60th birthdays as possible. Percentages refer to the number of subjects who are still living.

intelligence tests sharply differentiate the two groups of men. For example, 76 percent of the College sample but only 2 percent of the Core City sample had attended graduate school. At the same time, in more socially egalitarian outcome variables such as the warmth of childhood environment and adult mental health, the men were not so different.

If according to Erik Erikson's conception of the life cycle, 41 percent of the College men could be deemed "generative," so could 31 percent of the Core City men (Vaillant and Milofsky 1980). If 28 percent of the Core City men were psychiatrically impaired (scored below 70) on the Health Sickness Rating Scale (Luborsky 1962), so were 20 percent of the College men. (Measurement instruments are described in Chapter 7 and in the Appendix.)

The College men spent their young adulthood in World War II and were last interviewed at the height of the Vietnam War. The Core City men had childhoods blighted by the Great Depression, were too young for World War II, and were last interviewed during the calmer era of Gerald Ford's presidency. However, with the exception of the College men's greater "generation gap" anxiety over their war-protesting, pot-smoking adolescent children, no specific cohort effects were identified in the two samples born almost a decade apart.

TABLE 6.2. Comparison of Core City and College samples.

Characteristic	Core City	College
Age when childhood assessed	14±2	19±1
Year of birth	1929±2	1921±2
Parents attended high school	33%	94%
Parents in social class IV or V	89%	4%
Parents in social class I or II	1%	80%
Average score on childhood environmental strengths scale[a]	9.2±5	9.5±5
Average I.Q.	95±12	c.125–140
High school graduates	48%	100%
Attended Graduate School	2%	76%
Social class I or II at age 47	9%	98%
Social class IV or V at age 47	49%	0%
Health-Sickness Rating (HSRS)[b] < 70	28%	20%

a. See Appendix and Vaillant 1977.
b. Luborsky 1962.

The Core City and College samples of the Study of Adult Development possess three advantages for the longitudinal study of interrelationships between psychopathology and alcoholism. First, the subjects were all originally selected, interviewed, rated, and conceptually viewed as nondeviant, while at the same time each youth was systematically investigated in a manner usually reserved for studies of psychopathology and deviance. Most other available studies of normative development have paid relatively little attention to psychopathology. Second, since the Core City and the College men entered the study so young, they comprise a far more complete clinical universe than would a sample drawn from patients at alcohol or psychiatric clinics, which of necessity would oversample repeaters and undersample those who remit or who die without coming to clinic attention. Third, the men have all been followed through time without significant attrition due to loss, geographic mobility, or withdrawal from study.

On the negative side, the Core City and College samples provide a very narrow sampling of human beings (male, white, American, and born between 1919 and 1932). But if a narrow sampling is a failing of most longitudinal studies, the Study of Adult Development at least provides two very different samples that may be fruitfully contrasted with each other.

7 ～ The Measures

This chapter will orient the reader to the ways in which the Core City sample was studied and contrast it with the College sample. The methodology of the College sample follow-up has been fully described elsewhere (Vaillant 1977). This chapter will review all the major psychosocial Core City ratings with the exception of the scales used to assess alcohol use and abuse, which are discussed in Chapter 1.

A guiding principle of the follow-up of the Core City sample was to make maximum use of the study's prospective design. Thus, one set of raters blinded to all events after junior high school rated the men's childhoods. Both the person who interviewed the men at 47 and a second set of raters blinded to all events before 30 judged each man's current adjustment and use or abuse of alcohol. A second guiding principle, which is the focus of this chapter, was to identify those premorbid variables which most powerfully predicted midlife mental health, on the one hand, and social deviance, on the other. The question of whether these variables also predict alcoholism is addressed in Chapters 1 and 2.

Childhood Premorbid Variables

On the basis of social service records extending over three generations and of interviews with each boy, his parents, and his teacher, clinicians who were blind to all information after the boys' adolescence rated them on the scales listed below. Because of the vicissitudes of longitudinal study, the number of men for whom each variable was available varied somewhat; the number is given with the description of each variable. In many instances, the same scales that had been used to assess the College sample (Vaillant 1977) were used for the Core City sample. These scales are indicated with an asterisk.

Ethnicity (n = 456)

When a boy was first admitted to the study, his ethnicity was determined. The Gluecks (1950) observed the following rules: If both parents were foreign born in the same country, ethnicity was assigned to that country. If both parents were foreign born but in two different countries, ethnicity was assigned to the place of birth of the father. If only one parent was foreign born, ethnicity was assigned to the country of birth of that parent. If both parents were born in the United States, ethnicity was assigned to the birth-place of the paternal grandparents. While this system of classification may be controversial, and in individual cases misleading, the intent was statistically to identify cultural attitudes that might affect future behavior.

As a further means of assessing the effect of culture upon alcoholism, cultures were ranked according to their dominant attitude toward the use of alcohol. Cultures assigned the highest rank number tend to sanction drinking by children and proscribe drunkenness in adults. The Irish culture, assigned the lowest rank, shows the opposite pattern of attitudes. (The single Chinese subject was excluded.)

1 = Irish (n = 84)
2 = United States (n = 36) or Canada, Great Britain (n = 145)
3 = Poland, Russia, Germany, other northern European countries (n = 41)
4 = Italian (n = 115), other "Mediterranean" countries (Portuguese, Spanish, Greek, Syrian, Turkish, Armenian) (n = 26), Jewish (n = 8).

*Childhood Environmental Strengths Scale (n = 453)

On the basis of all available childhood data, each man was rated on the 20-point childhood environmental strengths scale, described in detail else-where (Vaillant 1974; 1977). The intent of the scale was to focus on what went right rather than what went wrong. The scale assigned points for the absence of childhood problems with physical, social, and mental health and for the presence of parental relationships and a home atmosphere conducive to "development of basic trust, autonomy, and initiative." In 1975 raters made judgments by clinically assessing the entire childhood record rather than depending solely on ratings of the Gluecks' original items. Rater reliability among three raters ranged from .70 to .89.

This 20-point scale was made up of subscales measuring childhood emotional problems, childhood health, home atmosphere, the mother-child relationship, the father-child relationship, sibling relationships, school social adjustment, and the rater's overall, global impression of the childhood environment. Details of these subscales are given in the Appendix. On each subscale, points were assigned for the presence or absence of problems, with more points for fewer problems. For example, under the category "childhood emotional problems," an unusually social child would receive 2 points, an average child 1 point, and an unusually dissocial or troubled child 0 points. The points from the subscales were summed to get the childhood environmental strengths scale.

This scale could have been altered to reflect better the data available in the Gluecks' records and to contrast more sharply with the childhood environmental weaknesses scale. However, in order to be directly comparable with the previous assessment of the College sample, the childhood environmental strengths scale was applied to the Core City sample in the same form.

The men whose childhood environmental strengths score fell in the top quartile were characterized as coming from *warm childhoods*. Those whose scores fell in the bottom quartile were said to come from *bleak childhoods*.

Childhood Environmental Weaknesses Scale (n = 453)

A second way of looking at the men's childhoods was in terms of weaknesses rather than strengths. The 25-item childhood environmental weaknesses scale (which is described fully in the Appendix) was made up of five subscales measuring lack of a cohesive home, lack of maternal supervision, lack of maternal affection, lack of paternal supervision, and lack of paternal affection. On the basis of objective information, this scale was constructed by redefining the Gluecks' Delinquency Prediction Table (Glueck and Glueck 1950), which consists of subjective assessments of home cohesiveness and of maternal and paternal supervision and affection. The new scale was designed to use available, prospectively gathered, unambiguous data in the original case records. Rater reliability was .94.

Sixty-two of the men, or 14 percent, had grown up in families manifesting 10 or more of the 25 problems in the childhood environmental weaknesses scale; these families were labeled *multiproblem families*. The childhoods of another 25 percent of the men manifested two or fewer weaknesses. The men from the multiproblem families contributed a disproportionate number of deaths and drops, so that at age 47, 21 of the 62 men from multiproblem families could not be personally interviewed. In contrast, all but 8 of the 66 men whose families had one or no problems were interviewed. Thus, because of selective attrition, the proportion of boys from multiproblem families is smaller among the 400 well-studied men than in the original sample.

The two childhood scales, environmental strengths and environmental weaknesses, correlated with each other with an *r* of only −.61. Some Core City men grew up in environments that were not grossly disrupted and yet were devoid of positive attributes; others experienced home environments with both great defects and great strengths. Ten of the men from the 160 families with the fewest weaknesses still experienced childhoods classified as bleak, or in the bottom quartile. Conversely, six of the 93 men with six or more problems on the childhood weaknesses scale had childhoods classified as warm, or in the top quartile.

Table 7.1 illustrates the midlife consequences of growing up in childhoods classified as warm, bleak, or multiproblem. What is most noteworthy about the men who grew up in multiproblem families was that they turned out so well. These men from families with 10 or more problems (n = 62) represented a more extreme group than did the men with bleak childhoods (n = 124) but with the exception of experiencing less stable first marriages, they actually turned out better. For example, the childhood strengths scale correlated with mental health (HSRS) with an *r* of .21 ($p < .001$), while the childhood weaknesses scale correlated with an *r* of only −.10 (not significant). In brief, it appeared more damaging to a child's later development to have nothing go right than to have many things go wrong (Vaillant and Milofsky 1980; Vaillant and Vaillant 1981).

Table 7.1 illustrates that, however subjective or arbitrary these judgments of childhood, they predicted future mental health and object relations 35 years later. Perhaps the cruelest prediction of a bleak childhood was early mortality. Six men from the bleakest childhoods and only one from the warmest childhoods died before age 40. The excess deaths were from suicide or violence. Had these men survived, they would most likely have increased the disparity in mental health between the men with bleak and warm childhoods. Surprisingly, scores on the childhood environmental strengths scale were roughly the same for both the College and the Core City samples. The childhood environmental weaknesses scores, however, were 20 times greater

TABLE 7.1. Relationship of extreme childhood environments to adult outcome.

Outcome variable	Warm childhood (n = 93)[a]	Bleak childhood (n = 124)[a]	Multiproblem childhood (n = 62)[a]
Mental health in bottom third			
(HSRS 0–70)	22%	47%	41%
Sociopath (5+ on Robins scale)	2	12	11
Ever diagnosed mentally ill	20	42	42
Social competence in bottom quartile	19	34	33
Income < $10,000/year	11	30	26
Four years or more unemployed	12	34	28
Social class V	2	17	15
Dead	5	10	10
Mental health in top third			
(HSRS 81–100)	48	23	32
Still enjoys first marriage	57	33	45
Enjoys his children	56	35	33
Social class I–III	71	43	38

a. These n's represent the number of boys out of the original 456 in each childhood category. Since the outcome variables could only be ascertained for 400±25 men, the percentages in the table are based on somewhat smaller n's.

for the Core City sample. In other words, if loving parents are not the prerogative of the socially privileged, freedom from multiproblem households is such a benefit.

Boyhood Competence Scale: Success at Erikson's Stage Four Tasks (n = 451)

This eight-point scale, defined more fully in the Appendix, reflects what the boys did—not what they said or felt. The items reflect assessment of systematically recorded observations made when the boys were between the ages of 11 and 16; their average age was 14±1.

The boyhood competence scale included the following objective measures: regular part-time job, regular household chores, participation in extracurricular clubs or sports, school grades relative to I.Q., regular school participation in activities, and coping capacity—the ability to plan, to make the best of the environment.

Assessment of these tasks was made by raters blind to the men's futures. Each rater had access to transcripts of interviews with the boy and with his parents, school reports, teachers' evaluations, Wechsler Bellevue I.Q. scores, and reports of truancy, school problems, and class behavior. Possible total scores for Stage Four tasks ranged from 0 to 8 and the mean ($\pm$SD) score was 4 ± 1. (Twenty-five men were assessed by all three raters and the Spearman-Pearson correlation coefficients for the ratings among the three possible pairs of judges were .78, .79, and .91.)

Boyhood competence was perhaps the most interesting of the childhood predictors. However, this effort to quantify success at Erikson's Stage Four requires justification. In *Childhood and Society*, Erikson set forth an eight-stage schema of human development. The first three stages embraced issues and tasks associated with preschool development, and the fourth stage embraced the life issues confronting the grammar-school child. Erikson called his fourth stage of the life cycle "Industry vs. Inferiority," and described the dominant virtue of that stage as "competence": "Industriousness involves doing things beside and with others, a first sense of the division of labor . . . Competence, then, is the free exercise . . . of dexterity and intelligence in the completion of serious tasks. It is the basis for cooperative participation in some segment of the culture" (1968, pp. 289–290).

Efforts to translate Erikson's conceptual framework into a numerical score at best are reductionistic and at worst rate real human beings in a Horatio Alger look-alike contest. At the same time, like the art of politics, the study of lives must be based upon existing and not upon ideal circumstances. Thus, the testing of hypotheses does involve reductionistic thinking, and the justification of the boyhood competence scale must lie in whether the scale can predict future adaptation better than can other available childhood variables.

Common sense was used in making the ratings of boyhood competence. For example, the requirements for being given credit for a part-time job were more stringent for older boys, and such jobs reflected both after-school and vacation employment. The most subjective item in the scale was "coping capacity." The purpose of this item was to give special credit to the boys who, in spite of very disorganized homes, were coping particularly well. To make this judgment, the rater took into account all available data from the psychiatric interviews with the boy and his mother as well as multiple reports from social service agencies. Assessment included how well the boy was coping and how realistic were both his views of himself and his plans for the future. A major source of bias was that the same rater also assessed childhood strengths

TABLE 7.2. Relationship of boyhood competence to adult outcome.[a]

	Rating on boyhood competence	
Outcome variable	Best (7–8) (n = 45)[b]	Worst (0–2) (n = 74)[b]
Mental health in bottom third (HSRS 0–70)	24%	43%
Sociopath (5+ on Robins scale)	0	13
Ever diagnosed mentally ill	16	33
Social competence in bottom quartile	17	34
Four or more years unemployed	2	32
Social class V (age 47)	0	11
Dead	2	12
Mental health in top third (HSRS 81–100)	51	30
Still enjoys first marriage	58	34
Enjoys his children	53	34
Income > $20,000/year (1978 dollars)	53	11

a. Since these comparisons represent the contrast of extreme groups, citing statistical significance is not really appropriate. Table 2.3 makes it clear, however, that boyhood competence scores are correlated with most of these variables at $p < .001$.

b. These n's represent the number of boys out of the original 456 in each childhood category. Since the outcome variables could only be ascertained for 400±25 men, the percentages in the table are based on somewhat smaller n's.

and weaknesses; this may have produced halo effects between boyhood competence and childhood environment.

Forty-five of the youths received very high scores (7–8), and 67 received very low scores (0–2). Table 7.2 contrasts the outcome of these two extreme groups more than 30 years later. By the age of 47 the men who were most successful at the Stage Four tasks of boyhood competence were twice as likely to have warm relations with a wide variety of people, and 5 times more likely to be well paid for their adult work. The boys with the highest scores on Stage Four tasks were also 16 times less likely to have experienced significant unemployment. Conversely, sociopathy, premature death, and mental illness were the fate of a disproportionate number of boys who had trouble mastering the arbitrary tasks measured by the boyhood competence scale. In summary, as tables 7.1 and 7.2 illustrate, extremes in premorbid childhood

TABLE 7.3.   Relationship of boyhood competence to other childhood variables.[a]

	Rating on boyhood competence	
Variable	Best (7–8) (n = 45)[b]	Worst (0–2) (n = 74)[b]
Warm childhood	69%	7%
Childhood emotional problems	16	57
Multiproblem family	4	27
I.Q. < 90	20	42
Parents' social class II or III	13	10
Ever attended college	22	12

a. Since these comparisons represent the contrast of extreme groups, citing statistical significance is not really appropriate. Table 2.2 provides the significance and strength of association among most of these variables.

b. Full data sets were not available for all individuals; thus the number of men in each category varied slightly.

adjustment correlate strongly with extremes in adult outcome. As we have seen, however, these same variables are much less useful in predicting alcoholism.

Table 7.3 reveals that boyhood competence was by no means independent from the other important premorbid variables in the environmental weaknesses scale. Development of boyhood competence was most highly associated with warm childhoods and the absence of emotional problems. Parental social class and intelligence appeared relatively unimportant. In other words, boyhood competence appeared to be more a measure of emotional well-being than of intellectual endowment or social good fortune.

*Parents' Social Class (n = 453)

Social class was evaluated by the five-point classification devised by Hollingshead and Redlich (1958), which is derived by assigning separate weights to scales for education, residence, and prestige of occupation and then summing the three scores. This scale is fully defined in the Appendix. In general, Social Class I included managers and professionals with college degrees who owned their own houses in prosperous suburbs. Social Class V included unskilled laborers with less than 10 grades of schooling who lived in deteriorating rented housing. Class III mostly included skilled blue-collar workers with high school educations who owned houses in working-class neighborhoods, but Class III could also include men with a year of college who owned small stores and lived in apartments in middle-class suburbs, or, as was true for some Core City fathers, men who were educated as lawyers but lived in slum housing.

Thirty-three years later this same rating of social class was assigned to the subjects themselves at age 47 by a rater blind to the past. As is illustrated by Table 7.4, there was considerable upward mobility. Perhaps more surprising was the fact that within this sample there was little correlation between the social class of the men and that of their parents.

School Problems and Truancy (n = 429)

A dichotomous rating (present or absent) was made from childhood records of school behavior problems and of truancy by a rater who was not blind to later outcome. A total of 22 men were noted to engage in repeated truancy and/or received repeated complaints concerning discipline from teachers and/or fought often with other students.

Intelligence (n = 451)

I.Q. was assessed by means of the Wechsler Bellevue. At the beginning of the study, each Core City subject was given an individual test by a research psychologist. Because the Core City subjects were matched with delinquents remanded to reform school, they were selected for low I.Q. Twelve percent had tested I.Q.'s below 80, 30 percent between 80 and 89, 38 percent between 90 and 99, 24 percent between 100 and 109, and only 9 percent (39 subjects) between 110 and 130. Because of troubled home lives and inner-city schooling, it seems certain that many of these I.Q. scores underestimate the intellectual potential of the Core City men. In many of their childhoods English was not spoken at home.

*Alcohol Abuse in Relatives (n = 454)

Three scales were used to measure the presence or absence of alcohol abuse in relatives. The first scale, alcohol abuse in parents, reflected alcoholism in the child's environment. Points were assigned as follows: 1 = Neither parent (or surrogate) abused alcohol. 2 = One parent (or surrogate) with minor evidence of alcohol abuse (two arrests for drunkenness or mention of alcohol abuse in official records or strong suspicion of alcohol abuse in case record). 3 = One parent (or surrogate) with major evidence (two or more criteria for

TABLE 7.4. Upward social mobility of the Core City men.[a]

Parents' social class in 1943±2	Subject's social class in 1976±2					
	I	*II*	*III*	*IV*	*V*	*Total*
II	0	0	3	0	0	3 (1%)
III	2	3	20	10	3	38 (9%)
IV	2	22	108	94	22	248 (58%)
V	2	7	49	60	17	135 (32%)
Total	6(1%)	32(8%)	180(42%)	164(39%)	42(10%)	424(100%)

a. Association between parents' (1943) and subject's (1976) social class not significant ($p = .17$, chi-square test, 12 degrees of freedom).

minor evidence *and* evidence of chronicity) or two parents with minor evidence of alcohol abuse. 4 = Both parents (or surrogate) abused alcohol—major evidence for at least one.

The second scale, alcohol abuse in ancestors, reflected alcoholism in the child's heredity (in known ancestors prior to 1945). Parents and siblings were excluded but other first- and second-degree relatives—if known—were included. 1 = No evidence of alcohol abuse in family. If no reliable judgment was possible due to ambiguous or absent familial data, rating was left blank. 2 = One relative with minor evidence of alcohol abuse (defined as above). 3 = Two relatives with minor evidence of alcohol abuse or one relative with major evidence (defined as above). 4 = Three relatives with minor evidence or two relatives with major evidence of alcohol abuse.

The third scale, alcohol abuse in heredity, was made when the men were 47 by a rater blind to their alcohol use or abuse. The rater used information from a three-generation search of public records (Glueck and Glueck 1950), from the original interviews with the subject's parents, and from the subsection of the age-47 interview that concerned relatives. Thus, the rating combined ratings of alcoholism in ancestors and in biological parents; the rating also included fresh data obtained over the intervening three decades on parental alcohol abuse and on alcohol abuse by siblings.

Parental Delinquency (n = 456)

Parental delinquency was measured by the following four-point scale: 1 = Neither parent (or if parents absent, parental surrogate) delinquent. 2 = One parent with minor evidence (documented criminal arrest or child neglect or multiple arrests for nonsupport, driving offenses, etc., or an illegal profession). 3 = One parent with major evidence (more than a year in jail and chronic serious criminal behavior), or both parents with minor evidence.

*Heredity for Mental Illness (n = 454)

This was assessed in the same way as alcoholism in ancestors. To minimize the effect of environment, parents and siblings were excluded. The Department of Mental Health records were searched for all relatives in Massachusetts. Points were assigned as follows: 1 = No known mental illness in any relative. 2 = One relative with minor evidence (occupationally disabled for emotional reasons, markedly paranoid, eccentric, or depressed, received a clinician's diagnosis of neurosis or personality disorder, or psychiatric hospitalization of less than a year). 3 = Two relatives with minor evidence or one relative with major evidence (definite diagnosis of schizophrenia or more than a year of psychiatric hospitalization) or two non-alcohol-related psychiatric hospitalizations. 4 = Three relatives with minor or two relatives with major evidence of mental illness.

(In the light of modern psychiatric epidemiology, such a scheme seems very crude, but it made the most of the evidence available in our records. This was the only premorbid variable that has been mentioned so far that significantly correlated with none of the major outcome variables that we studied.)

Hyperactivity (n = 456)

Hyperactivity was a composite variable that was assessed on a 0–28 scale (see Appendix). Ratings were obtained by retrospectively searching the men's records for evidence of hyperactivity, employing the scale devised by Wender and co-workers (Wood et. al. 1976): restlessness, impulsivity, short attention span, fidgeting, low frustration tolerance, tantrums, and rapid mood changes. However, as already noted, one of the problems with prospective studies is that they do not permit redesign and thus they fail to keep up with scientific progress. Therefore, our estimate of hyperactivity was undoubtedly very crude, and, since the Core City subjects were relatively old (12–16), perhaps not even age-appropriate.

Midlife Outcome Variables

The major outcome variables obtained for the Core City sample at age 47 were rated by judges who were blind to the individuals' adjustment prior to their second reinterview at age 31. An asterisk indicates which midlife outcome ratings were also available for the College sample.

Health Sickness Rating Scale (HSRS) (n = 378)

Luborsky's (1962) Health Sickness Rating Scale (HSRS) was used to assess global mental health. On the basis of graded ratings, illustrated by 34 case examples, the HSRS assigns points along a continuum from 1 (totally incapacitated) to 100 ("an ideal state of resiliency in the face of stress, of happiness and social effectiveness"). From 18 published studies, Luborsky and Bachrach (1974) have summarized the reliability and validity data of the HSRS. They conclude that global mental health can be judged by clinicians along a single continuum with surprisingly good reliability. In the present study we obtained reliability of .89.

The HSRS is based on a single overall rating of seven facets of psychological functioning: (1) the individual's need to be protected and/or supported versus his ability to function autonomously; (2) the degree to which an individual's psychiatric symptoms—if any—reflect personality disorganization, and their severity; (3) the extent of the subject's objective discomfort and at the same time the extent of his inner peace of mind; (4) the individual's effect on his environment for good or for ill; (5) the warmth, intimacy, closeness versus the distortions in his interpersonal relationships; (6) the breadth and depth of his interests; and (7) the degree to which he can utilize his abilities, especially at work. Since the assessment of global mental health required the most complete data base, fewer men (378) could be rated on the HSRS than on any other major variable.

Subjects who scored above 80 on the HSRS not only were without significant psychopathology but also exhibited many traits that reflected positive mental health: 138 men or 37 percent fell in this category. Those who scored under 60 had clear evidence of disability in their everyday functioning attributable to emotional instability; 44 men or 12 percent fell in this category. Those between 70 and 80 showed neither significant emotional problems in living nor particular strengths, and those between 60 and 70 showed evidence of personality disorder or significant neurotic symptoms but nevertheless were functioning independently.

Endicott and her colleagues (1976) have justifiably criticized the HSRS for confusing diagnostic categories with severity of symptoms. To shift the emphasis from diagnosis to severity of disability, they devised a closely related scale: the global assessment scale. In sympathy with this viewpoint we asked our raters to assess the subjects' average functioning for the previous 10 years. They were instructed to pay attention to the behavioral impairment reflected by Luborsky's illustrative cases and to ignore diagnosis. Thus, a once-hospitalized schizophrenic patient who had been functioning autonomously for several years with few symptoms and regular employment received a higher HSRS score than an unemployed loner who had lived all his life with his mother but had never required psychiatric attention.

In the assignment of HSRS scores, the effects of physical illness upon psychological functioning (unless the central nervous system was involved) were discounted. Rating the effects of a subject's alcoholism, which can be construed as a physical illness but which also affects the brain, was very problematic; a clear solution was not possible. In a desire to determine which was cart and which was horse, we wished to separate the syndrome of alcohol abuse from preexisting psychiatric dysfunction. Thus, no individual was given a low HSRS solely because he had lost control of his use of alcohol. In actual fact, however, over time, personality disorder and severe alcoholism are so intertwined that the distinction between primary psychiatric disability and disability caused by alcohol abuse became blurred. Thus, an unemployed alcoholic living on welfare probably would have received a higher HSRS than had he been schizophrenic but a lower HSRS than had he been disabled from polio or an industrial accident but making the best of it. Such vagueness is unsatisfactory. In order to elucidate the degree to which alcohol abuse develops independently of psychiatric vulnerability, psychiatric assessment prior to alcohol abuse (see Chapter 2) is necessary.

Table 7.5 presents the proportion of men in the entire sample who manifested each of selected midlife outcome variables that later will be referred to in relationship to alcohol abuse. The table also depicts the association of these outcomes with extremes in global mental health (the 44 men with ratings of 60 or less and the 138 men with ratings of over 80 on the HSRS). The distinction between the two groups of men at the extremes of global mental health is striking—both in terms of achievement of social competence and happy marriage and in terms of regularity of employment and income.

TABLE 7.5. Frequency of major outcome variables among the total Core City sample and among the men with the highest and lowest HSRS scores.[a]

		HSRS	
	Total sample (n = 378–442)	0–60 (n = 44)	81–100 (n = 138)
Psychosocial variables			
Ever received psychiatric diagnosis	29%	82%	9%
Sociopathy 5+ symptoms	7	27	1
Social competence in top quarter	22	0	44
Social competence in bottom quarter	23	84	1
Happy first marriage	49	0	75
Unemployed 4+ years	21	75	4
Income > $20,000 (1978 dollars)	24	0	46
Income < $10,000 (1978 dollars)	19	70	3
Social class I–III	51	9	77
Social class V	10	45	1
Chronic physical illness, or dead	27	48	20
Alcohol variables[b]			
Lifelong abstainer	20	34	20
Lifelong social drinker	53	23	69
Alcohol abuser (PDS)	27	43	11
Alcohol dependent (DSM III)	18	28	9

a. See Table 7.6 for strength of statistical association between the HSRS and outcome variables.
b. Defined in Chapter 1.

Elsewhere it has been shown that although global mental health in these men was also highly correlated with social upward mobility, social class was cart and not horse (Vaillant and Milofsky 1980; Vaillant and Vaillant 1981).

After 30 years of observation, 82 percent of the 44 men with the poorest mental health had received a psychiatric diagnosis; this was true for only 9 percent of the best outcomes. This lends support to an observation made for the College sample (Vaillant 1977) as a result of similar data; namely, in spite of the vagueness and subjectivity of our psychiatric diagnoses, in naturalistic studies of male life spans clinicians appear to have assigned psychiatric diagnoses with surprising discrimination.

Between the two extremes of mental health, differences in alcohol dependence were less marked than the differences in likelihood of receiving a psychiatric diagnosis. But men at the most pathologic end of the HSRS continuum were far more likely to be lifelong teetotalers. What distinguished

TABLE 7.6. Correlation between HSRS and other theoretically important variables.[a]

Variable	HSRS
Psychosocial maturity[b]	.78
Maturity of ego defenses[c]	.78
Social competence	.68
Percentage of adult life unemployed	−.64
Sociopathy	−.55
Earned income	.54
Enjoys his children	.52
Social class at age 47	.52
Percentage of adult life married	.49
Parental social class	.08
I.Q.	.15

a. Correlations greater than .15 are significant at $p < .001$ (Pearson product-moment correlation coefficient).

b. An estimate of maturation based on Erikson's stages of development (See Vaillant and Milofsky 1980).

c. An estimate of ego maturity based on the men's tendency to use defenses associated with personality disorder (such as projection and passive aggression) or defenses associated with mental health (such as suppression and sublimation). See Vaillant 1977.

the alcohol consumption of the two groups most clearly was that 63 percent of the most mentally healthy men in contrast to only 9 percent of the least healthy men managed to use alcohol regularly all of their lives without any problems.

When mental health was defined in alternative ways—by psychosocial maturity or maturity of ego defenses or capacity for object relations—the correlations with mental health as defined by the HSRS remained very high, as shown in Table 7.6. Of considerable theoretical interest is the observation that, although adult social class, employment, and income were highly correlated with HSRS, ratings of global mental health seemed quite independent of I.Q. and parental social class. In a sample confined to white urban males, mental health appeared to exert greater influence upon social class than social class exerted upon mental health.

Having defined and validated the HSRS as a measure of global mental health, it is possible to examine the relationship of mental health to premorbid variables. Table 7.7 presents the frequency of occurrence of major premorbid variables within the whole sample and also with respect to the extreme groups in global mental health. Ethnicity, heredity positive for alco-

TABLE 7.7. Frequency of major premorbid variables among total sample and among men with highest and lowest HSRS scores.[a]

		HSRS	
Premorbid variable	Total sample (n = 44)	0–60 (n = 44)	81–100 (n = 138)
Childhood environmental strengths 14–20 (warm)	21%	5%	28%
Childhood environmental strengths 0–5 (bleak)	27	52	17
Childhood emotional problems	30	52	24
Boyhood competence (top quarter)	24	9	33
Parents' social class V	32	32	24
Less than 10 years of school	34	45	27
I.Q. 57–89	30	36	20
I.Q. 100–120	33	22	41
Multiproblem family	14	16	9
More than one alcoholic relative	42	34	33
Irish ethnicity	19	20	20
Mediterranean ethnicity	33	34	34
Truant and school problems	4	5	2
Poor infant health	9	23	7
Hyperactivity	3	0	4

a. The statistical significance and strength of association of the HSRS with premorbid variables are defined in table 2.3.

holism, multiproblem family membership, and truancy or school problems were relatively weak predictors of future mental health—although as documented in Chapter 2, these are the variables that predicted alcohol abuse. Rather, the variables that were most significantly associated with subsequent mental health were warmth of childhood, boyhood competence, and freedom from emotional problems in childhood.

Psychopathology (n = 399)

To assess psychopathology, the severity of all psychiatric diagnoses received by the men during their adult lives was assessed on an arbitrary five-point scale: one point if no mental illness was ever formally diagnosed (n = 285); two if a diagnosis had been assigned on an outpatient basis by either a physician or a psychiatrist (n = 86); three if the subject had been hospitalized for emotional problems but was not psychotic (n = 15); four if the individual was hospitalized for psychosis but was never labeled schizophrenic (n = 2); five if the individual was hospitalized and diagnosed "schizophrenic" (n = 11).

Sociopathy Scale (n = 430)

The 19 criteria used by Robins (1966) for the diagnosis of sociopathic personality were looked for in all of our subjects. The scale is described in full in the Appendix and discussed in Chapter 2. These criteria were equally weighted. If 5 or more criteria were identified, the individual was categorized as a "sociopath." The sociopathy scale depended upon the redundancy of deviant behavior and included variables like school problems, impulsive behavior, multiple suicide attempts, poor armed service records, vagrancy, use of aliases, and reckless youth. Being frequently arrested or in "repeated trouble with the law" was only one of the 19 items; and thus, illegal behavior per se could not lead to a diagnosis of sociopathy. One of the 19 items was "school problems and truancy" which was treated also as an independent premorbid variable.

*Social Competence (n = 384)

Capacity for human relations was measured by a 9-item social competence scale that reflected success at a wide variety of human relationships. Each of the 8 items was assessed by the interviewer on a 3- or 4-point scale; these totals were then summed. The 8 items reflected the previous 10 years and included whether the subject enjoyed his children, his parents and siblings, and his friends, and whether he got along with workmates, enjoyed membership in social organizations, entertained nonrelatives, participated in community activities, and engaged in pastimes that included others. The scale is described in full in the Appendix. Because stable marriage is thought by many to reflect twentieth-century middle-class morality rather than an enduring facet of mental health, marital success or failure was not included in the scale of social competence but was treated as a separate variable.

*Enjoyment of Children (n = 384)

The fifth variable was one of the 8 items from the social competence scale: enjoyment of children. One point was assigned if the subject had a positive relationship with all of his children, spent time with them, maintained open communication, and spoke of them positively; 2 points if the subject had either a good relationship with some of his children and poor with others or a mediocre relationship with all of them; 3 points if the subject allowed his wife to take major responsibility for the children and shared little interest in them, or if after a divorce the subject had less contact with his children than was possible; 4 points if the subject had consistently poor relationships with his children and frankly neglected or avoided them. Men who had no children or children less than 15 years old were scored 2 on this variable for the purpose of computing their social competence scores.

Marital Happiness and Stability (n = 436)

This scale was a composite of three ratings. Each man's present marriage was assessed in terms of stability over the previous few years; in terms of whether enjoyment was clear, uncertain, or absent; and in terms of how seriously divorce had been considered. This variable was highly correlated with HSRS, $r = .48$.

Percentage of Adult Life Married (n = 427)

This simpler and more reliably assessed marital variable was obtained by calculating the percentage of time since age 21 that the men had spent married and living with a spouse. Percentage of adult life married was significantly correlated ($p < .0001$) with the percentage of time unemployed ($r = -.38$), with income ($r = .35$), with social competence ($r = .38$), and with the HSRS ($r = .49$).

Percentage of Adult Life Unemployed (n = 420)

After global mental health, employment stability proved to be one of the most potent correlates of mental health in the study (Vaillant and Vaillant 1981). As with marriage, this variable was computed by the number of months an individual was known to have been unemployed, divided by the total number of months that had elapsed since his 21st birthday.

Annual Earned Income (n = 405)

Individual earned income was calculated in terms of 1978 dollars: subjects who were interviewed in 1975, 1976, and 1977 had their coded annual incomes increased by 15 percent, 10 percent, and 5 percent respectively. In general income was assessed as the average highest income that the individual had received over any of the preceding five years. The annual income of 15 percent of the men was less than $8,000 and that of 15 percent more than $22,000. Mean annual income was $16,000.

Adult Social Class (n = 426)

Social class for the men at age 47 was calculated in the same way that social class of their parents had been calculated.

**Educational Attainment (n = 435)*

Educational attainment was included as an outcome variable rather than as a premorbid variable because it included the men's total educational experience, which often continued well into adulthood. Many of these men received the benefits of the G.I. Bill. For purposes of computer analysis, education was divided into 7 arbitrary sections: 1 = some graduate education (n = 7); 2 = college graduates (n = 23); 3 = 1–2 years of college or a post-high-school technical school course (n = 38); 4 = high school diploma or equivalency certification (n = 142); 5 = 10–11 grades (n = 74); 6 = 7–9 grades (n = 145); 7 = less than 7th-grade education (n = 6).

**Physical Health (n = 409)*

This rating on a five-point scale was based on the men's own description of their physical health, and for slightly over half of the men was complemented by recent hospital records or physical exam reports. 1 = Good health—an essentially normal physical exam; this could include a current illness that was fully reversible (n = 150). 2 = Minor but chronic complaints (such as back problem, mild emphysema, gout, kidney stones, borderline hypertension, chronic ear problems) (n = 149). 3 = Chronic illness without disability which would not fully remit and would probably progress (such as hypertension requiring treatment, emphysema with cor pulmonale, diabetes) (n = 62). 4 = Irreversible chronic illness with disability (such as severe angina, disabling back trouble, high blood pressure plus extreme obesity, multiple sclerosis) (n = 34). 5 = Deceased (n = 14). (In addition, 19 men had died before the age of 40 and were excluded from this book's consideration of the life course of alcoholism.)

TABLE 7.8. Thoroughness of follow-up at age 47.

Follow-up group	% of total sample	Number of men	Number abusing alcohol	
Included in most analyses				
Personally interviewed	80%	367	95	
Relative interviewed	5	22[a]	10	
Questionnaire and telephone	1	4	0	27%
Not interviewed but much				
data	2	7[b]	5	
Excluded from most analyses[c]				
Withdrew from study	6	27	6	
Alive but not contacted	2	10[d]	2	22%
Died before age 40	4	19	2	
Total	100	456	120	

a. Nine of these men had died after age 40.

b. Three of these men had died after age 40.

c. Too little was known about 14 of the 56 men in this group to assess alcohol use; the figure of 10 alcohol abusers or 22 percent probably represents a minimum estimate.

d. One of these men had died after age 40.

Attrition

In following up the 500 controls originally interviewed in 1940–1945, the Gluecks made the decision in the 1950s (because of budgetary constraints) to ignore the 44 men born after July 1, 1932. Since this decision was based solely on birthdate, it should introduce no bias. Table 7.8 describes the thoroughness of follow-up for the remaining 456 men at age 47±2. The table also reports the percentage of observed alcohol abuse in the different follow-up categories. (Alcohol abuse was defined as four or more symptoms on the Problem Drinking Scale described in Chapter 1.)

Lifetime records were relatively complete for 400 men; this is the group that will be included in most of the analyses in this book. (The number of men for whom any single variable was available varied considerably, however, from 385 in the case of some clinical judgments to 456 in the case of some childhood variables.) Of these 400 men, 367 were personally interviewed for roughly two hours as close to their 47th birthday as possible. In 22 cases a cooperative relative was interviewed instead of the subject; in 9 such cases, relatives were interviewed because the subjects had died after age 40 and in the others the subject was geographically inaccessible or too ill medically or psychiatrically to be interviewed. Finally, 7 of the 400 men were not interviewed but fairly complete records were pieced together from relatives, institutional records, and telephone conversations; 5 of these men were known to be serious alcohol abusers, which may explain their own reluctance and that of their relatives to submit to a complete interview.

All of the 19 men who died before age 40 were arbitrarily excluded from most analyses. Since this study focuses on the natural history of alcoholism, it seemed inappropriate to include men who died before the age of maximum risk for alcoholism. However, death certificates could be obtained for 16 of these men and arrest records and psychiatric records were obtained for all of them. Seven of the 19 men survived long enough to be interviewed at age 25 and 32. Only 2 men were known to have abused alcohol (and died alcohol-related deaths); but 2 out of 19 may be an underestimate. Data from old interviews, information from relatives, and criminal records led us to classify as alcohol abusers 6 of the 27 men who when personally contacted asked to withdraw from the study.

There were 10 surviving men who by the end of the study had not been personally contacted. Recently, interviews have been obtained of four of these men and confirmed lifelong absence of alcohol abuse. One man had died at age 41 and his relatives were not available for interviews. The remaining 5 men are known to be still alive but have eluded any kind of direct contact; their relatives cannot or will not reveal their whereabouts. Recent information has been obtained on 2 of these 5 and indicates that one is an alcohol abuser. Two men, one a heavy drinker, have been reported by their relatives to be living somewhere in the South with uncertain recent addresses. The fifth man was known to be alive by a public agency that forwarded our correspondence but could not reveal his address; he did not reply to our letters.

In summary, adequate information was obtained on 400 (92 percent) of the 437 men who survived until age 40, and at some point in their lives 110 (27 percent) of these men abused alcohol. This book focuses upon these 110 men. For 42 of the remaining 56 men the presence or absence of alcohol abuse could be estimated; 10 (24 percent) probably abused alcohol. For 14 men (3 percent of the sample) information regarding alcohol use was lacking.

Tables 7.9 and 7.10 contrast the 400 men for whom it was possible to obtain complete information with the 56 men who died young or asked to withdraw from the study or for whom there was incomplete data. Table 7.9 indicates that the two groups of men did not differ significantly on most of

TABLE 7.9 Insignificant premorbid differences between completely and incompletely followed-up cases.[a]

Premorbid variable	Completed cases (n = 400)	Drops, little data, or dead (n = 56)
Unfavorable Rorschach	32%	35%
Excellent childhood health	19	26
Childhood emotional problems	29	38
No delinquent ancestors	53	49
No delinquent parents or sibs	69	59
Parents' marriage unhappy	34	41
Bleak childhood	27	32
No alcoholic ancestors	54	48
No alcoholic parents	61	59
No mentally ill ancestors	82	86
No mentally ill parents	87	79
Irish ethnicity	19	16
Mediterranean ethnicity	32	36

a. Eighty-three percent of the 400 completed cases and 76 percent of the survivors among the other 56 cases had been personally interviewed at age 32. In most other cases relatives have been interviewed.

the variables in Table 2.18 that predicted future mental health or alcoholism. Within the limitations of our data there is no evidence that alcoholism was a major factor in the attrition experienced by this study.

However, the men who withdrew, died prematurely, or eluded contact were at much greater risk for social deviance. As Table 7.10 illustrates, the 56 men who were lost to follow-up were less intelligent, tended to grow up in multiproblem families, truanted more, and dropped out of school sooner than the subjects who took part in the study. As adolescents they were viewed as far less competent, and as adults they were more likely to manifest sociopathy and go to jail.

To take a different tack, how could so many men from the inner city—27 percent of whom abused alcohol, 19 percent of whom had been in jail, and 7 percent of whom had been hospitalized for mental illness—be followed for almost 35 years without anyone being completely lost? Originally, Eleanor Glueck had seen to it that each record contained a complete address list for each of the men's relatives. Ninety percent of the men or their close relatives had been reinterviewed at ages 25 and 31. As already mentioned, the inde-

TABLE 7.10. Significant differences between completely and incompletely followed-up cases.

Variable	Completed cases (n = 400)	Drops, little data, or dead (n = 56)
I.Q. < 90	29%	42%
< 10 grades of school	34	47
Some college	17	0
Subject in social class IV–V	47	75[a]
Parents in social class V	30	46
Worst boyhood competence	14	36
Multiproblem family (10+ problems)	12	30
Truant or school problems	5	13
5+ signs sociopathy	7	16[b]
Ever in prison	18	27

a. Percentage of the 28 men for whom the Hollingshead-Redlich scale could be applied.
b. Percentage of the 31 men for whom the Robins scale could be applied.

fatigable thoroughness with which the Gluecks' staff (especially their resourceful social investigator, John Burke) followed the men made all the difference.

In the 1970s, armed with these clues, the Study of Adult Development staff used city directories, voters' lists, and the sort of staff persistence described in the following case histories to locate most of the men. In about 10 cases it was necessary to ask large public agencies that had helped the Gluecks in the past either to forward letters or to check whether men were living or dead. In perhaps 10 additional cases, our limited access to criminal records at least confirmed identity, survival, and a plausible reason why the men chose to ignore both their relatives and our letters. Of the original sample, 30 percent continued to live in the city of Boston and only 13 percent had left New England—half of these had moved to Florida or California. This limited geographic mobility facilitated follow-up.

Nevertheless, even in Boston, persistence was required. The case of James Ryan (all names are changed) illustrates both problems and solutions. Initially, we found a Lena Ryan at Center Street, Charlestown—the same address where James Ryan's brother Fred had lived. Lena was, indeed, the sister-in-law of the subject, but, now divorced, she had lost touch with her ex-husband's side of the family. We next phoned the ex-mother-in-law of our subject, but she stated that she had lost touch with her daughter (this turned out not to be true) and suggested we try James Ryan's sisters. With her help we located and telephoned Rose Ryan, a sister of the subject. Rose sounded vague—almost as if she knew where the subject was, but would not tell. Almost immediately after talking with her we received a phone call from James himself who said that he feared we were bill collectors—a number of whom were pursuing him. James Ryan gave us his telephone number and address in Everett and was quite willing to fill out a preliminary questionnaire, which he returned to our office.

On August 17 our interviewer telephoned James Ryan for an interview; he readily agreed to Friday, August 20. At the appointed time, his wife answered the door and cordially invited the interviewer in, apologizing that her husband unexpectedly was working, replacing his son for two days driving a truck. Her parlor was filled with nine children watching *I Love Lucy* on TV. Mrs. Ryan accepted our explanation of the study, seemed interested in our work, and was quite willing to answer some questions while the interviewer waited for her husband.

After 30 minutes James Ryan came in. He was quite friendly and apologetic, but he wanted to know if 20 minutes would do for the interview. It was explained that it would take longer, and he readily agreed to 4:30 P.M. on Tuesday, August 24. At the appointed time on August 24 his wife again answered the door and said James had to work overtime and that she had tried to cancel without success. She said her husband was "awfully sorry" that he had had to break the appointment.

On August 26 the interviewer talked on the phone with the subject, who apologetically set up another appointment for Wednesday, September 1, at 4:30 P.M. On August 31 we telephoned the subject to confirm an appointment for the next day. His wife reported that Mr. Ryan had been called to work in the western part of the state. On September 1 we called back in the afternoon. A daughter answered the phone and said her father was in New York working and suggested we call back in two weeks. On October 5 we reached his wife on the phone, and she said her husband was away working and probably would be back in two weeks.

On October 23 we spoke by phone with the subject's daughter, who said her father was in the hospital for an ulcer operation and "some tests." On October 28 we reached Mr. Ryan by phone, and he said he was better after his operation. Since he would be busy the rest of the week, he suggested that we call back the following week. On November 2 we again talked with the subject on the phone. He sounded very concerned and said that something had happened to one of his kids. He asked if he could put off the interview for a week or two. He sounded distressed but cooperative. On November 16, James Ryan told us by phone that he was presently unemployed and free to see us, and offered November 19 at 1 P.M. He said he had a house full of kids and suggested we talk in the car.

On November 19, 3 months after he first agreed to see us, the interviewer arrived at the Ryans' house to find nobody home. Five minutes later, Mr. Ryan drove up in his car and indicated that the interviewer should climb in. He gave us a cooperative interview.

Another example illustrates the persistence required to obtain information on the alcohol abusers. We had expected Bill Smith to be discharged from the Cambridge Detoxification Center on Wednesday, February 3. On February 2 we called the Center to find out if we could interview Mr. Smith during visiting hours. This request was refused on the grounds that our visiting would interrupt Mr. Smith's treatment. Accordingly, our interviewer visited the subject's home on February 4 in hopes that he would be there. No one was home so the interviewer returned three hours later. A short man came out of Mr. Smith's apartment carrying a large bag of trash to the hallway. He was a disheveled man in his late forties with a head of curly grey hair and appeared to be cleaning out the apartment. He was unshaven and moved slowly. Asked if he was Bill Smith, the man replied that Bill was due to be discharged from the Detoxification Center on the next day at around 3 P.M. On February 5 our interviewer returned; there was no one home.

On February 6 our interviewer visited Mr. Smith's home once more. This time a tall dark-haired man answered the door; a few other men were visible inside watching TV. Asked if he was Mr. Smith, the tall man said no. After determining who the interviewer was, he called Bill Smith to the door. The short, grey-haired man who came to the door was the same man who had brought the trash into the hallway on February 4, only now he had had a haircut and a shave. Without reference to the prior meeting, he acknowledged that he was indeed Mr. Smith. He said that he had just gotten home from the hospital, did not feel well, was still on medication, and did not want to risk answering the questions incorrectly. When he suggested that the interviewer come back in a couple of weeks, the interviewer observed that the check the study had made out for Mr. Smith was back-dated and that perhaps waiting too long was not a good idea. (Although in most cases participation in the study was not recompensed and in many cases money was vigorously refused, we paid about 20 men $10 an hour for their cooperation.) Mr. Smith brightened at the mention of the check and agreed to the interview. Then he recalled that his friends were present and decided that he was too weak after all. He proposed Sunday, February 8, at 2 P.M.

To the interviewer's surprise, Mr. Smith himself answered the door at 2 P.M. on February 8. He was dressed in a clean but somewhat worn pair of trousers and an old T-shirt. He took a final moment to reconsider. "How long will this take?" The interviewer promised to expedite things.

The inside of Mr. Smith's apartment was shabby but clean. The tall, dark-haired man sat in one of the living-room chairs watching TV. Mr. Smith led the interviewer into the kitchen, made him coffee, and gave a cooperative interview for two hours. Sounds of cowboys, Indians, and cartoons from the living room provided the background music.

However hard the interviewers might have to work for the interviews, the men themselves deserve great credit for making a reciprocal effort to cooperate. Their collective loyalty to the study over its forty years of existence has been extraordinary.

Limitations

I must acknowledge and examine the potential pitfalls of longitudinal study identified by Baekeland and colleagues (1975) and Baltes (1968). First, bias due to selective attrition was not a significant problem in the present study. The distorting effects of selective losses by drops and death were diminished by the fact that no subjects were completely lost and that much was known about the drops and the dead. The lifetime pattern of alcohol use was quite unknown in only 2 College and 14 Core City men.

Second, the distorting effect of selective sampling (for example, studying only alcoholics who came to a clinic) was avoided by studying an entire community cohort. A subject could not volunteer for either study, and only about 15 percent of those originally selected for either the College or the Core City study refused to participate.

Third, longitudinal studies tend to be locked into one point in history, so that comparability with other studies is difficult. The present study is no exception. I have attempted to facilitate the comparison of the Study of Adult Development with other studies by using multiple definitions for subjective outcome variables like mental illness and alcoholism. However, our efforts, after the fact, to define variables like hyperactivity were clearly hampered by the longitudinal design. In 1945 neither the diagnosis of hyperactivity (minimal brain damage) nor the underlying criteria for making such a diagnosis existed.

Fourth, in any long-lived longitudinal study the effects of repeated testing, of being studied ("Western Electric" or "Hawthorne" effects), and halo effects affect both subject and observer. In the present study repetitive testing was avoided, and to reduce halo effects ratings at different times were made by different observers. Nevertheless, many of the College—if very few of the Core City—men were acutely aware of being studied and felt special as a result. How this may have distorted the results remains uncertain.

Fifth, longitudinal studies assume but do not effect continuous observation. The Core City men were interviewed only four different times and the College men only three. Such frequency of follow-up is commendable when compared to other prospective studies of alcohol abuse (see Chapter 2), but it is still far from ideal. Much data is inevitably retrospective. For example, the men reported both drinking problems and paths into abstinence more vividly if they had occurred recently rather than many years in the past. To ensure that all subjects are in the same state of disease or recovery at follow-up requires a cross-sectional design.

Sixth, perhaps the most serious limitation of this study (and of most longitudinal studies) is that it is by no means a panel study. The sample members were all white males chosen from a narrow birth cohort, from one country, and reflecting a truncated range of social class and intelligence. There were two facts, however, that mitigated this limitation. Conclusions were drawn only by comparing the subjects with one another; and because many confounding variables could be held constant, in some respects the uniformity of each sample enhanced the validity of such comparison. It is no accident that biological laboratories strive to obtain uniformity among their experimental animals. Nevertheless, until the findings in this book are supported by replication, their relevance to other alcoholic populations must remain in question.

Seventh, of necessity longitudinal studies of humans are naturalistic; the observer lacks experimental control over his subjects or what happens to them, and controlled study is impossible. And lastly, as in the case of depicting a landscape through aerial photography, in a longitudinal study much fine detail escapes observation.

IV ~ Lessons for Treatment

8 ～ The Doctor's Dilemma

While writing this book, I received an invitation to a conference on alcohol treatment from Griffith Edwards, director of the Addiction Research Unit of the Institute of Psychiatry at the Maudsley Hospital in London. He noted that for seven years I had been codirector of an alcohol treatment program about which I was enthusiastic. He also noted that for many years I had been keen on long-term follow-up research. Keeping these facts in mind, Professor Edwards presented me with a dilemma:

> What we are hoping is that you will try to portray the picture of the research-minded treatment man, who jolly well knows that much of the evidence isn't there to support his treatment methods, or who feels that the evidence may even contradict his practices. Nonetheless, he may sense that the research often in some ways goes blindly past what is seen in the clinic, and that he may choose to trust his own nose rather than what the papers say. Is he a fool, or a knave, or a sensible man? . . . How do we retain open-mindedness without losing confidence to deal with the next patient who is certainly expecting our help?

This chapter represents my efforts to resolve that dilemma.

Thomas Szasz (1972) would have us believe that alcoholism, like the dilemma, is a mythical beast. Unfortunately, sometimes mythical beasts are endowed with real horns. One horn of my dilemma is that Szasz, Al-Anon, and the best follow-up research instruct would-be caregivers that they are powerless over alcoholism. To try too hard to *cure* an alcoholic is to break one's heart, and many follow-up studies suggest that elaborate treatment may be no better than brief sensible advice (Orford and Edwards 1977). The other

347

horn of my dilemma is that to ignore a chronic malady as painful to the individual, as damaging to his health, as destructive to his family, and as refractory to willpower, to motivation, and to common sense as alcoholism— for doctors to ignore such a malady—is unconscionable. What are we to do?

The Clinic Sample as an Illustration of the Dilemma

My own awareness of Edwards's dilemma began 10 years ago, when I was asked by the relatives of an alcoholic friend for help. The friend, aged 55, was quietly drinking himself to death. He had exhausted the patience of probably the wisest family doctor in Boston; he had frustrated the staff at perhaps Boston's finest teaching hospital; he had managed to spend several weeks in an excellent Boston psychiatric hospital as a "bipolar depression" without noticeable improvement. His relatives pointed out that I was considered knowledgeable about addictions. What or whom could I suggest? I called a few very senior colleagues and then reported back that no one on the faculty of my medical school was expert in the treatment of alcoholism and that, as best I knew, modern medicine had little to offer.

Shortly afterwards, as part of the trend in both America and England to acknowledge the enormity of the problem of alcohol abuse, the Cambridge and Somerville Program for Alcohol Rehabilitation (CASPAR), was started at the Cambridge-Somerville Mental Health Center. Since the sister cities of Cambridge and Somerville contained an estimated 20,000 alcoholics, the decision was made to redeploy present services so as to offer much less intensive help to many more people. The single staff member, who, by appointment, had offered therapy and counsel to these 20,000 souls was replaced by a much better staffed walk-in clinic.

Caught up in the historical moment and because private specialists and academic medicine had been found wanting, my friend turned to this public clinic. He found hopeful paraprofessionals who were willing to meet his needs as he saw them and who discussed alcoholism as if it were a disease—neither a psychological symptom nor some vague unnamed metabolic riddle waiting to be deciphered. The CASPAR staff invited him to groups that they led, with other alcoholics. In part, these groups were designed as stepping stones between the walk-in clinic of a municipal hospital and eventual use of the cheaper, more accessible resources of Alcoholics Anonymous. But my friend had often previously refused to consider Alcoholics Anonymous a viable alternative. He was no joiner; he rarely went to church; he was an artist; and he was much too sophisticated—both socially and intellectually—to get involved in AA. After two years of clinic contact in the acceptable "medical" environment of CASPAR, he found his way into AA. Two years later he became a group chairman, and to the best of my knowledge his family relationships and health have been gradually restored.

Supported by the generous infusion of government funds into community-based mental health programs for the treatment of alcoholism, I too, was caught in the historical moment. Two years after I had told my friend that I knew of no treatment for alcoholism, I joined the staff at Cambridge Hospital as a psychiatric consultant to CASPAR. This program was designed on a medical model, was based in a general hospital, and was directed by an internist. The program included round-the-clock walk-in counseling to patients and relatives, "wet" and "dry" shelter, groups, and immediate access to detoxification and to medical and psychiatric consultation. CASPAR offered alcohol consultation to the medical, surgical, and psychiatric wards of the hospital; it provided halfway houses for homeless men and women and a comprehensive alcohol education program to an entire city school system. At present, CASPAR sees 1000 *new* clients a year, carries out 2500 detoxifications (50 percent directly referred from the police), and receives 20,000 outpatient visits a year. Annually, the program costs about a million dollars including educational personnel; and no one is denied treatment because of multiple relapses, poor motivation, poverty, criminal history, or skid-row lifestyle. At the same time, because skilled and hopeful consultation is always available, the rich have come as well as the poor.

When I joined the staff at Cambridge Hospital, I learned about the disease of alcoholism for the first time. My prior training had been at a famous teaching hospital that from past despair had posted an unwritten sign over the door that read "alcoholic patients need not apply." Next, I had worked for years at a community mental health center that, in spite of a firm commitment to meeting the expressed mental health needs of the community, ignored alcoholism—which, after all, was untreatable and might overwhelm the clinic. At Cambridge Hospital I learned for the first time how to diagnose alcoholism as an illness and to think of abstinence in terms of "one day at a time." Instead of pondering the sociological and psychodynamic complexities of alcoholism, while at the bedside I learned how to keep things simple. (If the oversimplification inherent in Jellinek's disease model works mischief in research, too much doubt and vagueness wreak havoc in the clinic.) My ability to interview alcoholics improved. To me, alcoholism became a fascinating

TABLE 8.1.   Comparison of selected two-year follow-up studies.

Study	n in original sample	n followed up	Duration of follow-up (years)	Abstinent or social drinking	Improved	Abusing alcohol
Clinic sample	106	100	2	20%	13%	67%
Three pooled "no treatment" studies[a]	245	214	2–3	17	15	68
Four treatment studies[b]	963	685	2	21	16	63

a. These are studies by Orford and Edwards (1977), Kendell and Staton (1966), and Imber et al. (1976). Because at 1 year there was no difference between Orford and Edwards's treated and control populations and because at 2 years their report did not clearly separate the two populations, all 85 of their subjects on whom they had 2-year follow-up are included.

b. These are the studies by Belasco (1971), Bruun (1963), Robson, Paulus, and Clarke (1965), and van Dijk and van Dijk-Koffeman (1973).

disease. It seemed perfectly clear that by meeting the immediate individual needs of the alcoholic, by using multimodality therapy, by disregarding "motivation," by turning to recovering alcoholics rather than to Ph.D.'s for lessons in breaking self-detrimental and more or less involuntary habits, and by inexorably moving patients from dependence upon the general hospital into the treatment system of AA, I was working for the most exciting alcohol program in the world.

But then came the rub. Fueled by our enthusiasm, I and the director, William Clark, tried to prove our efficacy. Our clinic followed up our first 100 detoxification patients, the Clinic sample described in Chapter 3, every year for the next 8 years. Initially we created a control group comprising the patients we rejected because our beds were full, but after a few months this seemed pointless. Our treatment network was sufficiently widespread that eventually controls reapplied and were accepted for treatment.

Table 8.1 shows our treatment results. After initial discharge, only 5 patients in the Clinic sample *never* relapsed to alcoholic drinking, and there is compelling evidence that the results of our treatment were no better than the natural history of the disease. In Table 8.1, the outcomes for the Clinic sample patients are contrasted with two-year follow-ups of four treatment programs that analyzed their data in a comparable way and admitted patients similar to ours. The Clinic sample results are also contrasted with three studies of equal duration that purported to offer no formal treatment. Although the

TABLE 8.2. Long-term follow-up of treated and untreated alcoholics.

Study	n in original sample	n followed up	Duration of follow-up (years)	Abstinent or social drinking	Improved	Abusing alcohol or dead	Dead	Gamma alcoholics
Clinic sample	106	100	8	38%	7%	55%	29%	95%
Myerson and Mayer 1966	101	100	10	22	24	54	20	100
Bratfos 1974	1179	478	10	12	25	63	14	87
Goodwin, Crane, and Guze 1971	123	93	8	26	15	59	5	c.75
Voetglin and Broz 1949	?	104	7	22	13	65	?	?
Lundquist 1973	200	200	9	27	20	53	22.5	c.75

treatment populations differ, the studies are roughly comparable; in hopes of averaging out major sampling differences, the studies are pooled. Costello (1975), Emrick (1975), and Hill and Blane (1967) have reviewed many more disparate two-year outcome studies and have noted roughly similar proportions of significantly improved and unimproved alcoholics. Not only had we failed to alter the natural history of alcoholism, but our death rate of three percent a year was appalling. How was I to answer Griffith Edwards's Socratic inquiry? However, if our death rate was rather inconsistent with a mythical affliction, it was all too consistent with the medical model of alcoholism as a disease.

The CASPAR treatment program was open-ended. A majority of the unremitted Clinic alcoholics continued to return to our treatment program and, as illustrated in Chapter 3, improvement continued.

In Table 8.2, the results of the Clinic sample at eight years are compared with five rather disparate follow-up studies in the literature which are of similar duration but which looked at very different patient populations. Once again, our results were no better than the natural history of the disorder. Admittedly, Kissin has warned us that "Perhaps negative results should be reported even more cautiously, since almost everyone tends to view positive ones with a jaundiced eye and to take negative ones at their face value" (1977, p. 1087); but I did not find this warning comforting. Edwards's dilemma seemed a real enough beast.

Natural Healing Forces in Alcoholism

Recently the *Annals of Internal Medicine* editorialized that "the treatment of alcoholism has not improved in any important way in twenty-five years" (Gordis 1976). Alas, I am forced to agree. Perhaps the best that can be said for our exciting treatment effort at Cambridge Hospital is that we were certainly not interfering with the normal recovery process. How can I, a clinician, reconcile my enthusiasm for treatment with such melancholy research data?

The answer derives from addressing the second horn of the dilemma. The problem of alcoholism is too immense and the pain it causes too severe to suggest that hospitals once again hang out signs that read "alcoholics need not apply." The demands alcoholism places on the health-care delivery system are too pervasive to tell government bodies that it is useless to fund large-scale treatment programs. It is not a step forward to say that alcoholism is the sole responsibility of families, of the church, and of the police. Therefore, if treatment as we currently understand it does not seem more effective than natural healing processes, then we need to understand those natural healing processes. We need also to study the special role that health-care professionals play in facilitating those processes.

Consider tuberculosis as an analogy. In 1940 a well-known textbook of medicine advised, "Since there is no known specific cure for tuberculosis, treatment rests *entirely* on recognition of the factors contributing to the resistance of the patient" (Cecil 1940). In saying this the textbook did not recommend that the government and doctors get out of the business of treating tuberculosis; nor did it suggest that because genes and socioeconomic factors were etiologically just as important as contagion, tuberculosis was really *just* a social problem and not a medical disorder. Rather, the text suggested that doctors learn more about natural healing processes.

In concluding their exhaustive review of alcohol treatment programs, Baekeland and colleagues wrote: "Over and over we were impressed with the dominant role the patient, as opposed to the kind of treatment used on him, played both in his persistence in treatment and his eventual outcome" (1975, p. 305). Similarly, Orford and Edwards, introducing their pessimistic controlled study of treatment, wrote: "In alcoholism treatment research should increasingly embrace the closer study of natural forces which can be captured and exploited by planned, therapeutic intervention" (1977, p. 3).

Throughout history, physicians faced with disease that they can neither comprehend nor cure have played invaluable roles in capturing these natural forces. In his classic monograph, *Persuasion and Healing,* Jerome Frank, professor of psychiatry at Johns Hopkins University, offered a transcultural model for healing that is nonspecific for disease or patient; but Frank's model maximizes both the relief of suffering and—of special importance in alcoholism—attitude change. Frank acknowledges the paradox that demand for therapy may seem increasingly insatiable at the very time of mounting complaint that such therapy may represent expensive fraud. What feeds such demand is not the patient's need for cure as much as his need to elevate his morale.

First, alcoholics feel defeated, helpless, and without ability to change. If their lives are to change, they need hope as much as relief of symptoms. Second, alcoholics often have an ingrained habit that is intractable to reason, threat, or willpower. To change a maladaptive habit, be it smoking or getting too little exercise or drinking too much alcohol, we cannot "treat" or compel or reason with the person. Rather, we must change the person's belief system and then maintain that change. Time and time again, both evangelists and behavior therapists have demonstrated that if you can but win their hearts and minds, their habits will follow. In other words, if we can but combine the best placebo effects of acupuncture, Lourdes, or Christian Science with the best attitude change inherent in the evangelical conversion experience, we may be on our way to an effective alcoholism program. I shall describe Frank's view in general terms and then illustrate his points with four relatively successful programs.

Frank's prescription for an effective "placebo" therapy (that is, for a modern-day Lourdes) has as its goal to raise the patient's expectation of cure and to reintegrate him with the group. "At Lourdes, pilgrims pray for each other, not for themselves. This stress on service counteracts the patient's morbid self-preoccupation, strengthens his self-esteem by demonstrating that he can do something for others and cements the tie between patient and group" (Frank 1961, p. 63). Such therapy involves the sharing of suffering with a sanctioned healer who is willing to talk about the patient's problems in a symbolic way. The sanctioned healer should have status and power and be equipped with an unambiguous conceptual model of the problem which he is willing to explain to the patient. (Within the medical model of alcoholism, this is the strategy behind Jellinek's disease concept.) Enhancement of the patient's self-esteem and reduction of his anxiety are the inevitable consequences. The common ingredients of such a program include group acceptance, an emotionally charged but communally shared ritual, and a shared belief system. Such a ritual should be accompanied by a cognitive learning process that "explains" the phenomenon of the illness. The point is that if one cannot cure an illness, one wants to make the patient less afraid and overwhelmed by it.

Frank's prescription for attitude change is initially interrogation by and confession of sins to a high-status healer. This process involves four components: indoctrination, repetition, removal of ambiguity, and opportunity for identification. It has been demonstrated that the patient's active participation in such a process "increases a person's susceptibility especially if the situation requires him to assume some initiative" for his own attitude change (p. 112). In the Stanford Heart Disease Prevention Program, internist John Farquhar (1978) and his colleagues (Farquhar et al. 1977) have examined different models of reducing smoking, altering diet, and increasing exercise. In their efforts to reduce coronary risk in large populations of patients, they found that explanation of risk and rational advice by physicians are less useful than

TABLE 8.3. Two-year follow-up results of "special" treatment programs compared with results from "routine" treatment programs.

Treatment program	n in original sample	n followed up	Duration of follow-up (years)	Abstinent or social drinking	Improved	Continued trouble
Four pooled treat-ment studies[a]	963	685	2	21%	16%	63%
Emetine aversion (Shadel 1944)	?	300	2	60	5	35
Antabuse (Waller-stein 1956)	47	40	2	53%		47
AA (Beaubrun 1967)	57	57	7	37	16	47
Behavior modification (Sobell and Sobell 1976)	20	20	2	35	50	15

a. These are the studies cited in Table 8.1.

systematic *indoctrination* and *repetition* using mass media and *opportunity for identification* through peer support groups.

Frank writes: "the greatest potential drawback of therapy groups is their tendency not to supply sufficient support, especially in early meetings, to enable members to cope with the stresses they generate" (p. 190). One of the functions, then, of the medical-care system is to facilitate the transition of the isolated patient to group membership. Finally, if attitude change is to be maintained, repetition of group rituals and the group support that they engender must be sustained after clinic discharge.

Table 8.3 presents four alcohol treatment programs that fortuitously followed Frank's prescription and significantly facilitated remission from alcoholism. The table reflects the early treatment results reported by the Shadel clinic using emetine aversion (Shadel 1944; Voegtlin and Broz 1949), by the Menninger Clinic using disulfiram (Antabuse) and group therapy (Wallerstein 1956), by Beaubrun (1967) using an imaginative combination of indigenous paraprofessionals and medically sanctioned Alcoholics Anonymous, and by Sobell and Sobell using behavior modification (1973, 1976). Because they were adequately controlled, the Wallerstein and Sobell studies are especially convincing. Each program employed the newest method of its decade, was led by competent investigators, and found results that were clearly superior to those usually reported.

But what could emetine aversion conditioning in the 1940s, disulfiram coupled with group therapy in a world-famous clinic in the 1950s, the use of AA coupled with indigenous Calypso-singing ex-alcoholics in the 1960s, and behavior therapy to return to controlled drinking in the 1970s have in common? First, they all maximized the placebo effect of medical treatment and effected significant attitude change. As sanctioned powerful healers, each treatment staff brought hope and provided a rational explanation of mysterious suffering and then created a framework for sharing that suffering with others.

Second, consistent with Frank's suggestions, in each of these programs the illness of alcoholism was carefully explained to each patient. Although these explanations differed, they were consistent with the medical knowledge of each era. Although each patient was made responsible for his future involvement, alcoholism was represented as a clearly defined disorder, not as a symptom of moral or psychiatric incompetence. For example, each of Shadel's patients was given 10 rules. Rules #3 and #4 were "Do not look on alcoholism as a personal weakness. Remember that alcoholism is an illness . . . sensitivity to alcohol is inborn and you will always have it." Beaubrun wrote: "In any culture, where gamma alcoholism prevails the most helpful thing which the therapist can say to the alcoholic is that his problem is an illness. There is a world of difference between therapeutic and research orientations in this respect. The therapist knows that the semantic distinction between 'addiction' and 'disease' can make all the difference to his patient's sobriety. It is in the distinction between a criminal and a sick person" (1967, p. 656).

Third, consistent with altering ingrained behavior, all four treatments maximized attitude change in an emotionally charged setting. Each program indoctrinated its patients into a coherent ideology. In each case, a daily ritual was prescribed. For example, Wallerstein wrote: "In maintaining this sober state outside the hospital, the more compulsive the character of the patient and the more he could ritualize the Antabuse ceremony itself, the better his prognosis" (1956, p. 232). Shadel's patients had a sign—"There is one thing I cannot do"—which they were to hang by the mirror while they shaved. The Sobells' patients were given a wallet-sized card of Dos and Don'ts to keep with them at all times, and after leaving the hospital Beaubrun's patients had to continue to go to AA several times a week.

Fourth, rather than trying to alter attitude by threat or by rational advice, each program altered attitudes by affecting self-esteem. The Sobells' patients were shown videotapes of themselves drinking in control and out of control; they highly valued the mastery involved in their return to controlled drinking.

Shadel's rules #7 and #9 were "Develop other outlets" and "Get your strength for living from a desire to help yourself and others and not from the bottle. Help other alcoholics to master their problem." As they were encouraged in group activities, a comradeship developed among the patients. As well as taking disulfiram, Wallerstein's patients stayed in a psychodynamically oriented hospital for three months and attended therapy groups. Shadel wrote that as each alcoholic came into his clinic environment, "it is interesting to see how the gang of old patients goes to work on a new patient"; and Shadel's patients were encouraged to continue groups after leaving. As Beaubrun put it, "It was not enough to tell a patient to attend a meeting; someone was sent to bring him to the first few meetings until he got accustomed to the new group."

Why, then, has history been unkind to these individual treatment methods? Why, thus far, have none led to widespread replication? In the nineteenth century Sir William Osler wrote to a friend who had been treating tuberculosis, "That is a fine record . . . I'm afraid there is one element you've not laid proper stress upon—your own personality. Confidence and faith count so much in these cases" (Cushing 1925). Thus, because the clinicians listed in Table 8.3 brought the newest techniques of their decade to bear, they not only brought hope but also conveyed assurance to the alcoholics of their own power to cure. The Menninger Clinic in the 1950s was world renowned, and the Sobells' elaborate research unit at Patton State Hospital was an impressive stage set filled with scientific gadgetry.

Of course, with confidence and faith can come misleadingly enthusiastic evaluation of outcome data. Independent evaluation, especially after several years, is rarely as favorable as the initial report by the original treatment staff. Thus, the ten-year follow-up by Voegtlin and Broz (1949) suggested that Shadel's (1944) initial report of emetine aversion therapy was overly optimistic. The ten-year re-follow-up by Pendery and colleagues (1982) suggests that the Sobells' view of the value of training in controlled drinking was also too optimistic. Therapists must resign themselves to the fact that hope is unscientific.

The success of Alcoholics Anonymous—and its reasonable facsimiles, which are continuously being rediscovered—probably results from the fact that it conforms so well to the natural healing principles that Frank outlined and with Frank's general prescription for therapeutic group processes. Thus, the strategy behind our treatment of both the Clinic sample and the 8,000 other alcoholics who have sought help at CASPAR has been to involve them with Alcoholics Anonymous. As Table 8.4 illustrates, at Cambridge Hospital, if we have not cured all the alcoholics who were first detoxified over 8 years ago,

TABLE 8.4 Use of Alcoholics Anonymous over time in the Clinic and Core City samples.

	Core City sample	Clinic sample	
n in original sample	110	106	106
n followed up	103	106	100
Duration of follow-up			
(years)	10–25	1	8
Abstinent or social			
drinking	51%	15%	38%
Improved	17%	19%	7%
Continued trouble or dead	32%	66%	55%
% of those abstinent who			
became abstinent through AA	37%	31%	65%
Average number of meetings per			
abstinent AA attender	300	n.a.	600

the likelihood of members of the Clinic sample attending AA has been significantly increased. The table contrasts the AA use of the Clinic sample with that of the naturalistically derived Core City sample. In the Core City sample, 18 (or 37 percent) of the 49 men who achieved a year of abstinence became abstinent in part through AA. Each of these 18 men attended an average of 300 meetings. One year after treatment, 5 of the Clinic sample had achieved stable abstinence that had begun while regularly attending AA; but after 8 years, 19 patients—or 4 times as many—had attained a stable abstinence that began in part through AA. In the 8 years, these 19 patients, 65 percent of all those stably abstinent, had attended an average of 600 meetings. If one excludes the 3 highest attenders in each sample (who attended an estimated average of 1200 meetings each), then the 110 Core City alcohol abusers attended 3000 AA meetings and the 100 Clinic alcoholics attended 15,000—5 times as many meetings on a per capita basis. Admittedly, severity of alcohol abuse correlates with high AA utilization (Table 4.4).

In emphasizing the belief of the CASPAR program in Alcoholics Anonymous, I do not wish to suggest that Alcoholics Anonymous is the *best* answer; there are many paths to recovery in alcoholism, ranging from the diverse programs listed in Table 8.3 to the Anti-Bacchus and Amethyst Clubs in the

Soviet Union. We need to understand what is common to all of them. At the same time, we may need to recognize that the recovery process in alcoholism is best catalyzed not by a single episode of treatment but by fostering natural healing processes over time.

Resolution of the Dilemma

Let me now attempt to resolve my dilemma. First, and somewhat paradoxically, recognition of our limited ability to alter the course of alcoholism may lead to improved care, not chaos. Modern surgery took a giant stride forward when it realized that wounds healed best by natural methods and that wound healing could often be slowed, but could never be hastened, by zealous intervention. Modern medicine began when toward the end of the nineteenth century doctors gave up bleeding patients and abandoned virtually their entire pharmacopoeia. Today, psychiatry has a painful lesson to learn from the fact that schizophrenics have a better prognosis in underdeveloped countries than they do in developed ones (Sartorius et al. 1978). One of the few conclusions that Emrick (1975) drew from his scrutiny of 384 alcohol follow-up studies was that it may be easier for improper treatment to retard recovery than for proper treatment to hasten it. Once recovered, several of the College sample saw their psychotherapy as having retarded recognition of their alcoholism.

Second, we have much to learn from how medicine before 1950 learned to cope with tuberculosis. We do not wish to squander either our natural resources or our own time on just a few alcoholics. Rather, we want to reach as many patients as possible. By remembering the first step of Al-Anon, "And we admitted that we were powerless over alcohol," we protect ourselves from maintaining the guilty illusion that if we just try harder, we can *cure* the alcoholic. Indeed, a major task of any psychiatric consultant to an alcohol program is to remind the staff that they are not to blame for their patients' relapses. At the same time, we never want to ignore the problem. Not surprisingly, results reported by Kissin and colleagues (1968) suggest that openly ignoring alcoholics on a waiting list produced an improvement rate of only 4 percent—far worse than naturalistic studies in the literature. As Seligman (1975) reminds us, hopelessness kills.

Third, at the same time that Ambroise Paré gave us his humble epigram "I dressed him, God healed him," he had the wit to invent the surgical ligature to stop hemorrhage. In 1978, CASPAR provided medical and social assistance to twice as many alcoholics as the entire Connecticut Department of Mental Health provided in 1965 to a catchment population that was *10 times* as large (Shepard 1967). I have no doubt that by providing consultation, detoxification, welfare, and shelter, we stop hemorrhage.

Besides, the samaritan role is not to be sneezed at—especially in chronic disease. When large benefits are not forthcoming, patients will be especially grateful for small ones.

Fourth, I believe that honesty brings its own reward. We must remain alert to the limitations of our alcohol treatment programs. Otherwise, national health schemes may suddenly regard as cost ineffective *all* alcohol treatment, rather than just long hospital stays. Anyone familiar with the therapeutic milieu of a high-cost, high-intensity, high-morale two-to-four-week inpatient treatment unit will find the pessimism of this statement hard to believe and yearn for a controlled study. But when such studies have been undertaken, their findings have indicated that prolonged inpatient treatment appears to contribute nothing additional to outcome (Stinson et al. 1979; Costello 1980; Edwards and Guthrie 1966, 1967; Willems et al. 1973).

The 67 percent rate of improvement with treatment originally suggested in the Rand Report (Armor et al. 1978)—an illusion produced by attrition, by cross-sectional design, and by ignoring the law of initial values—will become dangerous if clinical staff and legislators discover that such hopeful results are a cruel cheat, and if doctors and public funding sources withdraw support that give hope and care to alcoholics.

Fifth, even if alcohol treatment does not indubitably alter the long-term course of alcoholism, it does help over the short term (McLellan et al. 1982). Far more concretely, outpatient alcohol treatment saves money. There have now been at least 12 controlled cost-benefit studies of health maintenance organizations and employee-based alcoholism programs (Jones and Vischi 1979; Reiff et al. 1981). The uniform conclusion of these studies is that the cost involved in providing outpatient alcoholism programs is more than repaid by the decline in medical care utilization, in sick days, and in sickness and accident benefits.

⮑ Alcoholism Treatment Revisited

The recent randomized trial by Walsh and colleagues (1991) has put all negative findings about the limitations of hospital treatment for alcohol abuse in question. The reason for the importance of this study is that it represents the most methodologically sophisticated and most carefully conducted test of hospitalization versus outpatient treatment that we have. The study was a completely randomized clinical trial that enrolled a consecutive cohort of 227 employees, identified by a joint company-union employee-assistance plan. Alcoholic employees were randomized to one of three treatments: hospitalization with AA as aftercare; AA only; and free choice of treatment modality. Of those employees who were offered choice, 41 percent elected to be treated in a hospital and 46 percent elected to go directly to AA. After two years of follow-up, the hospital/AA aftercare group fared best with an abstinence rate of 55 percent at one year and of 36 percent at two years. Subjects assigned to AA alone had the lowest abstinence rate (23 percent at one year, 16 percent at two years). Subjects offered a choice of treatments fell in between. A significant factor accounting for much of the advantage of hospitalization plus AA over AA alone was the fact that hospitalization proved particularly useful for individuals who abused both cocaine and alcohol.

In recent years, using increasingly sophisticated techniques, Holder and his associates have estimated the magnitude of the health care savings associated with alcoholism treatment. In one study Holder and Shachtman (1987) utilized the health care records of alcoholic patients enrolled with Aetna Insurance Company. The study group included 1,645 patients, from all 50 states, enrolled from 1980 to 1983. The offset savings by the end of the third year after an initial treatment for alcoholism were estimated at between $400 and $9,000, depending upon the assumptions of the predicting model. By the end of the third year after alcoholism treatment, the estimated net savings in general health care was $2,515 per person.

In a six-year study Holder and Hallen (1986) examined the health care costs not only for the alcoholics but also for their family members. They contrasted these costs with those for a matched group of comparison families with no alcoholic members. (There were 90 alcoholic families representing 245 individuals and 83 comparison families representing 291 individuals). They found that utilization and costs for all forms of inpatient medical care for both nonalcoholic and alcoholic family members dropped after alcoholism treatment began. Ultimately, costs reached a level similar to those for the matched comparison group. Total monthly costs fell in the final follow-up period to one-sixth the costs before alcoholism treatment began.

9 ~ Suggestions for Would-Be Helpers

It is not conscionable to write a book on the natural history of alcoholism without also discussing its treatment. It is not fair to suggest what may not be effective without sharing with the reader what may be very effective. What follows is advice intended for patient, relative, friend, and clinician alike. The advice reflects my own experience and represents opinion, not scientific fact.

The first step in treatment is hope. The fact that patients who fail treatment—and fail treatment often—are disproportionately represented in clinic waiting rooms means that the overall statistics of any clinical series—including those in Tables 8.2 and 8.3—are too pessimistic. Too often, treatment of alcoholics is not undertaken because of pessimism about the results. It is important to remember that half of all alcoholics achieve stable recoveries and that a significant number of alcoholics achieve stable remissions the very first time they seriously seek clinical treatment.

The second step in treatment is diagnosis. But diagnosis is difficult; as Table 1.7 illustrates, more than half the alcoholics seen by physicians go undiagnosed. One reason for this is that many would-be helpers recognize only stereotypic alcoholic drinkers. Different social groups regard alcohol abuse differently, and individual use and abuse patterns differ. The observer's own belief systems and patterns of alcohol use may interfere with his appraisal of those of others.

A second reason is that alcoholics are adept at concealing overt signs of intoxication, and the alcoholic's denial is often convincing. To overcome their own myopia and the alcoholic's denial, both relative and clinician must learn to conceive of alcoholism as a disease that *causes* depression, marital breakup, and unemployment, not as a symptom that *results from* such distressing

362

events. In other words, to decide if a person is drinking alcoholically, the clinician should ask diagnostic questions of the form, "Was your use of alcohol one of the reasons your wife left you?" rather than merely accepting the patient's explanation, "I did not drink really heavily until my wife ran off with another man."

As Chapter 1 underscores, no single symptom is sufficient to make the diagnosis. The diagnosis of alcoholism can be reached only after the considered integration of evidence from all available sources. Contrary to popular belief, a red nose, alcohol on the breath, psychological dependence on the before-dinner cocktail, drunkenness per se, and solitary drinking are not good indices of alcoholism. The observer must appreciate that individuals drinking alcoholically are very frightened and guilty about what is happening to them. They cannot be relied upon to divulge their symptoms freely. Thus, a series of questions that circumvent denial have been devised that can identify most people with alcoholism. The following list of questions provides the most useful single guide I know to the clinical interview:

1. Do you occasionally drink heavily after a disappointment or a quarrel, or when the boss gives you a hard time?
2. When you have trouble or feel under pressure, do you always drink more heavily than usual?
3. Have you noticed that you are able to handle more liquor than you did when you were first drinking?
4. Did you ever wake up on the "morning after" and discover that you could not remember part of the evening before, even though your friends tell you that you did not "pass out"?
5. When drinking with other people, do you try to have a few extra drinks when others will not know it?
6. Are there certain occasions when you feel uncomfortable if alcohol is not available?
7. Have you recently noticed that when you begin drinking you are in more of a hurry to get the first drink than you used to be?
8. Do you sometimes feel a little guilty about your drinking?
9. Are you secretly irritated when your family or friends discuss your drinking?
10. Have you recently noticed an increase in the frequency of your memory "blackouts"?
11. Do you often find that you wish to continue drinking after your friends say they have had enough?
12. Do you usually have a reason for the occasions when you drink heavily?

13. When you are sober, do you often regret things you have done or said while drinking?
14. Have you tried switching brands or following different plans for controlling your drinking?
15. Have you often failed to keep promises you have made to yourself about controlling or cutting down on your drinking?
16. Have you tried to control your drinking by making a change in jobs, or moving to a new location?
17. Do you try to avoid family and close friends when you are drinking?
18. Are you having an increasing number of financial and work problems?
19. Do more people seem to be treating you unfairly without good reason?
20. Do you eat very little or irregularly when you are drinking?
21. Do you sometimes have the "shakes" in the morning and find that it helps to have a little drink?
22. Have you recently noticed that you cannot drink as much as you once did?

These questions are indirect and are designed to minimize guilt and to maximize self-awareness. One does not ask an alcoholic how much he drinks but how often his drinking has caused him pain. The individual who answers yes to more than two or three of these questions is very likely to be an alcoholic.

A similar set of questions is useful for persons who are worried that a friend or relative may be an alcoholic. If an individual answers yes to five or more of the following questions, the friend or relative definitely has a serious drinking problem.

1. Do you worry about this person's drinking?
2. Have you ever been embarrassed by it?
3. Are holidays more of a nightmare than a celebration because of this person's behavior due to alcohol?
4. Are most of this person's friends heavy drinkers?
5. Does this person often promise to quit drinking, without success?
6. Does this person's drinking make the atmosphere tense and anxious?
7. Does this person deny a drinking problem because he drinks only beer?
8. Do you find it necessary to lie to employer, relatives, or friends in order to hide this person's drinking?
9. Has this person ever failed to remember what occurred during a drinking period?
10. Does this person avoid conversation pertaining to alcohol or problem drinking?

11. Does this person justify his or her drinking?
12. Does this person avoid social situations where alcoholic beverages will not be served?
13. Do you ever feel guilty about this person's drinking?
14. Has this person driven a vehicle while under the influence of alcohol?
15. Are children afraid of this person while he or she is drinking?
16. Are you afraid of physical or verbal attack when this person is drinking?
17. Do others comment on this person's unusual drinking behavior?
18. Do others fear riding with this person when he or she is drinking and driving?
19. Does this person have periods of remorse after a drinking occasion and apologize for unacceptable behavior?
20. Does drinking less alcohol bring about the same effects in this person as in the past required more?

It is far easier to treat alcoholism early in its natural history, before the drinker evolves an elaborate denial system to alleviate his despair. Early intervention can be achieved, however, only if the relative or clinician adopts single-minded attention to the possibility of the disease of alcoholism, even in its early stages. The observer must not let the ambiguity of the diagnosis or the patient's multitude of other complaints interfere with recognition of alcohol abuse.

No doctor should deem a patient possibly alcoholic without giving the patient a definite appointment to return. Once the clinician has made the diagnosis of alcoholism, *the diagnosis must be communicated to the patient.* But patients need to be shown, not told. In the early stages when the clinician, and especially the patient, are uncertain about the diagnosis, the patient may be instructed to drink alcohol ad lib but never to exceed three drinks in a given day, and to return in a few weeks. If the patient drinks moderately throughout a three-month period, that is a convincing piece of information that the patient is still in control of alcohol. A patient who cannot follow such a simple instruction may begin to appreciate his or her own loss of control. Thus, the task is to convince the patient not that he or she *is* an alcoholic, but that he or she is a decent person who has an insidious disease, a disease that is a primary *cause* of distress. Patients need to be Socratically taught that alcohol is foe, not friend.

Most alcoholics, when actively drinking and immediately following detoxification, suffer from a mild dementia ("wet brain") that may not fully clear for six months. Therefore, all instructions must be kept simple, unambiguous, and focused on alcohol as the primary problem. Because of the associated guilt, alcoholism is an intensely emotionally laden subject—a second reason to "keep it simple." During the first weeks after detoxification, I believe, the painfully simple Alcoholics Anonymous banners convey almost all the clinical pearls that a patient can hear: "Easy does it"; "It's the first drink that gets you drunk"; "Identify, don't compare"; "A day at a time."

Once both the doctor and the patient are impressed that the amount drunk often exceeds intent, that drinking is affecting physical, social, or financial well-being, it is useful to refer to alcoholism as a black-and-white disease. It is often useful to ignore the qualifiers that would be necessary if one were viewing alcohol abuse from a research perspective. Too often the patient will remember the qualifying adjectives and forget the noun, *alcoholism,* that the adjectives modify.

I believe it is important to explain to patients that their alcoholism, like a disease, has a life of its own and is not a moral or psychological problem. Repeated relapses that injure an alcoholic's loved ones generate enormous guilt and confusion. The ensuing shame further enhances denial. My experience has convinced me that the concept of disease facilitates rather than impedes patients' acceptance of responsibility for their illness and its treatment.

In conveying the concept that alcoholism is a disease to the patient, it is important also to underscore that alcoholism is a disease that is highly treatable, but that like the treatment of diabetes, treatment of alcoholism will require great responsibility from the patient. The clinician or family member may well add, "It's not as easy to stop drinking as some think" or "I don't believe anybody really enjoys heavy drinking; it creates more problems than it solves. But I can understand that alcohol sometimes seems like a friend."

Alcoholism distorts the family equilibrium, and the resulting group denial can reach extraordinary proportions. Thus, it is usually helpful for the would-be helper to discuss the problem with the whole family together. Supporting the family in gentle confrontation is effective and ensures that all members receive the same message. Such a family meeting, however, may require careful planning and preparation.

The process of conveying to another person the diagnosis of alcoholism is usually gradual—and the process is, in itself, therapeutic. Alcoholism is a syndrome, and there are no individual criteria that make the diagnosis. Initially, it is the would-be helper's task continuously to review with the patient the objective evidence (for example, through the 22 questions listed earlier) in order to remind the patient that his use of alcohol is putting him out of and not in control. The patient's anger at such confrontation should be construed as a manifestation of anxiety or cognitive dissonance, not lack of gratitude or motivation.

Only when doctor, family, and patient are all agreed that the patient has an illness that requires treatment can the third step of providing treatment begin. To achieve this end a flexible, multimodality approach appears to work best. Such a comprehensive alcohol treatment program must not just provide detoxification and outpatient counseling with the client and his family. It must also supply minimum nonpunitive shelter to the actively drinking client, alcohol-free halfway houses for the destitute client trying to stay sober, welfare counseling, emergency medical care, and child-oriented counseling and protective services for the minor children of alcoholic patients. Coordinated liaison services are needed between alcohol programs and the courts and psychiatric hospitals. Because of the inability of the most severely ill alcoholic patients to qualify for insurance programs, support often must come from directly publicly funded programs.

Actual detoxification should be kept as simple as possible. Patients who clearly need immediate psychiatric or medical care should be triaged to the appropriate service. The treatment of alcoholism should be directed toward altering an ingrained habit of maladaptive use of alcohol—and treatment should not be limited to focusing on the symptoms (such as alcohol withdrawal, homelessness, marital crisis, or enlarged liver), although such symptoms are important and may have to be addressed before more definitive treatment begins. The experimental evidence gleaned from Chapter 4 suggests that such an ingrained habit can best be changed by paying attention to four components: (1) offering the patient a nonchemical substitute dependency for alcohol, (2) reminding him ritually that even one drink can lead to pain and relapse, (3) repairing the social and medical damage that he has experienced, and (4) restoring his self-esteem.

Providing all four components at once is not easy. Disulfiram (Antabuse) and similar compounds that produce illness if alcohol is ingested are reminders not to drink, but they take away a cherished addiction without providing anything in return: they provide the second component but ignore the first. Prolonged hospitalization provides the first three components but ignores the fourth and eventually the first. Hospital patienthood destroys self-esteem, and when hospitalization ceases the patient loses his substitute dependency. Tranquilizing drugs provide the first component but ignore the other three. For example, providing the anxious alcoholic with tranquilizers will give temporary relief of anxiety but may also facilitate the chain of conditioned responses that lead to picking up a drink at the next point of crisis. Over the long term, providing alcoholics with pills only reinforces their illusion that relief of distress is pharmacological, not human.

Psychotherapy may provide the first and third components but not the second and not always the fourth. Because alcoholics abuse alcohol from habit and not to resolve conflict, the permissive, nondirective method of psychoanalytic psychotherapy is enormously limited. Besides, alcoholics need counseling at odd hours, not by appointment. By definition, a sustained therapeutic relationship and its accompanying transference present the therapist as a powerful and reliable figure. This process may actually worsen the alcoholic patient's already low self-esteem and exacerbate his contempt for his own incomprehensible unreliability. Alcoholics often learn to transform this self-contempt into contempt for the reliability, the tolerance, and the pious sobriety of their long-suffering therapists. A therapist can only experience such transformation as ingratitude, and sooner or later will betray anger. In response to such angry countertransference, the alcoholic may conclude that therapeutic alliance is impossible.

Self-help groups, of which Alcoholics Anonymous is one model, offer the simplest way of providing the alcoholic with all four components referred to above. First, the continuous hope, the gentle peer support, and the selected exposure to the most stable recoveries provide the alcoholic with a ritualized substitute dependency, and a substitute for lost drinking companions. Second, like the best behavior therapy, AA meetings not only go on daily, especially on weekends and holidays, but also singlemindedly underscore the special ways that alcoholics delude themselves. Thus, in a ritual manner, AA allows the alcoholic, who might unconsciously be driven to relapse, to remain conscious of this danger. Third, belonging to a group of caring individuals who have found solutions to the typical problems that beset the newly sober alcoholic alleviates loneliness. Fourth, the opportunity to identify with helpers who once were equally disabled and the opportunity to help others stay sober enhances self-worth.

As self-esteem goes up, the capacity to listen returns. As Edwards suggests, "Treatment is in part a matter of discovering strategies which will make the individual responsive again to the cues of his environment" (1974, p. 193). Thus, we have a paradox—psychotherapy encourages the patient to depend upon his doctor, encourages him to complain that he has little for which to be grateful, but insists that he be independent enough to pay for that privilege. Self-help groups care for the patient for nothing but show him that he is independent enough to help others and encourage gratitude for the smallest blessings. That such an approach involves an element of denial is true; but research into serious medical illness is slowly teaching us that selective denial can be life saving.

Acceptance of Alcoholics Anonymous is often a late, not an early, step in treatment. Unfortunately, clinicians or family members cannot simply refer an alcohol-dependent person to AA, any more than they could refer someone to a church or a hobby club. For one thing, people need to be introduced to AA by someone; few patients go to their first meeting by themselves. Second, AA is a "program of attraction," and required attendance is often not successful. Third, unlike attending a hobby club, attending AA may not be enjoyable. In recommending AA, the would-be helper should remember that regular attendance at meetings may be as unpleasant and as painful a prospect as applying iodine to a cut. At the same time, helpers should encourage patients not to judge AA on the basis of a few meetings. Like churches or college courses, AA groups are numerous and vary enormously. Patient experimentation may be needed to find a congenial group. It is a good practice for clinicians to schedule an office visit a few days after patients attend their first AA meeting and give them a chance to discuss their reactions.

There is no single, best, or only treatment for alcoholism, and it is easier to walk with two crutches than with one. Therefore, combinations of treatment, such as group therapy *and* renewed church attendance *and* disulfiram *and* vocational rehabilitation, may be employed to provide all of the four therapeutic components.

～ Pharmacotherapy and Psychotherapy Revisited

The past 15 years have seen continued research on the use of drugs to treat alcohol abuse. I will mention a few examples for their heuristic importance rather than attempt a coherent and comprehensive review of the literature. In a well-controlled study of consecutive, primary alcoholic admissions Schuckit (1985) has confirmed the long-term ineffectiveness of disulfiram. Of 348 men admitted for treatment, 172 agreed to take disulfiram and 176 refused. After a year of follow-up there was no significant difference in outcome. However, in his review of the literature, Schuckit also noted that patients who received either effective doses of disulfiram *or* a disulfiram placebo did significantly better than patients who were told that they were not receiving any drug. Hope continues to be an effective therapy for alcohol abuse.

So do external behavioral controls. Thus Azrin and colleagues (1982) observed that the reason traditional disulfiram treatment was ineffective was that clients stopped taking the drug. To remedy this they trained clients to take their disulfiram at a set time and place in the company of a significant other. They also provided relaxation training, behavioral training in how to refuse offered drinks, and rehearsals of difficult social situations that had led to drinking in the past. At the end of six months of follow-up, they had achieved perfect compliance: 14 out of 14 clients were still abstinent.

Lindström's (1992) discussion of Azrin's small and unreplicated study underscores what seems critical to so many successful treatments of alcohol abuse:

> The general approach was to rearrange the alcoholic's social environment in such a way that other reinforcing activities competed with drinking behavior. In order to be effective, reinforcers had to be valued, regularly occurring, and varied in nature. Furthermore, the newly developed 'natural' reinforcers (e.g., a good job, the wife's sustained attention, access to a social club) were contingent on the continued sobriety. Postponement of reinforcers as a result of alcohol intake was immediate. (p. 99)

The lesson is that disulfiram by itself only takes alcohol away. The alcohol must be replaced by something else. Two promising medications that offer to give as well as take away are Naltrexone and serotonin uptake inhibitors (such as fluoxitane). There have been many uncontrolled positive reports of the success of serotonin uptake inhibitors, and reports that such drugs are successful in inhibiting alcohol intake in experimental animals. In controlled clinical trials, however, serotonin uptake inhibitors seem no more effective than other antidepressants. For example, Naranjo and Sellers (1989) reported success, but when examined closely their statistically significant results were clinically insignificant. For example, in a sample of alcoholic men they increased the number of abstinent days from 1.5 to 3.7 over a two-week period, and they reduced the average number of daily drinks from 6.0 to 5.5. Gorelick (1989) also reported that "serotonin reuptake blockers offered a potentially promising treatment for alcoholism." However, Gorelick based such hope on a significant 14 percent decrease in ethanol consumption by chronic alcoholics during the first week of a four-week program. During this week, the men who received active medication reduced their average daily consumption from 25 ounces to 19 ounces of whiskey a day! Even this modest improvement was not maintained over the full four weeks.

In contrast, the use of Naltrexone in the treatment of alcohol dependence has proven genuinely promising (Volpicelli et al. 1992). Naltrexone is an effective opiate antagonist that is also a partial agonist (a stimulator of opiate receptors). Naltrexone dramatically decreases rats' preference for alcohol. When investigators administered 50 milligrams a day of Naltrexone to 70 alcohol-dependent men under double-blind-placebo controlled conditions, the relapse rate was 54 percent for the placebo-treated subjects but only 23 percent in the Naltrexone-treated subjects. Ninety-five percent of the 20 placebo-treated clients relapsed after they sampled alcohol, while only 8 of the 16 Naltrexone-treated patients who exposed themselves to alcohol relapsed. Numerous efforts are under way to replicate these findings.

Additional Guidelines

There are some useful additional guidelines for counseling the alcoholic patient in the early stages of treatment. First, once a would-be helper is sure that the use of alcohol puts the user out of control, he should *not* prescribe controlled drinking. An analogous situation is the futility of advising a two-pack-a-day smoker to cut down to five cigarettes. Obviously, the non-dependent individual whose drinking is truly reactive or merely excessive for good health may be helped by good advice to cut down to moderate drinking. But these individuals are rarely the ones who are a source of concern to themselves, their relatives, or their clinicians.

Second, the would-be helper should avoid making proclamations that the alcoholic should never take another drink. If too harsh, threats of death or chronic illness from alcohol abuse may add to the alcoholic's denial. If abstinence is suggested, it should be prescribed gently and only *one day at a time.* The helper should remember that nobody wishes to be asked to give up forever a substance that he truly, albeit ambivalently, loves and values.

Lastly, those who care about alcoholics are often unable to disguise their disappointment and resentment when the alcoholic seemingly willfully relapses. Clinicians and relatives alike need to take the first "step" of Al-Anon seriously: they must admit their own "powerlessness over alcohol." In alcoholism, as in much of medicine, we dress the wound; the individual's own resources heal it. To take an alcoholic's drinking personally, to see it as evidence of transference, spitefulness, or poor motivation, is to miss the point. A tuberculosis patient does not relapse to coughing bouts just because he resents his family, is resisting his therapist, or is poorly motivated. To a large extent relapse to and remission from alcoholism remain a mystery.

When and how a clinician or family member responds to a plea for help from an alcoholic is always problematic. Alcoholism is a disorder with unexpected relapses and intense needs for help at unexpected times. The alcoholic, like the unconscious, has little sense of time. Unexpected relapses tend to be destructive to any ongoing relationship, including the most selfless therapeutic alliance or loving relationship. A reasonable rule of thumb is that any alcoholic who asks for help for the first time should be responded to immediately—even if it puts the clinician or relative to considerable inconvenience. Once the diagnosis is established, it is important to convey to the patient the fact that the alcoholic cannot be helped by superficial band-aid measures or by caregivers who are made helpless or asked for help that they resent giving. Actively drinking alcoholics should be instructed that only institutions, not individuals, are powerful enough to meet their great needs. Alcoholics Anonymous, skid-row shelters, and hospital emergency rooms are available and willing to help 24 hours a day. By contrast, requests for loans or late-evening telephone calls to friends will only underscore the fact that the latter are powerless to change the patient's drinking and will lead to mutual guilt, anger, and rejection. Since such consequences can hardly be in the alcoholic's best interest, very inconvenient individual requests for help should be reflected back to the patient as evidence of the severity of the *disease* and of the patient's need to enter some systematic and more effective mode of treatment.

The alcoholic literally is not under control, but must be helped to bear responsibility for regaining control. One of the advantages of a walk-in clinic, a hotline, or a church is that, unlike individuals, such institutions do not expect the patient to be in control. If the would-be helper treats alcoholism by trying to sustain a therapeutic individual alliance, he comes to expect that the alcoholic's symptoms will be dynamically determined, controllable through insight, and affected by the state of "transference" or the sincerity of gratitude. Once a helper feels that there is a dynamic relationship between his response and the patient's drinking, he may develop superstitious and magical ideas about his own powers. This leads to hypervigilance, then mistrust, and, finally, rupture of the alliance. Rather than engendering therapeutic nihilism, the motto of Al-Anon, "We admitted we were powerless over alcohol," paradoxically becomes the cornerstone of effective work with alcoholics both by relatives and by clinicians.

There is no easy answer to a relapsing patient's request for repeated hospitalization. Certainly, a relapsing alcoholic should not be excluded from treatment. The results from the Clinic sample described in Chapter 3 suggest that many of the best eventual outcomes experienced multiple prior relapses.

Hospitalization not only helps to alleviate the secondary physical complications of alcoholism but also allows withdrawal medication to be administered more systematically than does outpatient management.

Alcoholism affects the entire family. In the past, social workers and psychiatrists have viewed alcoholism as symptom and not disease, and they have sometimes come to believe that the spouse was the *cause* of the alcoholic's illness and needed treatment. Such an approach is rarely productive and magnifies guilt that is already excessive.

The alcoholic's relatives need help, not treatment; and they can obtain help in many ways. They will gain strength and comfort if they understand that their relative by himself cannot control his drinking, that he has a treatable disease, that no one understands the cause of the disease, and that alcoholism certainly is not caused by relatives. Professional family counseling can be very comforting, as can the family or group approaches employed by many clinics. Al-Anon is a self-help organization in which the spouses of alcoholics assist each other in understanding the "disease," learn how not to interfere with the recovery process, and, most important, discover how to obtain comfort for themselves. Alateen is a self-help organization in which troubled adolescents in alcoholic families help each other to understand their painful home life. Its members are enormously grateful to each other. The times and places of such meetings can be obtained by calling the number listed after Alcoholics Anonymous in any telephone book.

Finally, follow-up is just as essential in the disease called alcoholism as it is in any chronic illness. The value of a sustained, nonjudgmental interest in the alcoholic by both the clinician and relative cannot be stressed too much. Periodic letters and recontact of alcoholics who have experienced trouble sustaining a treatment plan are useful. The implied message of forgiveness is most welcome. When a would-be helper acknowledges that recovery from alcoholism is the patient's own responsibility and that he is as powerless over another's alcoholism as he is over another's measles, the helper does not render himself useless. Instead of advice, would-be helpers can offer to the alcoholic their strength, their hope, and their experience.

⌁ A Summing Up

Much in this book is at variance with common suppositions about alcoholism. That is to be expected from a prospective study. Sixty years ago, Sigmund Freud wrote, "So long as we trace the development from its final outcome backwards, the chain of events appears continuous and we feel that we have gained an insight which is completely satisfactory or even exhaustive. But if we proceed the reverse way, if we start from the premises informed from the analysis; and try to follow them up to the final result, then we no longer get the impression of an inevitable sequence of events" (1920, p. 167).

By proceeding in the "reverse way" this prospective study of alcoholism has yielded surprises, and much of what we have learned retrospectively about alcoholism appears to be illusion. I have presented data from unique data sets; but that does not mean that I have better knowledge, only knowledge viewed from a fresh perspective—that of life-span development. In chronic illness time is such an important dimension.

In the world literature, besides our College sample, there have been only two other middle-class samples of adolescents followed into late middle life (Terman and Oden 1959; Eichorn et al. 1981); and neither of those studies really focused upon alcohol abuse. Besides the work of McCord (1979), our Core City sample is the only prospective study that has followed working-class adolescents into their mid-forties. And our Clinic sample is the only group of alcohol clinic patients who have been repeatedly followed for as long as eight years.

The seven questions I posed in the introductory chapter were: Is alcoholism a symptom or a disease? If alcoholism is a disease, is it progressive? Are alcoholics premorbidly different from other people? Are alcoholics when ab-

375

stinent often worse off than they were when drinking? Is return to asymptomatic drinking possible for alcoholics? How does clinical intervention alter the natural history of alcoholism? And lastly, in treating alcoholism, what is the relevance of Alcoholics Anonymous?

My answers to these questions are based on the life histories of 600 "normal" men—the 200 socially privileged men of the College sample and the 400 socially underprivileged men of the Core City sample, who have been followed from adolescence into middle life. Chapters 6 and 7 describe these samples and the design of their study in detail. In addition, as reported in Chapter 3, 100 hospitalized alcoholics, the Clinic sample, have been prospectively studied for eight years. If in discussing the seven questions about alcoholism I give the impression that I have definitive answers, I am in error. Throughout the text, I have tried to point out the limits of my evidence.

Alcoholism: Symptom or Disease?

The answer to the first question is examined and tentatively answered in Chapter 1. Tables 1.7 and 1.9 suggest that the number and the frequency of alcohol-related problems, rather than the specificity of such problems, best define the clinical phenomenon known as alcoholism. No single set of traits invariably defines alcoholism. Just as light can consist of both waves and particles, just so alcoholism can exist both as one end of a continuum of drinking problems and as a specific disorder. Alcoholism can simultaneously reflect both a conditioned habit and a disease; and the disease of alcoholism can be as well defined by a sociological model as by a medical model (Table 1.8). Thus, alcoholism is a construct of a higher order of complexity than, say, pregnancy or measles.

Where along the continuum of alcohol-related problems one makes the cutting-off point for the diagnosis of alcoholism is obviously arbitrary. Nevertheless, as Table 1.7 and Figure 1.1 suggest, if most of the alcohol in the world is consumed by people who do not have a large number of alcohol-related problems, most of the alcohol-related problems in the world may be experienced by a very small number of people—those whom clinicians label "alcoholics."

While it is probably true that loss of control over the ingestion of alcohol is neither a necessary nor a sufficient criterion for diagnosing alcoholism, it is true that once individuals experience many alcohol-related problems, they perceive themselves and others perceive them as no longer in control of their use of alcohol. The diagnosis, alcoholism, is neither so frequently made as to endanger asymptomatic drinkers by incorrect labeling nor so bound up with individual variation as to be meaningless. Patterns of alcohol *use* vary enormously, but the further along the continuum of alcohol-related problems individuals find themselves, the more they resemble other alcoholics.

One reason for regarding alcoholism as a disorder with a life of its own is the prospectively documented observation that those alcoholics who have achieved stable abstinence were not premorbidly psychologically healthier than those whose alcoholism has followed a more chronic course (Table 3.15). In other words, prospective study does not suggest that alcohol dependence is merely a symptom of underlying personality disorder. However, the exact point at which minimal alcohol abuse (for example, being arrested once for drunken driving) merits the label of alcoholism (a pattern of maladaptive alcohol use that malignantly leads to multiple alcohol-related problems) will always be as uncertain as where in the spectrum yellow becomes green.

〜 Symptom or Disease Revisited

Over the past 15 years this controversy has continued unabated. Of the many critics of the disease concept, perhaps the most articulate has been Herbert Fingarette (1988), a professor of philosophy. Among his concerns has been, first, that the disease concept is bad science: that not only is the inexorable progression of alcohol abuse a myth but also the disease concept oversimplifies alcoholism, which like mental retardation needs the attention of social scientists even more than that of medical scientists. A second concern has been that the disease concept, by removing the moral stigma from alcoholism, not only reduces the individual's sense of responsibility but also allows judges, police, and employers to pass their own responsibility for alcohol-related problems to the medical profession. Third, and perhaps of greatest legitimacy, has been his concern that the disease concept has been heavily lobbied by the alcoholic beverage industry. By supporting the position that alcohol abuse lies in the individual, and not in the bottle, the disease concept has made it easier for industry to fend off higher taxes on alcoholic beverages, restrictions on aggressive marketing, and other public constraints upon the availability of alcohol.

The counterargument to Fingarette has been made effectively by Robert Rose (1988), a research psychiatrist:

> . . . becoming ill and suffering from many sicknesses is really not a product of either the medical model or the moral model . . . but rather some mixture

of the two. It is a product of what we are born with, what our genes determine we are susceptible to and what happens to us, or what we do to ourselves that determines if and when we become ill. It is apparent that this is true in varying proportions for cancer, don't eat the wrong things and don't smoke; for hypertension, keep the weight off, exercise, and watch the salt; and for alcoholism, have the right parents and take it easy on the sauce. I would submit that alcoholism really isn't that different from many other illnesses that we suffer . . . Ultimately, whether or not we suffer from its various symptoms is not totally under our own control any more or less than is true of most other illnesses. (p. 140)

Fingarette himself unwittingly offers the best reason of all for labeling alcoholism a disease rather than a moral failing, namely self-efficacy. He boldly proclaims:

It is not compassionate to encourage drinkers to deny their power to change . . . Alcoholics are not helpless; they can take control of their lives. In the last analysis, alcoholics must truly want to change and actively choose to change. To do so they must make many difficult daily choices . . . we must also make it clear that heavy drinkers must take responsibility for their own lives. The assumption of personal responsibility . . . is a sign of health, and needless submission to spurious medical authority is a pathology. (p. 436)

A fervent advocate of Alcoholics Anonymous could not have made the point any more forcefully. Alcoholics who label themselves ill—and not bad—will be less helpless; they will have higher self-esteem; and, most important, they, like diabetics, and in contrast to pickpockets, will try harder to change and to let others help them to change.

Is Alcoholism a Progressive Disease?

Whether alcoholism is viewed as a progressive disease depends very much on whether the spectrum of alcoholism is approached from the side of heavy drinking or from the side of clear alcohol dependence. As Chapter 3 and Table 3.9 illustrate, if one looks at those individuals whose alcoholism *has* been progressive (that is, relapsing alcohol-dependent individuals seen in alcohol clinics and emergency rooms), then alcoholism certainly appears to be progressive. In contrast, by following heavy alcohol *users* prospectively (say, individuals with a single alcohol-related traffic violation), one finds that many such individuals may occasionally abuse alcohol without exhibiting progression. The most dramatic evidence for alcoholism's being progressive was seen in Figure 3.7, where the life course of 100 consecutive admissions to an alcohol detoxification unit were depicted for the next eight years. At the end of that time span, only 24 patients were still abusing alcohol; almost all the rest had either died or become abstinent.

Once it develops, alcoholism is a chronic disorder. Insidious, fulminating, and intermittent courses are all common; so is recovery. Extrapolating from the data in this book, the course of alcoholism can be conceived broadly as comprising three linked stages. The first stage is heavy "social" drinking—frequent ingestion of two to three ounces of ethanol (three to five drinks) a day for several years. This stage can continue asymptomatically for a lifetime; or because of a change of circumstances or peer group it can reverse to a more moderate pattern of drinking; or it can "progress" into a pattern of alcohol abuse (multiple medical, legal, social, and occupational complications), usually associated with frequent ingestion of more than four ounces of ethanol (eight or more drinks) a day. At some point in their lives, perhaps 10–15 percent of American men reach this second stage. Perhaps half of such alcohol abusers either return to asymptomatic (controlled) drinking or achieve stable abstinence. In a small number of such cases (the "atypical" cases described in Chapter 3) such alcohol abuse can persist intermittently for decades with minor morbidity and even become milder with time.* Perhaps a quarter of all cases of alcohol abuse (as defined by the criteria of the DSM III) will lead to chronic alcohol dependence, withdrawal symptoms, and the eventual need for detoxification. This last stage is reached by perhaps 3–5 percent of American adults, with men probably outnumbering women three or four to one. This last stage is much less plastic than the earlier stages and most commonly ends either in abstinence or in social incapacity or death (Figure 3.7).

Table 3.2 suggests one reason that short-term epidemiological studies have found alcohol abuse so plastic. In a drinking culture many individuals who in cross-section are identified as abstinent in fact include many alcoholics who have discovered that they cannot drink in safety and have become temporary or permanent teetotalers.

Figures 3.2, 3.3, and 3.4 suggest that alcoholics do not develop the disorder

---

*Continued follow-up of the alcohol abusers in both samples over the past 15 years has revealed that alcohol abuse can remain chronic for decades without either progression or improvement.

after the first few drinks but that the disorder requires many years to evolve. In some sociopathic individuals who use alcohol to alter consciousness, to obliterate conscience, and to defy social canons, dependence and apparent loss of control may appear in only a few months to a few years. For the majority of alcoholics, however, the time from the first drink to an inability consistently to control their drinking is a process of habit formation that takes from 5 to 30 years.

This general picture of the natural history of alcoholism summarizes the findings from this book, which may or may not be confirmed by other prospective studies. It is intended as a "first draft," not as gospel.

Are Alcoholics Premorbidly Different?

Chapter 2 suggests three areas in which alcoholics appear to be premorbidly different from asymptomatic drinkers. First, future alcoholics are more likely to come from ethnic groups that tolerate adult drunkenness but that discourage children and adolescents from learning safe drinking practices (such as consumption of low-proof alcoholic beverages at ceremonies and with meals). Thus, parents and grandparents of the alcoholics in our samples were more likely to have been born in English-speaking countries than in Mediterranean countries (Table 2.5). Second, future alcoholics are more likely to be related to other alcoholics (Table 2.8), and this relationship holds even with ethnicity controlled. However, if the number of alcoholics in one's ancestry increases the likelihood of alcohol abuse, presumably for genetic reasons, it also increases the likelihood of lifelong abstinence, presumably for environmental reasons (Figure 2.1). Almost half of the 48 teetotalers of Anglo-Irish-American descent had an alcoholic parent. Third, compared to asymptomatic drinkers, alcoholics are more likely to be premorbidly antisocial (Table 2.13), perhaps more extroverted (Table 2.17), but not more dependent. However, if many antisocial adolescents initiate alcohol abuse as a symptom of their antisocial behavior, most alcoholics are not premorbidly antisocial.

Far more surprising, most future alcoholics do not appear different from future asymptomatic drinkers in terms of premorbid psychological stability. However, not until several prospective studies were available (Table 2.1) could such a hypothesis be seriously entertained. It was difficult to conceive that the "alcoholic personality" might be secondary to the disorder, alcoholism. It was difficult to discard the illusion that alcohol serves as successful self-medication for unhappy, diffident people. In actual fact, however, alcohol in high doses is the very opposite of a tranquilizer.

In dismissing unhappy childhoods, membership in multiproblem families, depression, and anxiety from major etiological consideration, I do not wish to say that these factors are of no importance in alcoholism. These factors will make any chronic disease worse. I simply wish to underscore that in a prospective design, when other more salient variables like culture and familial alcoholism per se were controlled, then premorbid family and personality instability no longer made a statistical contribution to the risk of alcoholism (Table 2.16). Thus, Core City subjects with an alcoholic parent but with an otherwise stable family were *five* times as likely to develop alcoholism as were subjects from clearly multiproblem families without an alcoholic parent.

In retrospect, individuals often rationalized their slowly developing loss of control over alcohol use by citing past psychological trauma. Prospectively studied, however, abuse of alcohol usually predated the alleged trauma, and reactive alcohol abuse was rarely observed to be a cause of alcohol dependence. When it occurred, frequent intoxication in response to emotional crisis often led to a few alcohol-related problems, but rarely to enough problems for a Core City subject to be categorized as an alcohol abuser. In other words, a difficult life was rarely a major reason why someone developed alcohol dependence.

In summary, alcoholics often come from broken homes because their parents abused alcohol, not because broken homes cause alcoholism; and alcoholics are selectively personality disordered as a consequence, not as a cause, of their alcohol abuse. Although the conscience may be soluble in alcohol, heavy alcohol use does not relieve anxiety and depression as much as alcohol abuse induces depression and anxiety.

However, although certain psychosocial variables were not predictive of future alcohol abuse, they were nevertheless very useful in predicting poor subsequent mental health (Table 2.18). The three childhood variables that most powerfully predicted positive adult mental health—boyhood competence, warmth of childhood, and freedom from childhood emotional problems—did not predict freedom from alcoholism; whereas the three variables that most powerfully predicted alcoholism—family history of alcoholism, ethnicity, and adolescent behavior problems—did not predict poor future mental health.

As a byproduct of this study of alcoholism, a finding emerged that is of interest to social science in general. Parental social class, I.Q., and multi-problem family membership may be more important to outcome in short-term studies than when these variables are studied over the life span. In our admittedly small Core City sample, confined as it was to 400 white urban males, childhood mental health appeared to be a better predictor of future social class and of adult employment or unemployment than was childhood intelligence, multiproblem family membership, or parental dependence upon welfare (Table 2.3). It may be more damaging to a child's later development to have nothing go right than to have many things go wrong.

Is the Cure Worse Than the Disease?

Chapters 3 and 4 suggest that the answer to this question is "virtually never." By this I mean that prospective study turned up no evidence that abstinence from alcohol is sometimes harmful to the alcoholic. For the Core City and College samples, less highly selected for coexisting psychopathology than the Clinic sample, Table 3.10 and Table 4.7 suggest that psychosocial recovery and abstinence from alcohol went hand in hand. There was no evidence that long-term abstinence led to individuals' becoming more depressed or socially isolated than they had been while abusing alcohol. When a group of remitted alcoholics were systematically compared to active alcoholics, abstinence appeared as closely associated with subjective satisfaction as with objective social health. Abstinent alcoholics in both the Clinic (Table 3.10) and Core City (Table 4.6) samples appeared significantly happier than alcohol abusers.

However, returning to best premorbid adjustment appeared to require a convalescence of years, not months. Table 4.7 pointed out that for recovered alcoholics the quality of eventual social adjustment cannot be reliably assessed during the first two years of abstinence.

Surprisingly, eventual stable abstinence was not seen only among alcoholics with good premorbid adjustment. In the Core City sample, stable abstinence occurred most often in untreated and severely alcohol-dependent individuals. Sociopathic Core City alcoholics (Figure 3.4), if anything, became abstinent younger and more frequently than did the College sample's upper-middle-class college graduates selected for mental health (Figure 3.3). The implication is that until an alcohol abuser becomes very symptomatic, the subjective pain (or cognitive dissonance) is not sufficiently severe to lead to the complete rupture of a long-established habit.

I do not wish to maintain that abstinence per se is good for anybody or that a puritanical attitude is the best approach to compulsive habits. What I wish to emphasize is not that abstinence is good but that alcohol abuse is painful. Over the long term, if abstinence or return to asymptomatic drinking did not guarantee psychosocial recovery, such recovery while continuing to drink heavily was impossible.

Can "Real" Alcoholics Ever Safely Drink Again?

The answer to this question provided by Chapter 5 is "Yes, but . . ." Return to asymptomatic drinking was common among the alcohol abusers in both the College and Core City samples. As the case examples in Chapter 5 suggest, however, resumption of asymptomatic drinking was achieved more often by return to *controlled* drinking rather than to the less structured drinking patterns of drinkers who have never experienced subjective loss of control.

As Figure 5.1 demonstrated, the broader the definition of alcohol abuse, the more common was return to asymptomatic drinking. Thus, when young alcohol abusers without dependence altered their peer groups, they often returned to asymptomatic drinking, whereas when middle-aged alcoholics who had required detoxification attempted to return to asymptomatic drinking, their situation was analogous to driving a car without a spare tire—disaster was usually only a matter of time. In other words, as suggested by Table 5.1 and Figure 3.7, by the time an alcoholic is ill enough to require clinic treatment, return to asymptomatic drinking is the exception, not the rule.

～ Abstinence versus Controlled Drinking Revisited

Over the past 15 years, a consensus has emerged. This consensus replaces the contentious therapeutic debates between the advocates of a goal of abstinence and the advocates of a goal of controlled drinking. The consensus is based on three interlocking strands of evidence. First, despite its promise 15–20 years ago, training alcohol-dependent individuals to achieve stable return to controlled drinking is a mirage. Hopeful initial reports have not led to replication. In Miller and colleagues' (1992) review of well-designed studies supporting behavioral training to allow individuals to return to controlled drinking, the nine studies cited were all 12–20 years old. Rychtarik and colleagues (1987), in a five-to-six-year follow-up of one of the most recent studies, found no observable effects of training in controlled drinking skills either at one year or at six years.

Second, virtually nobody any longer contests that severely alcohol-dependent individuals *can* on occasion return to problem-free drinking; the caveat is that it is a relatively unusual occurrence. Even as staunch an advocate of return to controlled drinking as Heather (1987) has acknowledged that "few workers now dispute that a controlled drinking outcome becomes less likely as severity of dependence increases."

Third, for alcohol abusers with only borderline or early alcohol abuse return to controlled drinking *is* a worthwhile goal (Tobin et al. 1993) and a more acceptable goal than one of unnecessary abstinence (Sanchez-Craig and Lei 1986). The shorter the period of abuse, the fewer the alcohol-related problems, the less dependent the individual, and the greater his or her social stability, the better the outcome. Repeatedly, investigators have demonstrated the impressive results that can be obtained over the short term by even brief interventions that advocate moderate drinking (Chick et al. 1985; Lindström 1992; Bien et al. 1993).

Which Clinic Treatments Help?

Chapter 8 concludes (but does not prove) that prolonged hospital treatment does little to alter the natural history of alcoholism. A similar conclusion was cogently expressed by McCance and McCance (1969, p. 198):

> The outcome in alcoholism depends very little on the treatment given, but largely upon individual factors relating to each patient and upon the natural history of the condition. The cost of establishing and running the type of special unit which caters mainly to the treatment of alcoholics with social and behavioral characteristics associated with good prognosis may not be justified. More attention should be given to the provision of a range of facilities to suit the management of alcoholics with less favorable attributes who are more likely to continue drinking in spite of psychiatric treatment.

Both Chapter 8 and Table 3.8 bear powerful witness that alcoholics recover not because we treat them but because they heal themselves. Staying sober is not a process of simply becoming detoxified but often becomes the work of several years or in a few cases even of a lifetime. Our task is to provide emergency medical care, shelter, detoxification, and understanding until self-healing takes place. In any treatment cohort of alcoholic patients, I have found that 10–20 percent never relapse after their first serious request for help; and that thereafter, depending upon the characteristics of the sample, 2–3 percent will achieve stable recovery each year.

Neither the efforts of dedicated clinicians nor the individual's own will-power appear to be able to cure an alcoholic's conditioned habit at a given time. This should not be a cause for despair but should spur the clinician to redirect therapeutic attention toward the individual's own powers of resistance. Not only is the patient's social stability (at the time of seeking treatment) important to sustained abstinence, but so are four other factors (Table 4.3). Namely, recovery is associated with the alcoholic discovering: (1) a substitute dependency; (2) external reminders (such as disulfiram ingestion or a painful ulcer) that drinking is aversive; (3) increased sources of unambivalently offered social support; and (4) a source of inspiration, hope, and enhanced self-esteem (such as religious activity). Chapter 4 suggests that Alcoholics Anonymous, or any reasonable facsimile, appears to be an effective means of bringing all these four factors to bear.

ᴄ⌢ Clinic Treatment Revisited

In the past 15 years, treatment researchers have increasingly come to somewhat similar conclusions, namely that effective treatment of alcohol abuse is analogous to effective treatment of diabetes or gingivitis. Effective treatment lies not so much in professional intervention for acute relapses as in training the individual in the prevention of relapse. Thus, cognitive therapies of the sort advocated by Marlatt and Gordon (1985), cognitive behavioral strategies of the sort advocated by Miller and Heather (1986) and by Rational Recovery, and maintenance pharmacotherapy with drugs like Naltrexone (Volpicelli 1992), in contrast to disulfiram, all work toward long-term relapse prevention. All offer serviceable alternatives to inform, to augment, and sometimes to replace the folk wisdom of the Alcoholics Anonymous self-help groups.

Reviews, both by the Institute of Medicine (1989) and by Lindström (1992), indicate that, for unselected groups of alcoholics, the empirical evidence overwhelmingly supports three conclusions. First, inpatient treatments of a few weeks to a few months produce no better outcomes than a brief inpatient stay. Second, day treatment or partial hospitalization is as effective as inpatient treatment. Third, in general, outpatient treatment produces long-term results comparable to those of inpatient treatment.

These generalizations, based on the synthesis of a large number of studies, were recently dramatically confirmed in an evaluation of three treatment programs for alcoholism with an 18-month follow-up (Chapman and Huygens 1988). The authors contrasted a six-week *inpatient* treatment program, a six-week *outpatient* treatment program, and a *single* confrontational interview. They achieved good treatment results: at the end of follow-up almost half of their subjects reported that they either were abstinent or were drinking moderately. However, none of the three modalities proved significantly better than the others.

However, if, in fact, severe alcohol dependence is difficult to affect by several weeks of intensive hospital intervention, brief outpatient interventions such as suggested by Chapman and Huygens (1988) and by Chick and colleagues (1988) have proved surprisingly effective in helping individuals with mild alcohol abuse (Babor et al. 1986). This progress has been achieved by two means: improved early detection and clinical interventions that use behavioral techniques that facilitate self-monitoring.

Let me address improved detection first. Detection has improved because of the increasing recognition that it is problem drinking and loss of plasticity of drinking behavior, not heavy drinking in itself, that characterize alcohol abuse. Until recently, screening for alcohol abuse had been retarded by misconceptions. For example, questioning clinical patients about frequency and quantity of alcohol ingestion is much less informative than questioning patients about frequency and quantity of cigarette consumption. Just as the obese underestimate food consumption (Lichtman et al. 1992), alcohol abusers consistently underestimate the amount of alcohol they consume by a factor of perhaps 50 percent (Smith et al. 1990). In addition, because both alcohol consumption and liver damage show poor correlation with alcohol-related problems, biochemical tests have consistently provided too little sensitivity and specificity. However, by using the MAST (Selzer 1971), a problem-based measure, the simpler CAGE (Ewing 1984), and even by simply asking individuals "Have you ever had a drinking problem?" and "When was your last drink?" clinicians have achieved much greater sensitivity and specificity of diagnosis (Cyr and Wartman 1988).

In a study of 518 men and women Bush and colleagues (1987) employed the CAGE (Have you tried to Cut down your drinking? Do you get Angry when people discuss your drinking? Do you feel Guilty about things you have done while drinking? Do you ever have an Eye-opener?). A positive answer to one or more of the four questions provided a sensitivity of 85 percent and a specificity of 89 percent in distinguishing alcohol abusers. Only 63 percent of the alcohol abusers they identified were known to their physicians as alcohol abusers. In contrast, Bush and his co-workers found that elevated gamma-glutamyl transpeptidase (GGT) and/or increased mean corpuscular volume (MCV) of red blood cells produced a sensitivity of only 70 percent and a specificity of 65 percent, or a positive predictive value only half as good as a single positive answer on the CAGE. Unfortunately, such improved methods of identifying alcohol abuse are not yet routine. The likelihood that in a general hospital alcohol abusers will be correctly identified is still only somewhere between 25 and 50 percent (Moore et al. 1989).

∽ Behavioral Approaches Revisited

Next let me examine behavioral approaches to early alcohol abuse. Such interventions involve four interrelated activities that are all designed to increase awareness of drinking behavior. These four activities are practicing self-observation, setting achievable drinking goals, appreciating the antecedents and the consequences of maladaptive drinking, and devising coping alternatives to heavy drinking. Among others, Sanchez-Craig at the Addiction Research Foundation in Toronto has been instrumental in developing and assessing the efficacy of these methods (Sanchez-Craig 1984, Sanchez-Craig 1990, Sanchez-Craig et al. 1991). The value of teaching such self-monitoring to mild alcohol abusers is heightened by the fact that lasting abstinence is rarely achieved except by individuals with severe alcohol abuse. This point was clearly illustrated by the natural history of the College sample in Chapters 3 and 4.

First, for self-monitoring, the problem drinker is asked to record his or her daily number of drinks and the circumstances under which they were consumed, thereby making both the quantity and the risk of the drinking situation more conscious. Second, achievable short-term goals are set; for example, two weeks of abstinence. This trial abstinence in turn elucidates the last two goals—to understand the purposes that the drinking episodes serve in the individual's life, and to begin to uncover and develop individualized strategies for controlling or abstaining from alcohol. In other words, self-observation for the antecedents and consequences of drinking is developed and reinforced.

A major difference between such a behavioral approach and more traditional counseling approaches is that alcohol abuse is seen as the cause rather than as the result of the patient's problems. Unfortunately, Sanchez-Craig, like other investigators of behavioral-modification treatment, reports results that have not been demonstrated to be stable over long periods of time. However, over a few months, such interventions have reduced alcohol consumption in one study of alcohol abusers from 51 drinks a week to 13

(Sanchez-Craig et al. 1984). The obvious advantage of such methods is that they are also applicable as a first step in treating alcohol abusers who have not yet become convinced of the necessity of abstinence as a goal.

Is Recovery Through AA the Exception or the Rule?

The College sample and the Core City sample were two relatively unselected groups of individuals from two very different socioeconomic groups and with two very different levels of education. Nevertheless, more recovered alcoholics from both groups began stable abstinence while attending Alcoholics Anonymous than while attending alcohol treatment centers.

If one starts with a clinic sample rather than with alcoholics drawn from community samples, then over the short term many more individuals, through self-selection, will recover through clinical intervention. After all, they have sought help from a clinic, not from AA. When the 100 Clinic patients were followed for eight years, however, then perhaps an equal number of individuals achieved stable abstinence through AA as through detoxification and clinic treatment (Tables 3.12 and 8.4). Joining any club takes time.

The numbers of subjects in these studies are small, and these results, primarily drawn from middle-aged white males, must be interpreted with caution. The implication from the three samples, however, is that a great many severely alcohol-dependent Americans, regardless of their social or psychological makeup, find help for their alcoholism through Alcoholics Anonymous. (Some people have wondered if AA is as useful to women as to men, but the latest figures from AA suggest that the ratio of men to women in AA is two to one—a ratio no greater than occurs in the general population of alcoholics.)

A Final Reminder

The fact that we cannot easily alter the long-term course of alcoholism should be no reason for despair. If treatment as we currently understand it does not seem more effective than the natural healing processes, then we need to understand those natural healing processes better than we do. We also need to understand the special role that clinicians can play.

First, alcoholism produces enormous suffering, and to deny palliation to alcoholics because we are not certain how to effect long-range cure is as inhumane as denying palliation to hypertensives or to diabetics. Virtually all follow-up studies show alcoholics better off for several months after clinic treatment than they were just before treatment. Thus, even if clinics do not always cure, they do reduce mortality and suffering. Second, by understanding facts rather than illusions about alcoholism, we can learn to facilitate natural healing processes. Third, the factors that most powerfully affect the etiology of alcoholism can probably be modified by enlightened social policy. The future prevalence of alcohol abuse, like the future prevalence of heart disease, can be reduced by thoughtful education of children in our schools (Deutsch 1982) and in our homes. Informed legislation can modify risk factors, not by prohibition, but by public education and by careful *experimentation* with selectively raising the cost of high-proof alcohol and limiting availability in order to discourage drinking in the absence of food and to discourage drinking around the clock (Moore and Gerstein 1981).*

Finally, alcoholism costs the United States upwards of $50 billion a year. Indeed, if one multiplies the approximately 4 million alcohol-abusing wage earners in the United States by the $8000 annual difference between the income of active Core City alcohol abusers and that of asymptomatic drinkers (Table 4.6), then the lost earning power alone of alcoholics comes to $30 billion a year. The $100 million a year that the federal government has invested in alcohol treatment programs for the past decade (0.2 percent of the cost of the disease) hardly seems extravagant—especially when one considers that cost-benefit studies have repeatedly documented that alcohol outpatient clinics are cost-effective.

What is called for, then, is not despair but a redoubling of effort—and of financial outlay. The millions of alcoholics in the United States deserve the broad network of services outlined in Chapters 8 and 9; but we must coordinate such efforts with reality, not with illusions.

---

*To offer a single example, although beer is the least price-sensitive class of alcoholic beverages, states with the highest beer prices have the lowest rates of automobile fatalities for young adults (Saffer and Grossman 1985). In addition, increased taxation, warning labels, and counter-advertising—of the sort that have gradually become effective against smoking—must be developed to balance the efforts of the alcohol industry to increase consumption (Institute of Medicine 1989). At the present time U.S. government agencies spend a total of about $200 million annually for research and education to combat alcohol abuse. The alcohol industry spends ten times that much, $2 billion, in advertising and promotion to increase alcohol consumption (Knupfer 1989; Wallack 1992). Broad-based social interventions of the sort developed by the Stanford Five-City Project (Farquhar et al. 1990) must be directed against alcohol abuse.

Appendix: Measurement Scales

The following scales and interview schedules, used to assess the characteristics of the subjects in this study and discussed in the text, are presented in detail here:

Childhood Environmental Strengths Scale
Childhood Environmental Weaknesses Scale
Boyhood Competence Scale
Hollingshead-Redlich Social Class Scale
Social Competence Scale
Hyperactivity Scale
Robins's Sociopathy Scale
Interview Schedule for Alcohol Use
Cahalan Scale
DSM III Scale of Alcohol Abuse and Dependence

Childhood Environmental Strengths Scale

The score on this scale equals the sum of the points given for the following 8 items. ("Childhood emotional problems" is sometimes treated in the text as a separate item.)

1. Childhood emotional problems (age 0–10):
   0 = very shy, tics, phobias, bedwetting beyond age 8, dissocial, severe feeding problems, other noted problems.
   1 = average (no problems, but not quite 2).
   2 = good natured, normally social.

2. Child's physical health:
   0 = severe or prolonged illness, disability, handicapping deformity.
   1 = minor illnesses; childhood diseases not marked.
   2 = good physical health (childhood illnesses only minor; maximum of 2 of them reported).

3. Home atmosphere:
   0 = any noncongenial home, lack of family cohesiveness, parents not together, early maternal separation, known to many social agencies, many moves, financial hardship that imposed greatly on family life.
   1 = average home: doesn't stand out as good or bad; or lack of information.
   2 = warm, cohesive atmosphere, parents together, doing things as a family, sharing atmosphere, maternal and paternal presence, few moves, financial stability or special harmony in spite of difficulties.

4. Mother/child relationship:
   0 = distant, hostile, blaming others (such as father, teachers) for wrong methods of upbringing, overly punitive, overprotective, expecting too much, mother absent, seductive, not encouraging feeling of self-worth in child.
   1 = mostly for lack of information or lack of distinct impression about mother.
   2 = nurturing, encouraging of autonomy, helping boy develop self-esteem, warmth.

5. Father/child relationship:
   0 = distant, hostile, overly punitive, expectations unrealistic or not what son wants for himself, paternal absence, negative or destructive relationship.
   1 = lack of information, no distinct impression about father.
   2 = warmth, encouraging of autonomy in child, helping to develop self-esteem, does things with son, discusses problems, interested in child.

6. Relationship with siblings:
   0 = severe rivalry, destructive relationship, sibling undermines child's self-esteem.
   1 = no siblings, no good information, not mentioned as good though not particularly bad.
   2 = close to at least one sibling (mentioned).

7. School adjustment:
   0 = no sports, failures, marked social problems.
   1 = average, no competitive sports.

2 = does well at school, some competitive sports or extracurricular activities or above-average ratings by teacher. (All school ratings of grades are relative to I.Q. The following chart was used in helping to decide a school rating.)

0	Teacher's ratings less than average; no sports or clubs; behind class level; poor grades (I.Q. 90+)

1	Average teacher's ratings and

special class, or 2 grades behind and passing (I.Q. < 90)	1 grade behind and passing (I.Q. 90–100)	grade level and passing (I.Q. 100+)

2	Above-average teacher's ratings or active in sports and clubs and

1 grade behind and passing (I.Q. < 90)	grade level and passing (I.Q. 90–100)	grade level and at least B+ average (I.Q. 100+)

8. Global impression:
   0 = rater's overall hunch negative: nonnurturing environment.
   3 = neither negative nor positive feeling about subject's childhood.
   6 = positive, intact childhood; good relationships with parents, siblings, and others, environment seems conducive to developing self-esteem.

Childhood Environmental Weaknesses Scale

One point for each item; total score equals sum of the five five-item subscales.

1. Cohesive family—sum of the following 5 items:
    a. Boy made 8 moves or more.
    b. Parents together but incompatible, or separated.
    c. One parent absent more than 6 months before age 6.
    d. Raised for more than 6 months apart from both parents (or from surrogates if the surrogates were present since birth).
    e. 9 or more social service agency contacts or family chronically dependent. (Unless otherwise defined in an item, *mother* or *maternal* refers to biological mother or to a surrogate who assumed major and continued primary care of the child *before* 2 years of age. *Father* or *paternal* refers to biological father or to a surrogate who assumed major and continued care of the child for more than 50 percent of life before age 13.)

2. Maternal supervision—sum of the following 5 items:
    a. Boy says maternal supervision is inadequate.
    b. Mother either delinquent or alcoholic.
    c. Mother either suffering from severe physical ailment that interferes with normal activities or mentally retarded (strictly interpreted).
    d. When absent, mother does not provide surrogate supervision, or her own supervision is inadequate.
    e. Caseworkers describe housekeeping as substandard (2 observers).

3. Maternal affection—sum of the following 5 items:
    a. Boy describes maternal affection as inadequate.
    b. More than 2 years with surrogate mother after more than 2 years with real mother.
    c. Multiple observers describe affection as inadequate.
    d. Mother had mental illness severe enough to require and receive treatment.
    e. Boy describes self as indifferent to mother, or negative feelings.

4. Paternal supervision—sum of the following 5 items:
    a. Father described by observers as alcoholic on more than one occasion or as mentally retarded.
    b. Father arrested on more than one occasion (drunk arrests excluded).
    c. Father physically cruel toward subject or observers call discipline inadequate.

d. Boy describes discipline as inadequate, lax, or erratic.

e. Father or acceptable surrogate not present for 6 of the boy's first 12 years.

5. Quality of paternal affection—sum of the following 5 items:

a. Boy describes paternal affection as inadequate.

b. 2 or more observers describe affection as inadequate or father absent half or more of the time.

c. Father voluntarily absented self from son for more than 2 years.

d. Father had mental illness severe enough to require and receive treatment.

e. Boy describes self as indifferent to father, or negative feelings.

Boyhood Competence Scale

Score equals the sum of the following six items.

1. Job after school or during vacations (0–1).
2. Helps with chores at home (0–1).
3. Current participation in clubs, sports, extracurricular activities (0–1).
4. Grades in school—evaluated relative to I.Q. as in Childhood Environmental Strengths Scale (0–2).
5. Good adaptation to peer group; social life indicates friends, and good school adjustment (0–1).
6. Good adaptation to home life including relationship with siblings and parents; making the best of a poor home environment; sensible planning for the future (0–2).

Hollingshead-Redlich Social Class Scale

This same scale, dollar adjusted, was applied to the subjects at age 47 and to their parents 1940–1944. Final score is computed by multiplying residence scale by 6, occupation scale by 9, and education scale by 5. Score determines what social class an individual is assigned, as follows:

Range of Scores	Social Class
20–31	Class I
32–55	Class II
56–86	Class III
87–115	Class IV
116–134	Class V

A.　Residence scale:

1 = $75,000+ home.

2 = 6–8 room single-family home in a middle-range suburb such as Arlington and Winchester, Massachusetts.

3 = apartment in a middle-range suburb or a good neighborhood or owns a home in a working-class neighborhood, or owns a 2-family house.

4 = apartment in working-class neighborhood or owns a 3-family house in a rundown neighborhood or lives in a decent and well-kept-up housing project.

5 = lives in a run-down housing project or in a well-kept single room.

6 = derelict housing.

B.　Occupational scale:

1 = executives and proprietors of large concerns, and major professionals.

2 = managers and proprietors of medium-sized businesses, and lesser professionals.

3 = administrative personnel of large concerns, owners of small independent businesses, and semiprofessionals.

4 = owners of little businesses, clerical and sales workers, and technicians.

5 = skilled workers.

6 = semiskilled workers.

7 = unskilled workers.

C.　Educational scale:

1 = graduate professional training.

2 = a 4-year degree from a standard college or university.

3 = partial college training—at least 1 year.

4 = high school graduate.

5 = partial high school—finished 10th or 11th grade.

6 = junior high school—finished 7th, 8th, or 9th grade.

7 = less than a 7th grade education.

Social Competence Scale

The following 8 subscales were summed. (A score of 2 was given for any subscale that was inapplicable.) Marital success or failure was deliberately treated as a separate variable.

1.　Enjoyment of children:

1 = subject has a very positive relationship with all his children, has spent

time with them as they were growing up, and has good lines of communication with them. Subject speaks of children in a positive way.

2 = subject has a good relationship with some and not with others, or relationship clearly okay but not clearly "very positive," or no children.

3 = wife seems to have major responsibility for children, and subject seems to have spent little time with them *or* subject has some contact with children, though not as much as possible, who live with former spouse.

4 = relationship is consistently poor, or there is clear evidence of neglect or avoidance.

2. Friendship pattern (last 10 years):

1 = clear evidence of close friends sustained over time.

2 = evidence not clear, or distant friendship patterns.

3 = clear evidence that subject has no close friends at all.

3. Enjoyment of family of origin (includes foster parents, stepparents, and step siblings, but not in-laws or children):

1 = spends time with many of family of origin if possible, or is in mail or phone contact with them, and does this more for pleasure than out of duty.

2 = sees family members more from duty than fun, or relationship ambiguous.

3 = dislikes all his family, or does not see them except rarely—although it is perfectly feasible.

4. Work relationships:

1 = evidence of ability to get along with peers, subordinates, and boss.

2 = so-so.

3 = is a prickly or isolated employee and/or boss.

5. Frequency of contact with friends:

1 = goes out with and/or has nonrelatives in at least once a fortnight.

2 = goes out with or has nonrelatives in about once in every 3 to 10 weeks.

3 = little social activity with nonrelatives.

6. Social clubs or organizations:

1 = belongs to social clubs or organizations, is active, and attends meetings on a regular basis.

2 = belongs to clubs or organizations but is a rather inactive member and does not often attend meetings.

3 = no clubs or organizations.

7. Volunteer social service activities:

1 = actively participates in one or more community activities—including church, civic activities, and those involving his children.

2 = occasional participation.
3 = no volunteer activities.
8. Sports and interpersonal pastimes and hobbies:
    1 = active involvement in pastimes (sports, hobbies, etc.) with friends.
    2 = active involvement with relatives, if not with friends.
    3 = no involvement in shared recreational activities.

Hyperactivity Scale

This scale is modified from Wender's Temperament Questionnaire (Wood et al. 1976) for ages 6–10; unfortunately, our subjects were 12–16. Subjects were rated on 10 categories of behavior, with points assigned as shown below. (If an item was mentioned more than once, a point was given for each mention, but not more than 3 points were given in any one category.) The category scores were summed, and the total scores were interpreted as follows: 1–5 = No hyperkinesis; 6–9 = very little; 10–15 = ? hyperkinesis; 16–28 = hyperkinetic.

Category	Number of Points
1. Restless:	
Restlessness	2
Thoughtlessness	1
2. Excitable, impulsive:	
Interrupting	2
Destroying school property	1
Impatience	1
3. Disturbs other children:	
Quarrelsomeness	1
Disorderliness	1
Bullying	1
4. Short attention span:	
Fails to finish things he starts	1
Truancy	1
Unreliableness	2
5. Fidgeting:	
Attracting attention	1
Laziness	1
6. Inattentive, distractible:	
Whispering	1

Inattention	1
Carelessness	1
7. Easily frustrated:	
Lack of interest	1
Easily discouraged	2
8. Problems with birth (instead of Wender's "Cries")	1 (2 if multiple problems)
9. Mood changes quickly	1
10. Temper outbursts, explosive and unpredictable behavior:	
Tantrums	2
Impudence	1

Robins's Sociopathy Scale

One point was given for each item present. A score of 5 or more indicated a "sociopath." ("School problems and truancy" is treated as a separate item in the text.)

a. *Poor work history:* at least 6 of the following: 6+ jobs within 10 years, successive jobs at less pay or less prestige, fired for incompetence or personality conflict, unemployment for more than a month at a time, quitting because of fights or arguments, much time out for illness, chronic absenteeism, job troubles from drinking, no job of as much as 3 years' duration in the last 10 years.

b. *Poor marital history:* 2 or more divorces, marriage to wife with severe behavior problems, repeated separations.

c. *Excessive drugs:* addiction to barbiturates, tranquilizers, opiates, or stimulants, or a period of experimentation with drugs for nonmedical purposes.

d. *Heavy drinking:* medical complications, arrests, firing, or serious family complaints because of alcohol, or chronic intake of 3+ drinks at least 3 times a week or 7 drinks per sitting.

e. *Repeated arrests:* 3 or more nontraffic arrests.

f. *Physical aggression:* arrest record for fighting, reports of wife or child beatings, self-report of many fights.

g. *Sexual promiscuity or perversion:* arrests on charges pertaining to sex, interview claims of extreme promiscuity (e.g., 50 different sexual partners), interview reports of homosexuality.

h. *Suicide (attempts):* death by suicide, hospital or interview reports of suicide attempts.

i. *Impulsive behavior:* frequent moving from one city to another, more than one elopement, sudden army enlistments, unprovoked desertion of home.

j. *School problems and truancy:* 4 or more of the following plus repeated truancy: did not leave school at graduation point, 2 years older than average in the last year at school, attended 4 or more grammar schools, left school voluntarily before completing expected level, failed 1 full year or more, complaints *re* discipline from teachers, fights with students, expulsion or suspension.

k. *Public financial care:* totally or partially supported by relatives, friends, social agencies, or public institutions.

l. *Poor armed services record:* enlistment of less than 1 year's duration, demotions, repeated AWOL, court-martialed, punishments, desertion, dishonorable discharge.

m. *Vagrancy:* several months or more of travel around the country without prearranged employment.

n. *Many somatic symptoms:* at least 10 somatic symptoms scored from interview on medical-psychiatric inventory or fewer if severe and disabling.

o. *Pathological lying:* fantastic history given which does not apparently just serve the function of omitting or white-washing reports of antisocial behavior.

p. *Lack of friends:* does not participate in activities of any informal social group, sees friends less than once in 2 weeks, has no or only 1 close friend, sees fewer than 10 people socially.

q. *Use of aliases:* interview report or police record showing use of an assumed name.

r. *Lack of guilt about sexual exploits and crimes:* interviewer's impression from the way in which patient reports his history.

s. *Reckless youth:* age span of 18–20 years reported as characterized by 7 or more of these: feeling carefree, time spent almost entirely in social activity, little time spent at home, self-report as reckless or wild, drove fast, fought, drank excessively, changed jobs frequently, spent money extravagantly.

Interview Schedule for Alcohol Use

[Obtain dates and numbers for everything.]

1. We are very interested in how people use alcohol and its relation to health. Can you describe what and how much you drink during a week? When do you usually drink? [If on a weekend, find out how much.]
2. When did you first start to drink—at home, at parties, with friends?
3. Did you drink when you were younger?
   Did you drink more or less then?
4. Do you ever drink heavier than usual? How often? (For example, on Saturday night? When not feeling good or depressed?)
   Was this ever true in the past?
   Does drinking cheer you up when you are in a bad mood?
5. Do you ever go on binges? Last time tight?
6. Have you ever stopped drinking (gone on the wagon) for any period of time for any reason?
   When?
   For how long?
7. Has a doctor ever advised you to cut down or stop drinking for any reason?
8. Has anyone ever expressed concern or gotten angry with you about your drinking? Friends, relatives, neighbors?
   What did they usually say?
   Your wife?
   When did they start?
   Was this annoying to you?
9. Have you ever gotten into trouble with your boss or a fellow worker because of drinking?
10. Have you ever been late for work, say on a Monday morning because of the "night before"?
11. Have you ever been to an AA meeting? When? How many?
12. When did you have your first blackout, being unable to remember what happened to you the previous night, even though friends said you did not pass out?
13. When did you notice that after a hard night's drinking, you shook in the morning? Felt more anxious? Other symptoms?

14. When after a hard night's drinking did you start to drink the next morning to quiet your nerves?
15. Do you sometimes think you have a drinking problem? When did that begin?

[If at any point after #15 you are sure the person is an alcoholic, skip to #21.]

16. Have you often failed to keep the promise you have made to yourself about controlling or cutting down your drinking?
17. Do you sometimes feel a little guilty about your drinking?
18. Do you try to avoid family or close friends while you are drinking?
19. Do you sometimes have a drink or two at a party without letting others know? Or have a drink or two before you get there?
20. Do you often regret things you have done or said while drinking?
21. You mentioned that you stopped drinking once. What made you stop? [Praise and probe—other times, dates, be exact.]
22. Who may have helped? Were there any helping agencies?
    Halfway houses? When? How long?
    What were the substitutes for alcohol (e.g., religion)?
    Did you ever use Antabuse?
    When you wanted a drink, what did you do instead? [Probe for coping mechanisms.]
    Compulsory supervision (employer, legal)? [Expand.]
    What life changes were there (marriage, deaths, reunions, friends)?
23. Have you ever gone to a hospital for detoxification? [Probe.]
    When?
    Have you ever gone to a clinic for detoxification? [Probe.]
    When?

Cahalan Scale

One point for each of the following being true.

1. *Frequent intoxication:* 5 or more drinks once a week; or 8 or more drinks on 1 of the most recent 2 drinking occasions and twice in the last 2 months; or 12 or more drinks on one of the last 2 occasions and twice in the last year; or currently getting high or tight at least once a week.

2. *Binge drinking:* being intoxicated for at least several days at one time or for 2 days or more on more than one occasion.

3. *Symptomatic drinking:* more than one of the following: drinking to get rid of a hangover; having difficulty in stopping drinking; blackouts or lapses

of memory; skipping meals while on a drinking bout; tossing down drinks for a quicker effect; sneaking drinks; taking quick drinks in advance of a party to make sure one gets enough.

4. *Psychological dependence:* drinking to alleviate depression or nervousness or to escape from the problems of everyday living, i.e., a drink is helpful when depressed or nervous; an important reason for drinking is to forget everything, to help forget one's worries, to cheer one up when in a bad mood; a drink is needed when one is tense or nervous.

5. *Problems with spouse or relatives:* spouse leaves or threatens to leave the respondent or is chronically angry or concerned over the respondent's drinking; spouse or a relative asks the respondent to cut down on his drinking; the respondent himself feels his drinking has had a harmful effect on his home life.

6. *Problems with friends or neighbors:* friends or neighbors had suggested cutting down on drinking; respondent feels that drinking has been harmful to friendships and social life.

7. *Job problems:* respondent lost or nearly lost a job because of drinking; people at work suggest that he cut down on drinking; drinking has been harmful to work and employment opportunities.

8. *Problems with law, police, accidents:* trouble with law over driving after drinking; drunkenness; drinking contributed to an accident in which there was a personal injury.

9. *Health:* respondent feels that drinking is harmful to health and doctor advised cutting down.

10. *Financial problems.*

11. *Belligerence:* felt aggressive or cross after drinking; got into a fight or a heated argument.

DSM III Scale of Alcohol Abuse and Dependence

Diagnostic criteria for alcohol abuse: A, B, and C are required.

Diagnostic criteria for alcohol dependence: A, B, C, and D are required.

A. Continuous or episodic use of alcohol for at least one month.

B. Social complications of alcohol use: impairment in social or occupational functioning (e.g., arguments or difficulties with family or friends over excessive alcohol use, violent while intoxicated, missed work, fired), or legal difficulties (e.g., arrest for intoxicated behavior, traffic accidents while intoxicated).

C. Either (1) or (2). (1) *Psychological dependence:* compelling desire to use alcohol; inability to cut down or stop drinking; repeated efforts to control or reduce excess drinking by going on the wagon (periods of temporary abstinence) or restriction of drinking to certain times of the day. (2) *Pathological patterns of use:* (a) goes on binges (remains intoxicated throughout the day for at least 2 days); (b) occasionally drinks a fifth of spirits (or its equivalent in wine or beer); (c) has had 2 or more blackouts (amnesic periods for events occurring while intoxicated); (d) continues to drink despite a life-threatening disorder that he knows is exacerbated by alcohol.

D. Either (1) or (2). (1) *Tolerance:* increasing amounts of alcohol required to achieve desired effect, or diminished effect with regular use of same dose. (2) *Withdrawal:* development of alcohol withdrawal (e.g., morning "shakes" and malaise relieved by drinking) after cessation or reduction of drinking.

References

Aamark, C. 1951. "A Study of Alcoholism." *Acta Psychiatrica Scandinavica,* Supplement 70.

Allman, L. R., et al. 1972. "Group Drinking during Stress: Effects on Drinking Behavior, Affect, and Psychopathology." *American Journal of Psychiatry* 129(6):669–678.

American Psychiatric Association. 1980. *Diagnostic and Statistical Manual.* 3rd ed. Washington: APA.

———— 1987. Committee on Nomenclature and Statistics. *Diagnostic and Statistical Manual of Mental Disorders,* 3rd ed. rev. Washington: APA.

———— In press. Committee on Nomenclature and Statistics. *Diagnostic and Statistical Manual of Mental Disorders,* 4th ed. rev. Washington: APA.

Andreasson, S., A. Romelsjo, and P. Allebeck. 1991. "Alcohol, Social Factors, and Mortality among Young Men." *British Journal of Addiction* 86:877–887.

Anstie, F. E. 1864. *Stimulants and Narcotics, Their Mutual Relations: With Special Researches on the Action of Alcohol, Aether, and Chloroform on the Vital Organism.* London: Macmillan.

Armor, D. J., J. M. Polich, and H. B. Stanbul. 1978. *Alcoholism and Treatment.* New York: Wiley.

Ashley, M. J., and J. G. Rankin. 1980. "Hazardous Alcohol Consumption and Diseases of the Circulatory System." *Journal of Studies on Alcohol* 41:1040–1070.

Ashley, M. J., et al. 1977. "Morbidity in Alcoholics: Evidence for Accelerated Development of Physical Disease in Women." *Archives of Internal Medicine* 137:883–887.

Ashley, M. J. 1984. "Alcohol Consumption and Ischemic Heart Disease." In *Research Advances in Alcohol and Drug Problems,* ed. R. G. Smart et al., vol. 8, 99–47. New York: Plenum Press.

Asma, F. E., R. L. Eggert, and R. R. J. Hilker. 1971. "Long-Term Experience with Re-habilitation of Alcoholic Employees." *Journal of Occupational Medicine* 13:581–585.

Azrin, N. H., et al. 1982. "Alcoholism Treatment by Disulfiram and Community Reinforcement Therapy." *Journal of Behavior Therapy and Experimental Psychiatry* 13:105–112.

Babor, T. F., E. B. Ritson, and R. J. Hodgson. 1986. "Alcohol-related Problems in the Primary Health Care Setting: A Review of Early Intervention Strategies." *British Journal of Addiction* 81:23–46.

Bacon, S. D. 1957. "Social Settings Conducive to Alcoholism." *Journal of the American Medical Association* 164:177–181.

Baekeland, F., L. Lundwall, and B. Kissin. 1975. "Methods for the Treatment of Chronic Alcoholism: A Critical Appraisal." In *Research Advances in Alcohol and Drug Problems,* vol. 2, ed. R. J. Gibbons et al. New York: Wiley.

Baer, A. 1878. *Der Alcoholismus seine Verbreitung, und seine Wirkung auf den individu-ellen und socialen Organismus sowie die Mittel, ihn zu Bekämpfen.* Berlin: Hirschwald.

Bailey, M., and J. Stewart. 1967. "Normal Drinking by Persons Reporting Previous Problem Drinking." *Quarterly Journal of Studies on Alcohol* 28:305–315.

Bales, R. F. 1962. "Attitudes toward Drinking in the Irish Culture." In *Society, Culture, and Drinking Patterns,* ed. D. J. Pittman and C. R. Snyder. New York: Wiley.

Baltes, P. B. 1968. "Longitudinal and Cross-Sectional Sequences in the Study of Age and Generation Effects." *Human Development* 11:145–171.

Bandura, A. 1969. *Principles of Behavior Modification.* New York: Holt, Rinehart and Winston.

Barry, H. B., III. 1974. "Psychological Factors in Alcoholism." In *Clinical Pathology,* ed. B. Kissin and H. Begleiter. The Biology of Alcoholism, vol. 3. New York: Plenum Press.

Bean, M. 1975. "Alcoholics Anonymous." *Psychiatric Annals* 5:5–64.

Bean, M. H., and N. E. Zinberg, eds. 1981. *Dynamic Approaches to the Understanding and Treatment of Alcoholism.* New York: Free Press.

Beardslee, W. R., and G. E. Vaillant. 1984. "Prospective Prediction of Alcoholism and Psychopathology." *Journal of Studies on Alcohol* 45:500–503.

Beardslee, W. R., L. Son, and G. E. Vaillant. 1986. "Exposure to Parental Alcoholism During Childhood and Outcome in Adulthood: A Prospective Longitudinal Study." *British Journal of Psychiatry* 149:584–591.

Beaubrun, M. H. 1967. "Treatment of Alcoholism in Trinidad and Tobago, 1956–65." *British Journal of Psychiatry* 113:643–658.

Begleiter, H., and B. Porjesz. 1988. "Potential Biologic Markers in Individuals at High Risk for Developing Alcoholism." *Alcohol Clinical Experimental Research* 12:488–493.

Behar, D., G. Winokur, and C. J. Berg. 1984. "Depression in the Abstinent Alcoholic." *American Journal of Psychiatry* 141:1105–1107.

Belasco, J. A. 1971. "The Criterion Question Revisited." *British Journal of Addiction* 66:39–44.

Berglund, M. 1984. "Suicide in Alcoholism." *Archives of General Psychiatry* 41:888–891.

———— 1985. "Cerebral Dysfunction in Alcoholism Related to Mortality and Long-term Social Adjustment." *Alcoholism: Clinical and Experimental Research* 9:153–157.

Berkman, L. F., and S. L. Syme. 1979. "Social Networks Host Resistance and Mortality: A Nine-Year Follow-up of Alameda County Residents." *American Journal of Epidemiology* 109:186–201.

Bien, T. H., W. R. Miller, and J. S. Tonigan. 1993. "Brief Interventions for Alcohol Problems: A Review." *British Journal of Addiction* 88:315–336.

Bill C. 1965. "The Growth and Effectiveness of Alcoholics Anonymous in a Southwestern City, 1945–1962." *Quarterly Journal of Studies on Alcohol* 26:279–284.

Blane, H. T. 1968. *The Personality of the Alcoholic: Guises of Dependency.* New York: Harper and Row.

———— 1978. "Half a Bottle Is Better than None." *Contemporary Psychology* 23:396–397.

Block, J. 1961. *The Q-Sort Method in Personality Assessment and Psychiatric Research.* Springfield, Ill.: Charles C. Thomas.

———— 1971. *Lives through Time.* Berkeley, Calif.: Bancroft Books.

Blum, E. M. 1966. "Psychoanalytic Views of Alcoholism: A Review." *Quarterly Journal of Studies on Alcohol* 27:259–299.

Blume, S. B. 1986. "Women and Alcohol: A Review." *Journal of the American Medical Association* 256:1467–1470.

Boffetta, P., and L. Garfinkel. 1990. "Alcohol Drinking and Mortality among Men Enrolled in an American Cancer Society Prospective Study." *Epidemiology* 1:342–348.

Bohman, M. 1978. "Some Genetic Aspects of Alcoholism and Criminality." *Archives of General Psychiatry* 35:269–276.

Bourne, P., and R. Fox. 1973. *Alcoholism: Progress in Research and Treatment.* New York: Academic Press.

Bratfos, O. 1974. *The Course of Alcoholism: Drinking, Social Adjustment and Health.* Oslo: Universitet Forlaget.

Brenner, B. 1967. "Alcoholism and Fatal Accidents." *Quarterly Journal of Studies on Alcohol* 28:517–528.

Bromet, E., et al. 1977. "Posttreatment Functioning of Alcoholic Patients: Its Relation to Program Participation." *Journal of Consulting and Clinical Psychology* 45:829–842.

Brown, S. A., M. Irwin, and M. A. Schuckit. 1988. "Changes in Depression among Abstinent Alcoholics." *Journal of Studies on Alcohol* 49:412–417.

———— 1991. "Changes in Anxiety among Abstinent Male Alcoholics." *Journal of Studies on Alcohol* 52:55–61.

Brownell, K. D., et al. 1986. "Understanding and Preventing Relapse." *American Psychologist* 41:765–782.

Brugere, J., et al. 1986. "Differential Effects of Tobacco and Alcohol in Cancer of the Larynx, Pharynx and Mouth." *Cancer* 57:391–395.

Bruun, K. 1963. "Outcome of Different Types of Treatment of Alcoholics." *Quarterly Journal of Studies on Alcohol* 24:280–288.

Bruun, K., et al. 1975. *Alcohol Control Policies in Public Health Perspective.* Helsinki.

Bullock, K. D., and R. J. Reed. 1992. "Grant I: Reduced Mortality Risk in Alcoholics Who Achieve Long-term Abstinence." *Journal of the American Medical Association* 267:668–672.

Burch, G. E., and T. D. Giles. 1974. "Alcoholic Cardiomyopathy." In *Clinical Pathology,* ed. B. Kissin and H. Begleiter. The Biology of Alcoholism, vol. 3. New York: Plenum Press.

Burch, J. R., et al. 1988. "Chronic Ethanol or Nicotine Treatment Results in Partial Cross-tolerance between These Agents." *Psychopharmacology* 95:452–458.

Bush, B., et al. 1987. "Screening for Alcohol Abuse Using the CAGE Questionnaire." *American Journal of Medicine* 82:231–235.

Buydens-Branchey, L., M. H. Branchey, and D. Noumair. 1989. "Age of Alcoholism Onset: I. Relationship to Psychopathology." *Archives of General Psychiatry* 46:225–230.

Caddy, G. R., and S. H. Lovibond. 1976. "Self-Regulation and Discriminated Aversive Conditioning in the Modification of Alcoholics' Drinking Behavior." *Behavior Therapy* 7:223–230.

Cadoret, R. J., C. A. Cain, and W. M. Grove. 1980. "Development of Alcoholism in Adoptees Raised Apart from Alcoholic Biologic Relatives." *Archives of General Psychiatry* 37:561–563.

Cadoret, R. J., et al. 1985. "Alcoholism and Antisocial Personality: Interrelationships, Genetic and Environmental Factors." *Archives of General Psychiatry* 42:161–167.

Cahalan, D. 1970. *Problem Drinkers: A National Survey.* San Francisco: Jossey Bass.

Cahalan, D., I. H. Cisin, and H. M. Crossley. 1969. *American Drinking Practices: A National Survey of Behavior and Attitudes.* Monograph 6. New Brunswick, N.J.: Rutgers Center for Alcohol Studies.

Cahalan, D., and R. Room. 1972. "Problem Drinking among Men Aged 21–59." *American Journal of Public Health* 62:1472–1482.

——— 1974. *Problem Drinkers among American Men.* New Brunswick, N.J.: Rutgers Center for Alcohol Studies.

Camberwell Council on Alcoholism. 1980. *Women and Alcohol.* London: Tavistock.

Campbell, E. J. M., J. G. Scadding, and R. S. Roberts. 1979. "The Concept of Disease." *British Medical Journal* 2:757–762.

Cantwell, D. P. 1972. "Psychiatric Illness in the Families of Hyperactive Children." *Archives of General Psychiatry* 27:414–417.

Cappell, H., and J. Greeley. 1987. "Alcohol and Tension Reduction: An Update on Research and Theory." In *Psychological Theories of Drinking and Alcoholism,* ed. H. T. Blane and K. E. Leonard, pp. 15–54. New York: Guilford Press.

Carroll, J. F. X. 1978. "Proceedings of the 10th Annual Eagleville Conference on Alcoholism and Drug Addiction." *American Journal of Drug and Alcohol Abuse* 5:257–359.

Cassel, J. 1976. "The Contribution of the Social Environment to Host Resistance." *American Journal of Epidemiology* 104:107–123.

Castelli, W. P., J. T. Doyle, and T. Gordon. 1977. "Alcohol and Blood Lipids: The Cooperative Lipoprotein Phenotyping Study." *Lancet* 2:153–156.

Cecil, R. 1940. *Textbook of Medicine*. New York: Saunders.

Chapman, P. L. H., and I. Huygens. 1988. "An Evaluation of Three Treatment Programs for Alcoholism." *British Journal of Addiction* 83:67–81.

Chatham, L. R., et al. 1979. *Employed Alcoholic Women: The Right to Be the Same or Different*. Washington: National Council on Alcoholism.

Chick, J., G. Lloyd, and E. Crombie. 1985. "Counseling Problem Drinkers in Medical Wards: A Controlled Study." *British Medical Journal* 290:965–967.

Chick, J., et al. 1988. "Advice versus Extended Treatment for Alcoholism: A Controlled Study." *British Journal of Addiction* 83:159–170.

Clark, W. B. 1976. "Loss of Control, Heavy Drinking and Drinking Problems in a Longitudinal Setting." *Journal of Studies on Alcohol* 37:1256–1290.

Clark, W. B., and D. Cahalan. 1976. "Changes in Problem Drinking over a Four-Year Span." *Addictive Behaviors* 1:251–259.

Cloninger, C. R., M. Bohman, and S. Sigvardsson. 1981. "Inheritance of Alcohol Abuse: Cross-Fostering Analysis of Adopted Men." *Archives of General Psychiatry* 38:861–868.

Cloninger, C. R. 1987a. "Neurogenetic Adaptive Mechanisms in Alcoholism." *Science* 230:410–416.

———— 1987b. "A Systematic Method for Clinical Description and Classification of Personality Variants: A Proposal." *Archives of General Psychiatry* 44:573–588.

———— et al. 1988a. "Childhood Personality Predicts Alcohol Abuse in Young Adults." *Alcohol: Clinical and Experimental Research* 12(4):494–505.

———— et al. 1988b. "The Swedish Studies of the Adopted Children of Alcoholics: A Reply to Littrell." *Journal of Studies on Alcohol* 49(6):500–509.

Clyne, R. M. 1965. "Detection and Rehabilitation of the Problem Drinker in Industry." *Journal of Occupational Medicine* 9:265–268.

Coffey, T. G. 1966. "Beer Street: Gin Lane." *Quarterly Journal of Studies on Alcohol* 27:669–692.

Cohen, M., I. Liebson, and L. Faillace. 1973. "Controlled Drinking by Chronic Alcoholics over Extended Periods of Free Access." *Psychological Reports* 32:1107–1110.

Conger, J. J. 1956. "Alcoholism: Theory, Problem and Challenge, II: Reinforcement Theory and the Dynamics of Alcoholism." *Quarterly Journal of Studies on Alcohol* 17:296–305.

Costello, R. M. 1975. "Alcoholism Treatment and Evaluation, II: Collation of Two Year Follow-up Studies." *International Journal of Addictions* 10:857–867.

——— 1980. "Alcoholism Treatment Effectiveness: Slicing the Outcome Variance Pie." In *Alcoholism Treatment in Transition,* ed. S. G. Edwards and M. Grant. London: Croom Helm.

Cotton, N. S. 1979. "The Familial Incidence of Alcoholism." *Journal of Studies on Alcohol* 40:89–116.

Criqui, M. 1990. "The Reduction of Coronary Heart Disease with Light to Moderate Consumption: Effect or Artifact?" *British Journal of Addiction* 85:854–857.

Cross, G. M., et al. 1990. "Alcoholism Treatment: A Ten-Year Follow-up Study." *Alcoholism: Clinical and Experimental Research* 14:169–173.

Crowe, R. R. 1974. "An Adoption Study of Antisocial Personality." *Archives of General Psychiatry* 31:785–791.

Cushing, H. 1925. *The Life of Sir William Osler.* Oxford: Clarendon.

Cyr, M. G., and S. A. Wortman. 1988. "The Effectiveness of Routine Screening Questions in the Detection of Alcoholism." *Journal of the American Medical Association* 259:51–54.

Dahlgren, L. 1978. "Female Alcoholics III. Development and Pattern of Problem Drinking." *Acta Psychiatrica Scandinavica* 57:325–335.

D'Alonzo, C., and S. Pell. 1968. "Cardiovascular Disease among Problem Drinkers." *Journal of Occupational Medicine* 10:344–350.

Davies, D. L. 1962. "Normal Drinking in Recovered Alcohol Addicts." *Quarterly Journal of Studies on Alcohol* 23:94–104.

——— 1980. "The Treatment of Alcohol Dependence." In *Medical Consequences of Alcohol Abuse,* ed. P. M. S. Clark and L. J. Kricka, 263–275. Chichester: Ellis Horwood.

Davies, D. L., M. Shepherd, and E. Myers. 1956. "The Two-Years' Prognosis of 50 Alcohol Addicts after Treatment in Hospital." *Quarterly Journal of Studies on Alcohol* 17:485–502.

DeFrank, R. S., C. D. Jenkins, and R. M. Rose. 1987. "A Longitudinal Investigation of the Relationships among Alcohol Consumption, Psychosocial Factors and Blood Pressure." *Psychosomatic Medicine* 49:236–249.

DeLabry, L. O., et al. 1992. "Alcohol Consumption and Mortality in an American Male Population: Recovering the U-shaped Curve—Findings from the Normative Aging Study." *Journal of Studies on Alcohol* 53(1):25–32.

de Lint, J., and W. Schmidt. 1968. "The Distribution of Alcohol Consumption in Ontario." *Quarterly Journal of Studies on Alcohol* 29:968–973.

Deutsch, C. 1982. *Broken Bottles, Broken Dreams.* Totowa, N.J.: Teachers College Press.

Deykin, E. Y., J. C. Levy, and V. Wells. 1987. "Adolescent Depression, Alcohol and Drug Abuse." *American Journal of Public Health* 77 (2): 178–182.

Diamond, G. A., and J. S. Forrester. 1979. "Analysis of Probability as an Aid in Clinical Diagnosis of Coronary Artery Disease." *New England Journal of Medicine* 300:1350–1358.

DiFranza, J., and M. Guerrera. 1990. "Alcoholism and Smoking." *Journal of Studies on Alcohol* 51:130–135.

Ditman, K. S., et al. 1967. "A Controlled Experiment on the Use of Court Probation for Drunk Arrests." *American Journal of Psychiatry* 124(2):160–163.

Dorus, W., et al. 1989. "Lithium Treatment of Depressed and Nondepressed Alcoholics." *Journal of the American Medical Association* 162:1646–1652.

Drake, R. E., G. J. McHugo, and D. L. Noordsy. 1993. "Treatment of Alcoholism among Schizophrenic Outpatients: Four-year Outcomes." *American Journal of Psychiatry* 150: 328–329.

Drew, L. R. H. 1968. "Alcoholism as a Self-Limiting Disease." *Quarterly Journal of Studies on Alcohol* 29:956–967.

Dunn, F. 1988. "Are Women More Easily Damaged by Alcohol than Men?" *British Journal of Addiction* 83:1135–1136.

Dunner, D. L., B. M. Hensel, and R. R. Fieve. 1979. "Bipolar Illness: Factors in Drinking Behavior." *American Journal of Psychiatry* 136:583–585.

Dyer, A. R., et al. 1977. "Alcohol Consumption, Cardiovascular Risk Factors and Mortality in Two Chicago Epidemiological Studies." *Circulation* 56:1067–1074.

Earls, F., et al. 1988. "Psychopathology in Children of Alcoholic and Antisocial Parents." *Alcohol: Clinical and Experimental Research* 12:481–487.

Edwards, G. 1973. "Epidemiology Applied to Alcoholism: A Review and an Examination of Purposes." *Quarterly Journal of Studies on Alcohol* 34:28–56.

——— 1974. "Drugs, Drug Dependence and the Concept of Plasticity." *Quarterly Journal of Studies on Alcohol* 35:176–195.

——— 1984. "Drinking in Longitudinal Perspective: Career and Natural History." *British Journal of Addiction* 79:175–183.

——— 1985. "A Later Follow-up of a Classic Case Series: D. L. Davies' 1962 Report and Its Significance for the Present." *Journal of Studies on Alcohol* 46:181–190.

——— 1986. "The Alcohol Dependence Syndrome: Concept as Stimulus to Inquiry." *British Journal of Addiction* 81:171–184.

——— 1989. "As the Years Go Rolling By: Drinking Problems in the Time Dimension." *British Journal of Psychiatry* 154:18–26.

Edwards, G., and M. Grant, eds. 1980. *Alcoholism Treatment in Transition*. London: Croom Helm.

Edwards, G., and S. Guthrie. 1966. "A Comparison of Inpatient and Outpatient Treatment of Alcohol Dependence." *Lancet* 1:467–468.

——— 1967. "A Controlled Trial of Inpatient and Outpatient Treatment of Alcoholic Dependence." *Lancet* 1:555–559.

Edwards, G., C. Hensman, and J. Peto. 1972. "Drinking in a London Suburb, III: Comparisons of Drinking Troubles among Men and Women." *Quarterly Journal of Studies on Alcohol,* Supplement 6:120–128.

Edwards, G., E. Kyle, and P. Nicholls, 1974. "A Study of Alcoholics Admitted to Four Hospitals, I: Social Class and the Interaction of the Alcoholics with the Treatment System." *Quarterly Journal of Studies on Alcohol* 35:499–522.

Edwards, G., et al. 1967. "Alcoholics Anonymous: The Anatomy of a Self-Help Group." *Social Psychiatry* 1:195–204.

——— 1983. "What Happens to Alcoholics?" *Lancet* 2: 269–271.

——— 1988. "Long-term Outcome for Patients with Drinking Problems: The Search for Predictors." *British Journal of Addiction* 83:917–927.

Eichorn, D., et al., eds. 1981. *Present and Past in Middle Life.* New York: Academic Press.

Eiser, A. R. 1987. "The Effects of Alcohol on Renal Function and Excretion." *Alcohol: Clinical and Experimental Research* 11:127–138.

Emrick, C. D. 1974. "A Review of Psychologically Oriented Treatment of Alcoholism, I: The Use and Interrelationships of Outcome Criteria and Drinking Behavior Following Treatment." *Quarterly Journal of Studies on Alcohol* 35:523–549.

——— 1975. "A Review of Psychologically Oriented Treatment of Alcoholism, II: The Relative Effectiveness of Different Treatment Approaches and the Effectiveness of Treatment versus No Treatment." *Journal of Studies on Alcohol* 36:88–109.

——— 1989. "Alcoholics Anonymous: Membership Characteristics and Effectiveness as Treatment." In *Recent Developments in Alcoholism,* vol. 7, ed. M. Galanter, 37–53. New York: Plenum Press.

Endicott, J., et al. 1976. "The Global Assessment Scale: A Procedure for Measuring Overall Severity of Psychiatric Disturbance." *Archives of General Psychiatry* 33:766–770.

Erikson, E. 1950. *Childhood and Society.* New York: Norton.

——— 1968. "The Life Cycle." In *International Encyclopedia of the Social Sciences,* vol. 9. New York: Macmillan.

Eshbaugh, D. M., D. J. Tosi, and C. N. Hoyt. 1980. "Women Alcoholics: A Typological Description Using the MMPI." *Journal of Studies on Alcohol* 41:310–315.

Essen-Moller, E. 1956. "Individual Traits and Morbidity in a Swedish Rural Population." *Acta Psychiatrica Scandinavica,* Supplement 100.

Ewing, J. A. 1984. "Detecting Alcoholism: The CAGE Questionnaire." *Journal of the American Medical Association* 252:1905–1907.

Ewing, J. A., and B. A. Rouse. 1976. "Failure of an Experimental Treatment Program to Inculcate Controlled Drinking in Alcoholics." *British Journal of Addiction* 71:123–134.

Ewusi-Mensah, I., et al. 1983. "Psychiatric Morbidity in Patients with Alcoholic Liver Disease." *British Medical Journal* 287:1417–1419.

Falk, J. L., and M. Tang. 1980. "Schedule Induction and Overindulgence." *Alcoholism: Clinical and Experimental Research* 4:266–270.

Farquhar, J. 1978. "The Community-Based Model of Life Style Intervention Trials." *American Journal of Epidemiology* 108:103–111.

Farquhar, J., et al. 1977. "Community Education for Cardiovascular Health." *Lancet* 1:1192–1195.

——— 1990. "Effects of Communitywide Education on Cardiovascular Disease Risk Factors: The Stanford Five-City Project." *Journal of the American Medical Association* 214:359–365.

Fielding, J. W. 1985. "Smoking: Health Effects and Controls." *New England Journal of Medicine* 313:491–498, 555–561.

Fillmore, K. M. 1975. "Relationships between Specific Drinking Problems in Early Adulthood and Middle Age: An Exploratory 20-Year Follow-up Study." *Journal of Studies on Alcohol* 36:882–907.

——— 1987. "Women's Drinking across Adult Life Course as Compared to Men's: A Longitudinal and Cohort Analysis." *British Journal of Addiction* 82:801–812.

Fillmore, K. M., S. D. Bacon, and M. Hyman. 1979. "The 27-Year Longitudinal Panel Study of Drinking by Students in College, 1949–1976." Final Report to NIAAA. Contract no. ADM 281-76-0015.

Fingarette, H. 1988. *Heavy Drinking: The Myth of Alcoholism as a Disease.* Berkeley: University of California Press.

——— 1991. "Alcoholism: The Mythical Disease." In *Society, Culture and Drinking Patterns Reexamined,* ed. D. J. Pittman and H. R. White, 417–438. New Brunswick, N.J.: Rutgers Center for Alcohol Studies.

Finney, J., and R. Moos. 1991. "The Long-term Course of Treated Alcoholism, I: Mortality, Relapse and Remission Rates and Comparisons with Community Controls." *Journal of Studies on Alcohol* 52:44–54.

Finney, J. W., R. H. Moos, and C. R. Mewborn. 1980. "Posttreatment Experiences and Treatment Outcomes of Alcoholic Patients Six Months and Two Years after Hospitalization." *Journal of Counseling and Consulting Psychology* 48:17–29.

Frances, R. J., S. Timm, and S. Bucky. 1980. "Studies of Familial and Nonfamilial Alcoholism." *Archives of General Psychiatry* 37:564–566.

Frank, J. D. 1961. *Persuasion and Healing: A Comparative Study of Psychotherapy.* Baltimore: Johns Hopkins University Press.

Freud, S. 1920. "The Psychogenesis of a Case of Homosexuality in a Woman." In *The Complete Psychological Works of Sigmund Freud,* ed. J. Strachey, vol. 18. London: Hogarth Press, 1955.

Frezza, M., et al. 1990. "High Blood Alcohol Levels in Women." *New England Journal of Medicine* 322:95–99.

Gallant, D. M., M. A. Faulkner, and B. Stoy. 1968. "Enforced Clinic Treatment of Paroled Criminal Alcoholics—One Year Follow-up." *Quarterly Journal of Studies on Alcohol* 29:77–84.

Gelernter, J., D. Goldman, and N. Risch. 1993. "The A1 Allele at the D2 Dopamine

Receptor Gene and Alcoholism." *Journal of the American Medical Association* 269:1673–1677.

Gerard, D. L., and G. Saenger. 1966. *Out-Patient Treatment of Alcoholism: A Study of Outcome and Its Determinants.* Brookside Monograph no. 4. Toronto.

Gerard, D. L., G. Saenger, and R. Wile. 1962. "The Abstinent Alcoholic." *Archives of General Psychiatry* 6:83–95.

Gibbs, L., and J. Flanagan. 1977. "Prognostic Indicators of Alcoholism Treatment Outcome." *International Journal of Addictions* 12:1097–1141.

Gill, J. S., et al. 1986. "Stroke and Alcohol Consumption." *New England Journal of Medicine* 315:1041–1046.

Gitlow, S. E. 1973. "Alcoholism: A Disease." In *Alcoholism: Progress in Research and Treatment,* ed. P. B. Bourne and R. Fox. New York: Academic Press.

Glenn, S. W., and O. A. Parsons. 1989. "Alcohol Abuse and Familial Alcoholism: Psychosocial Correlates in Men and Women." *Journal of Studies on Alcohol* 50:116–127.

Glueck, S., and E. Glueck. 1950. *Unravelling Juvenile Delinquency.* New York: Commonwealth Fund.

——— 1968. *Delinquents and Nondelinquents in Perspective.* Cambridge, Mass.: Harvard University Press.

Glynn, R. J., et al. 1985. "Aging and Generational Effects on Drinking Behavior in Men: Results from the Normative Aging Study." *American Journal of Public Health* 75:1413–1419.

Gomberg, E. S. 1968. "Etiology of Alcoholism." *Journal of Consulting and Clinical Psychology* 32:18–20.

——— 1976. "The Female Alcoholic." In *Alcoholism,* ed. R. E. Tarter and A. A. Sugerman. Reading, Mass.: Addison-Wesley.

Gomberg, E. S. L. 1991. "Women and Alcohol: Psychosocial Aspects." In *Society, Culture and Drinking Patterns Reexamined,* ed. D. J. Pittman and C. R. Snyder, 263–284. New Brunswick, N.J.: Rutgers Center for Alcohol Studies.

Goodwin, D. W. 1973. "Alcohol in Suicide and Homicide." *Quarterly Journal of Studies on Alcohol* 34:144–156.

——— 1976. *Is Alcoholism Hereditary?* New York: Oxford University Press.

——— 1979. "Alcoholism and Heredity." *Archives of General Psychiatry* 36:57–61.

Goodwin, D. W., J. B. Crane, and S. B. Guze. 1971. "Felons Who Drink: An 8-year Follow-up." *Quarterly Journal of Studies on Alcohol* 32:136–147.

Goodwin, D. W., and C. K. Erickson. 1979. *Alcoholism and Affective Disorders.* New York: S. P. Medical and Scientific Books.

Goodwin, D., F. Schulsinger, and J. Knop. 1977. "Psychopathology in Adopted and Non-adopted Daughters of Alcoholics." *Archives of General Psychiatry* 34:1005–1009.

Goodwin, D. W., et al. 1969. "Why People Do Not Drink: A Study of Teetotalers." *Comprehensive Psychiatry* 10:209–214.

———— 1973. "Alcohol Problems in Adoptees Raised Apart from Biological Parents." *Archives of General Psychiatry* 28:238–243.

———— 1975. "Alcoholism and the Hyperactive Child Syndrome." *Journal of Nervous and Mental Disease* 160:349–353.

Gordis, E. 1976. "Editorial: What Is Alcoholism Research?" *Annals of Internal Medicine* 85:821–823.

Gordon, T., and J. T. Doyle. 1987. "Drinking and Mortality: The Albany Study." *American Journal of Epidemiology* 125: 263–270.

Gordon, T., and W. W. Kannel. 1983. "Drinking and Its Relation to Smoking, Blood Pressure, Blood Lipids and Uric Acid." *Archives of Internal Medicine* 143:1366–74.

Gorelick, D. A. 1989. "Serotonin Uptake Blockers and the Treatment of Alcoholism." *Alcoholism* 7:267–281.

Gottheil, E., et al. 1973. "Alcoholics' Patterns of Controlled Drinking." *American Journal of Psychiatry* 130:418–422.

Grant, I. 1987. "Alcohol and the Brain: Neuropsychological Correlates." *Journal of Consulting and Clinical Psychology* 3:310–324.

Greely, A., and W. C. McReady. 1980. *Ethnic Drinking Subcultures.* New York: Praeger.

Gruchow, H. W., et al. 1982. "Effects of Drinking Patterns on the Relationship between Alcohol and Coronary Occlusion." *Atherosclerosis* 43:393–401.

Guze, S. B., et al. 1963. "The Drinking History: A Comparison of Reports by Subjects and Their Relatives." *Quarterly Journal of Studies on Alcohol* 24:249–260.

———— 1986. "Alcoholism as a Medical Disorder." *Comprehensive Psychiatry* 27:501–510.

Haberman, P. W. 1966. "Childhood Symptoms in Children of Alcoholics and Comparison Group Parents." *Journal of Marriage and the Family* 28:152–154.

Haberman, P. W., and M. M. Baden. 1974. "Alcoholism and Violent Death." *Quarterly Journal of Studies on Alcohol* 35:221–231.

Haggard, H. W., and M. E. Jellinek. 1942. *Alcohol Explored.* New York: Doubleday.

Hagnell, O. 1966. *A Prospective Study of the Incidence of Mental Disorders.* New York: Humanities Press.

Hagnell, O., and L. Ojesjo. 1975. "A Prospective Study Concerning Mental Disorders of a Total Population Investigated in 1947, 1957, and 1972: The Lundy Study III (Preliminary Report)." *Acta Psychiatrica Scandinavica,* Supplement 263:1–11.

———— 1980. "Prevalence of Male Alcoholism in a Cohort Observed for Twenty-Five Years." *Scandinavian Journal of Social Medicine* 8:55–61.

Hagnell, O., and K. Tunving, 1972. "Prevalence and Nature of Alcoholism in a Total Population." *Social Psychiatry* 7:190–201.

Halikas, J. A. 1983. "Psychotropic Medication Used in the Treatment of Alcoholism." *Hospital and Community Psychiatry* 34:1035–1039.

Hall, R. C., and W. Malone. 1976. "Psychiatric Effects of Prolonged Asian Captivity: A Two Year Follow-up." *American Journal of Psychiatry* 133:786–790.

Hamburg, S. 1975. "Behavior Therapy in Alcoholism: A Critical Review of Broad-Spectrum Approaches." *Journal of Studies on Alcohol* 36:69–87.

Hampton, P. J. 1951. "A Psychometric Study of Drinkers." *Journal of Consulting Psychology* 15:501–504.

Harwood, H. J., D. M. Napolitano, P. L. Kristiansen, and J. J. Collins. 1984. "Economic Costs to Society of Alcohol and Drug Abuse and Mental Illness." Prepared for the Alcohol, Drug Abuse, and Mental Health Administration, RTI/2734/0001FR, Research Triangle Park, N.C.: Research Triangle Institute.

Hatsukami, D., and R. W. Pickens. 1982. "Posttreatment Depression in an Alcohol and Drug Abuse Population." *American Journal of Psychiatry* 139:1563–1566.

Haver, B. 1987. "Female Alcoholics. III. Patterns of Consumption 3–10 Years after Treatment." *Acta Psychiatrica Scandinavica* 75:397–404.

Heath, C. W. 1946. *What People Are.* Cambridge, Mass.: Harvard University Press.

Heath, D. B. 1975. "A Critical Review of Ethnographic Studies of Alcohol Use." In *Research Advances in Alcohol and Drug Problems,* vol. 2, ed. R. J. Gibbins et al. New York: Wiley.

Heather, N. 1987. "Misleading Confusion." *British Journal of Addiction* 82:253–255.

Heather, N., and I. Robinson. 1983. *Controlled Drinking.* 2nd ed. London: Methuen.

Helzer, J. E., and T. R. Pryzbeck. 1988. "The Co-occurrence of Alcoholism with Other Psychiatric Disorders in the General Population and Its Impact on Treatment." *Journal of Studies on Alcohol* 49:219–224.

Helzer, J. E., et al. 1985. "The Extent of Long-term Moderate Drinking among Alcoholics Discharged from Medical and Psychiatric Treatment Facilities." *New England Journal of Medicine* 312:1678–1685.

Henningfield, J. E., I. D. Chait, and R. R. Griffiths. 1984. "Effects of Ethanol on Cigarette Smoking by Volunteers without Histories of Alcoholism." *Psychopharmacology* 82:1–5.

Hesselbrock, M. N. 1981. "Women Alcoholics: A Comparison of the Natural History of Alcoholism between Men and Women." In *Implications for Research, Theory and Treatment,* ed. R. Myer et al. NIAAA Monograph Series. Washington: NIAAA.

Hesselbrock, V. M., M. N. Hesselbrock, and J. R. Stabenau. 1985. "Alcoholism in Men Patients Subtyped by Family History and Antisocial Personality." *Journal of Studies on Alcohol* 46:59–64.

Higley, J. D., et al. 1991. "Nonhuman Primate Model of Alcohol Abuse." *Proceedings of the National Academy of Sciences* 88:7261–7265.

Hill, M. J., and H. T. Blane. 1967. "Evaluation of Psychotherapy with Alcoholics: A Critical Review." *Quarterly Journal of Studies on Alcohol* 28:76–104.

Hodgson, R., H. Rankin, and T. Stockwell. 1979. "Alcohol Dependence and the Priming Effect." *Behavior Research and Therapy* 17:379–387.

Hodgson, R., T. Stockwell, H. Rankin, and G. Edwards. 1978. "Alcohol Dependence: The Concept, Its Utility and Measurement." *British Journal of Addiction* 73:339–342.

Hoffmann, H., R. G. Loper, and M. L. Kammeier. 1974. "Identifying Future Alcoholics with MMPI Alcohol Scales." *Quarterly Journal of Studies on Alcohol* 35:490–498.

Holder, H. D., and J. B. Hallen. 1986. "Impact of Alcoholism Treatment on Total Health Care Costs: A Six-year Study." *Advances in Alcohol and Substance Abuse* 6:1–16.

Holder, H. D., and R. H. Schachtman. 1987. "Estimating Health Care Savings Associated with Alcoholism Treatment." *Alcoholism: Clinical and Experimental Research* 11:66–73.

Hollingshead, A. B., and F. C. Redlich. 1958. *Social Class and Mental Illness*. New York: Wiley.

Hooton, E. 1945. *Young Man, You Are Normal*. New York: Putnam.

Hunt, G. J., and N. H. Azrin. 1973. "A Community Reinforcement Approach to Alcoholism." *Behavior Research and Therapy* 11:91–104.

Hutchings, B., and S. Mednick. 1975. "Registered Criminality in the Adoptive and Biological Parents of Registered Male Criminal Adoptees." In *Genetic Research in Psychiatry*, ed. R. R. Fieve, A. Brill, and D. Rosenthall. Baltimore: Johns Hopkins University Press.

Hyman, M. M. 1976. "Alcoholics 15 Years Later." *Annals of the New York Academy of Science* 273:613–623.

Imber, S., et al. 1976. "The Fate of the Untreated Alcoholic." *Journal of Nervous and Mental Disease* 162(4):238–247.

Institute of Medicine. 1980. *Alcoholism and Related Problems: Opportunities for Research*. Washington: National Academy of Sciences.

——— 1989. *Prevention and Treatment of Alcohol Problems: Research Opportunities*. Washington: National Academy Press.

Irwin, M., M. Schuckit, and T. Smith. 1991. "Clinical Importance of Age at Onset of Type 1 and Type 2 Primary Alcoholics." *Archives of General Psychiatry* 47:320–324.

Jackson, R., R. Scragg, and R. Beaglehole. 1991. "Alcohol Consumption and Risk of Coronary Heart Disease." *British Medical Journal* 303:211–216.

Jacob, T., et al. 1987. "The Alcoholic's Spouse, Children and Family Interaction." *Journal of Studies on Alcohol* 39:1231–1251.

Jacobson, G. R. 1976. *The Alcoholisms: Detection, Diagnosis and Assessment*. New York: Human Science Press.

Jacobson, R. 1986. "The Contribution of Sex and Drinking History to the CT Brain Scan Changes in Alcoholics." *Psychological Medicine* 16:547–559.

James, I. P. 1964. "Blood Alcohol Levels Following Successful Suicide." *Quarterly Journal of Studies on Alcohol* 27:23–29.

James, I. P., D. N. Scott-Orr, and D. H. Curnow. 1963. "Blood Alcohol Following Attempted Suicide." *Quarterly Journal of Studies on Alcohol* 24:14–22.

James, W. 1902. *The Varieties of Religious Experience*. London: Longmans Green.

Jellinek, E. M. 1952. "Phases of Alcohol Addiction." *Quarterly Journal of Studies on Alcohol* 13:673–684.

—— 1960. *The Disease Concept of Alcoholism.* New Haven: Hillhouse Press.

Jessor, R. 1987. "Problem-behavior Theory, Psychosocial Development and Adolescent Problem Drinking." *British Journal of Addiction* 82:331–342.

Jessor, R., and S. L. Jessor. 1975. "Adolescent Development and the Onset of Drinking." *Journal of Studies on Alcohol* 36:27–51.

Johnson, B. 1992. "Psychoanalysis of a Man with Active Alcoholism." *Journal of Substance Abuse Treatment* 9:111–123.

Jones, K. R., and T. R. Vischi. 1979. "Impact of Alcohol, Drug Abuse and Mental Health Treatment on Medical Care Utilization." *Medical Care,* Supplement 17:1–81.

Jones, M. C. 1968. "Personality Correlates and Antecedents of Drinking Patterns in Adult Males." *Journal of Consulting and Clinical Psychology* 32:2–12.

—— 1971. "Personality Antecedents and Correlates of Drinking Patterns in Women." *Journal of Consulting and Clinical Psychology* 36:61–69.

—— 1981. "Midlife Drinking Patterns: Correlates and Antecedents." In *Present and Past in Middle Life,* ed. D. Eichorn, J. Clausen, N. Haan, M. Honzik, and P. Mussen. New York: Academic Press.

Jushner, M. G., K. J. Sher, and B. D. Beitman. 1990. "The Relation between Alcohol Problems and Anxiety Disorders." *American Journal of Psychiatry* 147:685–695.

Kagle, J. 1987. "Women Who Drink: Changing Ages, Changing Realities." *Journal of Social Work Education* 3:21–28.

Kain, J. H. 1828. "On Intemperance Considered as a Disease and Susceptible of Cure." *American Journal of Medical Science* 2:291–295.

Kammeier, M. L., H. Hoffmann, and R. G. Loper. 1973. "Personality Characteristics of Alcoholics as College Freshmen and at Time of Treatment." *Quarterly Journal of Studies on Alcohol* 34:390–399.

Kamner, M. E., and W. G. DuPong. 1969. "Alcohol Problems: Study by Industrial Medical Department." *New York State Medical Journal* 69:3105–3110.

Kane, G. P. 1981. *Inner-City Alcoholism.* New York: Human Science Press.

Kaprio, J., et al. 1987. "Genetic Influences on Use and Abuse of Alcohol: A Study of 5,638 Adult Finnish Twin Brothers." *Alcohol: Clinical and Experimental Research* 11:349–356.

Keenan, R. M., et al. 1990. "The Relationship between Chronic Ethanol Exposure and Cigarette Smoking in the Laboratory and the Natural Environment." *Psychopharmacology* 100:77–83.

Keller, M. 1972. "On the Loss-of-Control Phenomenon in Alcoholism." *British Journal of Addiction* 67:153–166.

—— 1975. "Problems of Epidemiology in Alcohol Problems." *Journal of Studies on Alcohol* 36:1442–1451.

———— 1976. "The Disease Concept of Alcoholism Revisited." *Journal of Studies on Alcohol* 37:1694–1717.

Kendell, R. E. 1965. "Normal Drinking by Former Alcohol Addicts." *Quarterly Journal of Studies on Alcohol* 26:247–257.

Kendell, R. E., and M. C. Staton. 1966. "The Fate of Untreated Alcoholics." *Quarterly Journal of Studies on Alcohol* 27:30–41.

Kendler, K. S., et al. 1993. "Alcoholism and Major Depression in Women." *Archives of General Psychiatry* 50:690–698.

Kessel, N., and G. Grossman. 1961. "Suicide in Alcoholics." *British Medical Journal* 2:1671–1672.

Kish, G. B., and H. T. Hermann. 1971. "The Fort Meade Alcohol Treatment Program: A Follow-up Study." *Quarterly Journal of Studies on Alcohol* 32:628–635.

Kissin, B. 1977. "Comments on Alcoholism: A Controlled Trial of 'Treatment' and 'Advice'." *Journal of Studies on Alcohol* 38:1804–1808.

Kissin, B., and H. Begleiter, eds. 1974. *Clinical Pathology.* The Biology of Alcoholism, vol. 3. New York: Plenum Press.

———— 1977. *Treatment and Rehabilitation of the Chronic Alcoholic.* The Biology of Alcoholism, vol. 5. New York: Plenum Press.

Kissin, B., S. M. Rosenblatt, and S. Machover. 1968. "Prognostic Factors in Alcoholism." *Psychiatric Research Report* 24:22–60.

Klatsky, A. L., M. A. Armstrong, and H. Kipp. 1990. "Correlates of Alcoholic Beverage Preference: Traits of Persons Who Choose Wine, Liquor or Beer." *British Journal of Addiction* 85:1279–1289.

Klatsky, A. L., G. D. Friedman, and M. A. Armstrong. 1986. "The Relationships between Alcoholic Beverage Use and Other Traits to Blood Pressure: A New Kaiser-Permanente Study." *Circulation* 73:628–636.

Klatsky, A. L., et al. 1977. "Alcohol Consumption and Blood Pressure." *New England Journal of Medicine* 296:1194–1200.

Knight, R. P. 1937. "The Dynamics and Treatment of Chronic Alcohol Addiction." *Bulletin of the Menninger Clinic* 1:233–250.

Knupfer, G. 1972. "Ex-Problem Drinkers." In *Life History Research in Psychopathology,* ed. M. Roff, L. N. Robins, and H. Pollack, vol. 2. Minneapolis: University of Minnesota Press.

Knupfer, G. 1989. "The Prevalance in Various Social Groups of Eight Different Drinking Patterns, from Abstaining to Frequent Drunkenness: Analysis of Ten U.S. Surveys Combined." *British Journal of Addiction* 85:1305–18.

Kohlberg, L., J. LaCrosse, and D. Ricks. 1972. "The Predictability of Adult Mental Health from Childhood Behavior." In *Manual of Child Psychopathology,* ed. B. B. Wolman. New York: McGraw-Hill.

Kolb, L. C. 1973. *Modern Clinical Psychiatry.* Philadelphia: W. B. Saunders.

Krasner, N., et al. 1977. "Changing Pattern of Alcohol Liver Disease in Great Britain: Relation to Sex and Signs of Autoimmunity." *British Medical Journal* 1:1497–1500.

Kurtines, W. M., L. R. Ball, and G. H. Wood. 1978. "Personality Characteristics of Long-Term Recovered Alcoholics: A Comparative Analysis." *Journal of Consulting and Clinical Psychology* 46:971–977.

Lancet. 1977. "Editorial: W.H.O. and a New Perspective on Alcoholism." *Lancet* 1:1087–1088.

Lang, A. R., et al. 1975. "Effects of Alcohol on Aggression in Male Social Drinkers." *Journal of Abnormal Psychology* 84:508–518.

Längle, G., et al. 1993. "Ten Years After—The Post-treatment Course of Alcoholism." *European Psychiatry* 8:95–100.

Lau, H. 1975. "Cost of Alcoholic Beverages as a Determinant of Alcohol Consumption." In *Research Advances in Alcohol and Drug Problems*, vol. 2, ed. R. J. Gibbins et al. New York: Wiley.

Leach, B., and J. L. Norris. 1977. "Factors in the Development of Alcoholics Anonymous (AA)." In *Treatment and Rehabilitation of the Chronic Alcoholic*, ed. B. Kissin and H. Begleiter. New York: Plenum Press.

Ledermann, S. 1956. *Alcool, Alcoolisme, Alcoolisation. Donnés Scientifiques de Caractére Physiologique, Economique et Social.* Travaux et Documents, Cahier no. 29. Paris: Institut National d'Etudes Démographique.

Leighton, D. C., et al. 1963. "Psychiatric Findings of the Stirling County Study." *American Journal of Psychiatry* 119:1021–1026.

Lemere, F. 1953. "What Happens to Alcoholics." *American Journal of Psychiatry* 109:674–676.

Levine, J., and E. Zigler. 1973. "The Essential-Reactive Distinction in Alcoholism." *Journal of Abnormal Psychology* 81:242–249.

Lichtman, S. W., et al. 1992. "Discrepancy between Self-reported and Actual Caloric Intake and Exercise in Obese Subjects." *New England Journal of Medicine* 327:1893–1898.

Lindström, L. 1992. *Managing Alcoholism.* Oxford: Oxford University Press.

Lipscomb, T. R., et al. 1980. "Effects of Tolerance on the Anxiety-Reducing Function of Alcohol." *Archives of General Psychiatry* 37:517–582.

Lisansky-Gomberg, E. S. 1968. "Etiology of Alcoholism." *Journal of Consulting and Clinical Psychology* 32:18–20.

Lithell, H., et al. 1987. "Alcohol Intemperance and Sudden Death." *British Medical Journal* 294:1456–1458.

Littrell, J. 1988. "The Swedish Studies of the Adopted Children of Alcoholics." *Journal of Studies on Alcohol* 49:491–499.

Logue, P. E., et al. 1978. "Effect of Alcohol Consumption on State Anxiety Changes in Male and Female Nonalcoholics." *American Journal of Psychiatry* 135:1079–1081.

Lolli, G. 1952. "The Use of Wine and Other Alcoholic Beverages by a Group of Italians and Americans of Italian Extraction." *Quarterly Journal of Studies on Alcohol* 13:27–49.

Longnecker, M. P., et al. 1988. "A Meta-analysis of Alcohol Consumption in Breast Cancer." *Journal of the American Medical Association* 260: 652–656.

Loosen, P. T., B. W. Dew, and A. J. Prange. 1990. "Long-term Predictors of Outcome in Abstinent Alcoholic Men." *American Journal of Psychiatry* 147:1662–1666.

Loper, R. G., M. L. Kammeier, and H. Hoffmann. 1973. "M.M.P.I. Characteristics of College Freshman Males Who Later Became Alcoholics." *Journal of Abnormal Psychology* 82:159–162.

Lovibond, S. H., and G. Caddy. 1970. "Discriminated Aversive Control in the Moderation of Alcoholics' Drinking Behavior." *Behavior Therapy* 1:437–444.

Luborsky, L. 1962. "Clinicians' Judgments of Mental Health." *Archives of General Psychiatry* 7:407–417.

Luborsky, L., and H. Bachrach. 1974. "Factors Influencing Clinicians' Judgments of Mental Health." *Archives of General Psychiatry* 31:292–299.

Ludwig, A. M., and W. H. Lyle, Jr. 1964. "The Experimental Production of Narcotic Drug Effects and Withdrawal Symptoms through Hypnosis." *International Journal of Clinical Experimental Hypnosis* 12:1–17.

Ludwig, A. M., and A. Wikler. 1974. "Craving and Relapse to Drink." *Quarterly Journal of Studies on Alcohol* 35:108–130.

Ludwig, A. M., A. Wikler, and L. H. Stark. 1974. "The First Drink—Psychobiological Aspects of Craving." *Archives of General Psychiatry* 30:539–547.

Ludwig, A. M., et al. 1969. "A Clinical Study of LSD Treatment in Alcoholism." *American Journal of Psychiatry* 126:59–69.

Lundquist, G. A. R. 1973. "Alcohol Dependence." *Acta Psychiatrica Scandinavica* 49:332–340.

Mack, J. 1981. "Alcoholism, AA and the Governance of the Self." In *Dynamic Approaches to the Understanding and Treatment of Alcoholism,* ed. M. H. Bean and N. E. Zinberg. New York: Free Press.

Makela, K. 1991. "Social and Cultural Preconditions of Alcoholics Anonymous (AA) and Factors Associated with the Strength of AA." *British Journal of Addiction* 86:1405–1413.

Maltzmann, I. 1989. "A Reply to Cook, 'Craftsman versus Professional: Analysis of the Controlled Drinking Controversy'." *Journal of Studies on Alcohol* 50:466–472.

Manji, H. K. 1992. "G Proteins: Implications for Psychiatry." *American Journal of Psychiatry* 149:746–760.

Mann, M. 1968. *New Primer on Alcoholism.* 2nd ed. New York: Holt, Rinehart and Winston.

Mann, R. E., et al. 1991. "Reductions in Cirrhosis Deaths in the United States: Associations with Per Capita Consumption and AA Membership." *Journal of Studies on Alcohol* 52:361–365.

Margulies, R. Z., R. C. Kessler, and D. B. Kandel. 1977. "A Longitudinal Study of Onset of Drinking among High School Students." *Journal of Studies on Alcohol* 38:897–912.

Marlatt, G. A., B. Demming, and J. B. Reid. 1973. "Loss of Control Drinking in Alcoholics: An Experimental Analogue." *Journal of Abnormal Psychology* 81:233–241.

Marlatt, G. A., and J. R. Gordon. 1985. *Relapse Prevention: Maintenance Strategies in the Treatment of Addictive Behaviors.* New York: Guilford Press.

Marlatt, G. A., C. F. Kosturn, and A. R. Lang. 1975. "Provocation to Anger and Opportunity for Retaliation as Determinants of Alcohol Consumption in Social Drinkers." *Journal of Abnormal Psychology* 84:652–659.

Marlatt, G. A., and D. J. Rohsenow. 1980. "Cognitive Processes in Alcohol Use: Expectancy and the Balanced Placebo Design." In *Advances in Substance Abuse: Behavioral and Biological Research,* ed. N. K. Marlow. Greenwich, Conn.: JAI Press.

Marmot, M., and E. Brunner. 1991. "Alcohol and Cardiovascular Disease: The Status of the U-shaped Curve." *British Medical Journal* 303:565–568.

Marmot, M. G., and S. L. Syme. 1976. "Acculturation and Coronary Heart Disease." *American Journal of Epidemiology* 104:225–247.

Marmot, M. G., et al. 1981. "Alcohol and Mortality: A U-shaped Curve." *Lancet* 1:580–583.

Marshall, E. J., G. Edwards, and C. Taylor. 1994. "Mortality in Men with Drinking Problems: A 20 Year Follow-up." *Addiction* 89.

Masserman, J. H., and K. S. Yum. 1946. "An Analysis of the Influence of Alcohol and Experimental Neuroses in Cats." *Psychosomatic Medicine* 8:36–52.

McCabe, R. J. R. 1986. "Alcohol-Dependent Individuals Sixteen Years On." *Alcohol and Alcoholism* 21:85–91.

McCance, C., and P. F. McCance. 1969. "Alcoholism in Northeast Scotland: Its Treatment and Outcome." *British Journal of Psychiatry* 115:189–198.

McClelland, D. C., W. N. Davis, and R. Kahn. 1972. *The Drinking Man.* New York: Free Press.

McCord, J. 1979. "Some Child-Rearing Antecedents of Criminal Behavior in Adult Men." *Journal of Personality and Social Psychology* 37:1477–1486.

McCord, W., and J. McCord. 1960. *Origins of Alcoholism.* Stanford: Stanford University Press.

McDonnell, R., and A. Maynard. 1985. "Estimation of Life Years Lost from Alcohol Related Premature Death." *Alcohol and Alcoholism* 20:435–443.

McGinnis, J. M., and W. H. Foege. 1993. "Actual Causes of Death in the United States." *Journal of the American Medical Association* 270:2207–2212.

McGoldrick, E. J., Jr. 1954. *The Management of the Mind.* Boston: Houghton Mifflin.

McGregor, R. R. 1986. "Alcohol and Immune Disease." *Journal of the American Medical Association* 256:1474–1478.

McLellan, A. T., G. E. Woody, and C. P. O'Brien. 1979. "Development of Psychiatric Illness in Drug Abusers: Possible Role of Drug Preferences." *New England Journal of Medicine* 301:1310–1314.

McLellan, A. T., et al. 1982. "Is Treatment for Substance Abuse Effective?" *Journal of the American Medical Association* 247:1423–1428.

McNamee, H. B., J. H. Mendelson, and N. K. Mello. 1968. "Experimental Analysis of Drinking Patterns of Alcoholics: Concurrent Psychiatric Observations." *American Journal of Psychiatry* 124:1063–1069.

Mello, N. K. 1972. "Behavioral Studies of Alcoholism." In *Physiology and Behavior,* ed. B. Kissin and H. Begleiter. The Biology of Alcoholism, vol. 2. New York: Plenum Press.

——— 1975. "A Semantic Aspect of Alcoholism." In *Biological and Behavioral Approaches to Drug Dependence,* ed. H. D. Capell and A. E. LeBlanc. Toronto: Addiction Research Foundation.

Mello, N. K., H. B. McNamee, and J. H. Mendelson. 1968. "Drinking Patterns of Chronic Alcoholics: Gambling and Motivations for Alcohol." *Psychiatric Research Reports* 24:83–118.

Mello, N. K., and J. H. Mendelson. 1970. "Experimentally Induced Intoxication in Alcoholics: A Comparison between Programmed and Spontaneous Drinking." *Journal of Pharmacology and Experimental Therapeutics* 173:101–116.

——— 1972. "Drinking Patterns during Work—Contingent and Noncontingent Alcohol Acquisitions." *Psychosomatic Medicine* 34:139–164.

——— 1978. "Alcohol and Human Behavior." In *Handbook of Psychopharmacology,* ed. L. L. Iversen, S. D. Iverson, and S. H. Snyder, vol. 12. New York: Plenum Press.

Mello, N. K., et al. 1980. "Effects of Alcohol and Marihuana on Tobacco Smoking." *Clinical Pharmacology and Therapeutics* 27: 202–209.

Mendelson, J. H. 1980. "Biologic Concomitants of Alcoholism." *New England Journal of Medicine* 283:24–32, 71–81.

Mendelson, J. H., and N. K. Mello. 1979. "Biologic Concomitants of Alcoholism." *New England Journal of Medicine* 301:912–921.

Menninger, K. A. 1938. *Man Against Himself.* New York: Harcourt Brace.

Merikangas, K. R., and C. S. Gelernter. 1990. "Comorbidity for Alcoholism and Depression." *Psychiatric Clinics of North America* 13:613–632.

Merikangas, K. R., et al. 1985. "Familial Transmission of Depression and Alcoholism." *Archives of General Psychiatry* 42:367–372.

Merry, J. 1966. "The 'Loss of Control' Myth." *Lancet* 1:1257–1258.

Meyer, R. E., and S. M. Mirin. 1979. *The Heroin Stimulus.* New York: Plenum Press.

Miller, W. R., and N. Heather, eds. 1986. *Treating Addictive Behaviors: Processes of Change.* New York: Plenum.

Miller, W. R., and R. K. Hester. 1986. "The Effectiveness of Alcoholism Treatment: What Research Reveals." In *Treating Addictive Behaviors: Processes of Change,* ed. W. R. Miller and N. Heather, pp. 121–174. New York: Plenum Press.

Miller, W. R., and R. F. Munoz. 1982. *How to Control Your Drinking.* Rev. ed. Albuquerque: University of New Mexico Press.

Miller, W. R., et al. 1992. "Long-term Follow-up of Behavioral Self-control Training." *Journal of Studies on Alcohol* 53:249–261.

Monks, J. P. 1957. *College Men at War.* Boston: American Academy of Arts and Sciences.

Moore, M. H., and D. R. Gerstein, eds. 1981. *Alcohol and Public Policy: Beyond the Shadow of Prohibition.* Washington: National Academy Press.

Moore, R. A., and F. Ramseur. 1960. "Effects of Psychotherapy in an Open Ward Hospital on Patients with Alcoholism." *Quarterly Journal of Studies on Alcohol* 21:233–252.

Moore, R. D., L. Mead, and T. A. Pearson. 1990. "Youthful Precursors of Alcohol Abuse in Physicians." *American Journal of Medicine* 88:332–336.

Moore, R. D., et al. 1989. "Prevalence, Detection and Treatment of Alcoholism in Hospitalized Patients." *Journal of the American Medical Association* 261:403–407.

Moos, R. H., B. Mehren, and B. S. Moos. 1978. "Evaluation of a Salvation Army Alcoholism Treatment Program." *Journal of Studies on Alcohol* 39:1267–1275.

Morrison, J., and M. Stewart. 1971. "A Family Study of the Hyperactive Child Syndrome." *Biological Psychiatry* 3:189–195.

Morrison, J. R. 1974. "Bipolar Affective Disorder and Alcoholism." *American Journal of Psychiatry* 131:1130–1133.

———— 1975. "The Family Histories of Manic Depressive Patients with and without Alcoholism." *Journal of Nervous and Mental Disease* 160:227–229.

Morse, R. M., and D. K. Flavin. 1992. "The Definition of Alcoholism." *Journal of the American Medical Association* 268:1012–1014.

Morse, W. H., and R. T. Kelleher. 1970. "Schedules as Fundamental Determinants of Behavior." In *The Theory of Reinforcement Schedules,* ed. W. N. Schoenfeld. New York: Appleton Century Crofts.

———— 1977. "Determinants of Reinforcement and Punishment." In *Operant Behavior,* vol. 2, ed. W. K. Hornig and J. E. R. Studdan. Englewood Cliffs, N.J.: Prentice-Hall.

Mottin, J. L. 1973. "Drug Induced Attenuation of Alcohol Consumption." *Quarterly Journal of Studies on Alcohol* 34:444–472.

Mulford, H. A., and D. E. Miller. 1960. "Drinking in Iowa, IV." *Quarterly Journal of Studies on Alcohol* 21:279–291.

Muuronen, A., et al. 1989. "Influence of Improved Drinking Habits on Brain Atrophy and Cognitive Performance in Alcoholic Patients: A Five-year Follow-up Study." *Alcoholism: Clinical and Experimental Research* 13:137–141.

Myerson, D. J., and J. Mayer. 1966. "Origins, Treatment and Destiny of Skid-Row Alcoholic Men." *New England Journal of Medicine* 275:419–424.

Nace, E. P. 1992. "Alcoholics Anonymous." In *Substance Abuse, A Comprehensive Textbook,* ed. J. H. Lowinson, P. Ruiz, and R. B. Millman, 486–495. Baltimore: Williams and Wilkins.

Naranjo, C. A., and E. M. Sellers. 1989. "Serotonin Uptake Inhibitors Attenuate Ethanol Intake in Problem Drinkers." In *Alcoholism,* ed. M. Galanter, vol. 7, 255–266. New York: Plenum Press.

Nathan, P. E., et al. 1970. "Behavioral Analysis of Chronic Alcoholism." *Archives of General Psychiatry* 22:419–430.

National Council on Alcoholism. 1972. "Criteria for the Diagnosis of Alcoholism." *Annals of Internal Medicine* 77:249–258.

———— 1976. "Definition of Alcoholism." *Annals of Internal Medicine* 85:764.

National Institute of Alcoholism and Alcohol Abuse. 1972. *The Alcoholism Report.* Washington: NIAAA.

Nerviano, V. J. 1977. "Common Personality Patterns among Alcoholic Males: A Multivariate Study." *Journal of Consulting and Clinical Psychology* 44:104–110.

Newborn, O. W., et al. 1981. "Behavioral-Chemical Treatment of Alcoholism: An Outcome Replication." *Journal of Studies on Alcohol* 42:806–810.

Nicholls, P., G. Edwards, and E. Kyle. 1974. "A Study of Alcoholics Admitted to Four Hospitals, II: General and Cause-Specific Mortality During Follow-up." *Quarterly Journal of Studies on Alcohol* 35:841–855.

Nie, N. H., et al. 1975. *SPSS Statistical Package for Social Sciences.* New York: McGraw-Hill.

Nordstrom, G., and M. Berglund. 1987a. "Type 1 and Type 2 Alcoholics (Cloninger and Bohman) Have Different Patterns of Successful Long-term Adjustment." *British Journal of Addiction* 82:761–769.

Nordstrom, G., and M. Berglund. 1987b. "A Prospective Study of Successful Long-term Adjustment in Alcohol Dependence: Social Drinking versus Abstinence." *Journal of Studies on Alcohol* 48:95–103.

Norton, R., et al. 1987. "Alcohol Consumption and the Risk of Alcohol Related Cirrhosis in Women." *British Medical Journal* 295:80–82.

Norvig, J., and B. Neilsen. 1956. "A Follow-up of 221 Alcoholic Addicts in Denmark." *Quarterly Journal of Studies on Alcohol* 17:633–642.

Noyes, R., et al. 1978. "The Familial Prevalence of Anxiety Neurosis." *Archives of General Psychiatry* 35:1057–1059.

O'Briant, R. G., and H. L. Lennard. 1973. *Recovery from Alcoholism.* Springfield, Ill.: C. C. Thomas.

O'Connor, A., and J. Daly. 1985. "Alcoholics: A Twenty Year Follow-up Study." *British Journal of Psychiatry* 146:645–647.

O'Connor, J. 1979. *The Young Drinkers.* London: Tavistock.

Ogborne, A. 1987. "A Note on the Characteristics of Alcohol Abusers with Controlled Drinking Aspirations." *Drug and Alcohol Dependence* 19:159–164.

Ojesjo, L. 1981. "Long-Term Outcome in Alcohol Abuse and Alcoholism among Males in the Lundby General Population, Sweden." *British Journal of Addiction* 76(4):391–400.

Orford, J. 1973. "A Comparison of Alcoholics Whose Drinking Is Totally Uncontrolled and Those Whose Drinking Is Mainly Controlled." *Behavior Research and Therapy* 11:565–576.

Orford, J., and G. Edwards. 1977. *Alcoholism.* New York: Oxford University Press.

Ornstein, S. I. 1980. "Control of Alcohol Consumption Through Price Increases." *Quarterly Journal of Studies on Alcohol* 41:807–818.

Paffenbarger, R. S., M. C. Thorne, and A. L. Wing. 1968. "Chronic Disease in Former College Students, VIII: Characteristics in Youth Predisposing to Hypertension in Later Years." *American Journal of Epidemiology* 88:25–36.

Paolino, T. J., and B. S. McCrady. 1977. *The Alcoholic Marriage: Alternative Perspectives.* New York: Grune and Stratton.

Paredes, A., et al. 1973. "Loss of Control in Alcoholism: An Investigation of the Hypothesis, with Experimental Findings." *Quarterly Journal of Studies on Alcohol* 34:1146–1161.

Park, P. 1962. "Drinking Experiences of 806 Finnish Alcoholics in Comparison with Similar Experiences of 192 English Alcoholics." *Acta Psychiatrica Scandinavica* 38:227–246.

———— 1973. "Developmental Ordering of Experiences in Alcoholism." *Quarterly Journal of Studies on Alcohol* 34:473–488.

Park, P., and P. C. Whitehead. 1973. "Developmental Sequence and Dimensions of Alcoholism." *Quarterly Journal of Studies on Alcohol* 34:887–904.

Pattison, E. M. 1968. "A Critique of Abstinence Criteria in the Treatment of Alcoholism." *International Journal of Social Psychiatry* 14:268–276.

Pattison, E. M., M. B. Sobell, and L. C. Sobell. 1977. *Emerging Concepts of Alcohol Dependence.* New York: Springer.

Pattison, E. M., et al. 1968. "Abstinence and Normal Drinking: An Assessment of Changes in Drinking Patterns in Alcoholics after Treatment." *Quarterly Journal of Studies on Alcohol* 29:610–633.

Pell, S., and C. A. D'Alonzo. 1973. "A Five Year Mortality Study of Alcoholics." *Journal of Occupational Medicine* 15:120–125.

Pell, S., and W. E. Fayerweather. 1985. "Trends in the Incidence of Myocardial Infarction and in Associated Mortality and Morbidity in a Large Employed Population." *New England Journal of Medicine* 312:1005–1011.

Pendery, M. L., I. M. Maltzman, and L. J. West. 1982. "Controlled Drinking by Alcoholics? New Findings and a Reevaluation of a Major Affirmative Study." *Science* 217:169–175.

Peterson, W. L., et al. 1977. "Healing of Duodenal Ulcer with an Antacid Regimen." *New England Journal of Medicine* 297:341–345.

Pettinati, H. M. 1981. "Carrier Foundation: Following Alcoholics for Four Years." *Carrier Foundation Letter* 70:1–4.

Pettinati, H. M., A. A. Sugerman, and H. S. Maurer. 1982. "Four-year MMPI Changes in Abstinent and Drinking Alcoholics." *Alcoholism: Clinical and Experimental Research* 6:487–494.

Pickens, R. W., et al. 1991. "Heterogeneity in the Inheritance of Alcoholism." *Archives of General Psychiatry* 48:19–28.

Pittman, D. J. 1967. *Alcoholism.* New York: Harper and Row.

Pittman, D. J., and C. R. Snyder. 1962. *Society, Culture and Drinking Patterns.* New York: Wiley.

Plant, M. L. 1979. *Drinking Careers.* London: Tavistock.

Pokorny, A. D., T. Kanas, and J. Overall. 1981. "Order of Appearance of Alcoholic Symptoms." *Alcoholism: Clinical and Experimental Research* 5:216–220.

Pokorny, A. D., B. A. Miller, and S. E. Cleveland. 1968. "Response to Treatment of Alcoholism: A Follow-up Study." *Quarterly Journal of Studies on Alcohol* 29:364–381.

Pokorny, A. D., et al. 1971. "Dimensions of Alcoholism." *Quarterly Journal of Studies on Alcohol* 32:669–705.

Polich, J. M., D. J. Armor, and H. B. Braiker. 1981. *The Course of Alcoholism.* New York: Wiley.

Powers, E., and H. Witmer. 1959. *An Experiment in the Prevention of Delinquency.* New York: Columbia University Press.

Rakkolainen, V., and S. Turunen. 1969. "From Unrestrained to Moderate Drinking." *Acta Psychiatrica Scandinavica.* 45:47–52.

Regan, T. 1990. "Alcohol and the Cardiovascular System." *Journal of the American Medical Association* 264:377–381.

Regier, D. A., et al. 1990. "Comorbidity of Mental Disorders with Alcohol and Other Drug Abuse." *Journal of the American Medical Association* 264:2511–2518.

Reich, T., G. Winokur, and J. Mullaney. 1975. "The Transmission of Alcoholism." In *Genetic Research in Psychiatry,* ed. R. R. Fieve, D. Rosenthal, and H. Brill. Baltimore: Johns Hopkins University Press.

Reiff, S., B. Griffith, A. B. Forsythe, and R. M. Sherman. 1981. "Utilization of Medical Services by Alcoholics Participating in a Health Maintenance Organization Outpatient Treatment Program: Three Year Follow-up." *Alcoholism: Clinical and Experimental Research* 5:559–562.

Reinert, R. E., and W. T. Bowen. 1968. "Social Drinking Following Treatment for Alcoholism." *Bulletin of Menninger Clinic* 32:280–290.

Robertson, I. et al. 1987. "Is Controlled Drinking Possible for the Person Who Has Been Severely Alcohol Dependent?" *British Journal of Addiction* 82:235–255.

Robins, L. N. 1966. *Deviant Children Grown Up: A Sociological and Psychiatric Study of Sociopathic Personality.* Baltimore: Williams and Wilkins.

———— 1974. *The Viet Nam Drug User Returns*. Special Action Office Monograph Series A, no. 2. Washington: U.S. Government Printing Office.

Robins, L. N., W. N. Bates, and P. O'Neal. 1962. "Adult Drinking Patterns of Former Problem Children." In *Society, Culture and Drinking Patterns*, ed. D. J. Pittman and C. R. Snyder. New York: Wiley.

Robins, L. N., and E. M. Smith. 1980. "Longitudinal Studies of Alcohol and Drug Problems: Sex Differences." In *Alcohol and Drug Problems in Women*, ed. O. J. Kalant. New York: Plenum Press.

Robins, L. N., et al. 1988. "Alcohol Disorders in the Community: A Report from the Epidemiological Catchment Area." In *Alcoholism: Origins and Outcome*, ed. R. M. Rose and J. Barrett, 15–29. New York: Raven Press.

Robinson, D. 1972. "The Alcohologist's Addiction: Some Implications of Having Lost Control Over the Disease Concept of Alcoholism." *Quarterly Journal of Studies on Alcohol* 33:1028–1042.

———— 1979. *Talking out of Alcoholism*. London: Croom Helm.

Robson, R. A., I. Paulus, and G. G. Clarke. 1965. "An Evaluation of the Effect of a Clinic Treatment Program on the Rehabilitation of Alcoholic Patients." *Quarterly Journal of Studies on Alcohol* 26:264–278.

Roe, A. 1944. "The Adult Adjustment of Children of Alcoholic Patients Raised in Foster Homes." *Quarterly Journal of Studies on Alcohol* 5:378–393.

Rohan, W. P. 1978. "Comment on 'The N.C.A. Criteria for the Diagnosis of Alcoholism; an Empirical Evaluation Study.'" *Journal of Studies on Alcohol* 39:211–218.

Roizen, R., D. Cahalan, and P. Shanks. 1978. "'Spontaneous Remission' among Untreated Problem Drinkers." In *Longitudinal Research on Drug Use*, ed. D. B. Kandel. New York: Wiley.

Roman, P. M., and H. M. Trice. 1968. "The Sick Role, Labelling Theory and the Deviant Drinker." *The International Journal of Social Psychiatry* 14:245–251.

Room, R. 1977. "Measurement and Distribution of Drinking Patterns and Problems in General Populations." In *Alcohol Related Disabilities*, ed. G. Edwards et al. WHO Offset Publication no. 32. Geneva: World Health Organization.

Room, R., and N. Day. 1974. "Alcohol Mortality." In *Alcohol and Health: New Knowledge*. Second Report to the U.S. Congress. Washington: U.S. Government Printing Office.

Room, R., and T. Greenfield. 1993. "Alcoholics Anonymous, Other 12-step Movements and Psychotherapy in the U.S. Populations." *Addiction* 88:555–562.

Rose, R. M. 1988. "Blaming the Patient." In *Alcoholism: Origins and Outcome*, ed. R. M. Rose and J. E. Barrett, 127–141. New York: Raven Press.

Rosenberg, C. M., et al. 1973. "The Hill House Fire: Response of Alcoholics to Crisis." *Quarterly Journal of Studies on Alcohol* 34:199–202.

Rutter, M. 1992. "Nature, Nurture and Psychopathology." In *Vulnerability and Resilience in Human Development*, ed. B. Tizard and R. Varma, 21–38: London: Jessica Kingsley.

Rychtarik, R. G., et al. 1987. "Five-to-six-year Follow-ups of Broad Spectrum Behavioral Treatment for Alcoholism: Effects of Training Controlled Drinking Skills. *Journal of Consulting and Clinical Psychology* 55:106–108.

Saffer, H., and M. Grossmann. 1985. "Effect of Beer Prices and Legal Drinking Ages on Youth Motor Vehicle Fatalities." New York: National Bureau of Economic Research.

Sanchez-Craig, M. 1984. *Therapist Manual for Secondary Prevention of Alcohol Problems: Procedures for Teaching Moderate Drinking and Abstinence.* Toronto: Addiction Research Foundation.

———— 1990. "Brief Didactic Treatment for Alcohol and Drug-related Problems: An Approach Based on Client Choice." *British Journal of Addiction* 85:169–177.

Sanchez-Craig, M., and H. Lei. 1986. "Disadvantages to Imposing the Goal of Abstinence on Problem Drinkers: An Empirical Study." *British Journal of Addiction* 81:505–512.

Sanchez-Craig, M., K. Spivak, and R. Davila. 1991. "Superior Outcome of Females over Males after Brief Treatment for the Reduction of Heavy Drinking: Replication and Report of Therapist Effects." *British Journal of Addiction* 86:867–876.

Sanchez-Craig, M., et al. 1984. "Random Assignment to Abstinence and Controlled Drinking: Evaluation of a Cognitive-Behavioral Program for Problem Drinkers." *Journal of Consulting and Clinical Psychology* 52:390–403.

Sartorius, N., A. Jablensky, and R. Shapiro. 1978. "Cross-Cultural Difference in the Short-Term Prognosis of Schizophrenic Psychoses." *Schizophrenia Bulletin* 4:102–113.

Saunders, J. B. 1987. "Alcohol: An Important Cause of Hypertension." *British Medical Journal* 294:1045–1046.

Schacter, S., et al. 1977. "Studies of the Interaction of Psychological and Pharmacological Determinants of Smoking." *Journal of Experimental Psychology: General* 106:3–40.

Schilder, P. 1941. "The Psychogenesis of Alcoholism." *Quarterly Journal of Studies on Alcohol* 2:277–292.

Schlesser, M. A., G. Winokur, and B. M. Sherman. 1980. "Hypothalamic-Pituitary-Adrenal Axis Activity in Depressive Illness." *Archives of General Psychiatry* 37:737–743.

Schmidt, C., L. Klee, and G. Ames. 1990. "Review and Analysis of Literature on Indicators of Women's Drinking Problems." *British Journal of Addiction* 85:179–192.

Schmidt, W. 1968. "The Prevalence of Alcoholism and Drug Addiction in Canada." *Addictions* 15:9–13.

Schmidt, W., and J. deLint. 1972. "Causes of Death of Alcoholics." *Quarterly Journal of Studies on Alcohol* 33:171–185.

Schmidt, W., and R. E. Popham. 1975. "Heavy Alcohol Consumption and Physical Health Problems: A Review of the Epidemiological Evidence." *Drug and Alcohol Dependence* 1:27–50.

———— 1978. "The Single Distribution Theory of Alcohol Consumption." *Quarterly Journal of Studies on Alcohol* 39:400–419.

Schnall, C., and J. S. Weiner. 1958. "Clinical Evaluation of Blood Pressure in Alcoholics." *Quarterly Journal of Social Psychiatry* 19:432–446.

Schuckit, M. 1973. "Alcoholism and Sociopathy—Diagnostic Confusion." *Quarterly Journal of Studies on Alcohol* 34:157–164.

Schuckit, M. A. 1985. "A One-year Follow-up of Men Alcoholics Given Disulfiram." *Journal of Studies on Alcohol* 46:191–195.

———— 1986. "Genetic and Clinical Implications of Alcoholism and Affective Disorder." *American Journal of Psychiatry* 143:140–147.

———— 1992. "Advances to Understanding the Vulnerability to Alcoholism." In *Addictive States,* ed. C. P. O'Brien and J. H. Jaffe. New York: Raven Press.

———— 1994. "A Clinical Model of Genetic Influences in Alcohol Dependence." *American Journal of Psychiatry* 151:184–189.

Schuckit, M. A., D. W. Goodwin, and G. Winokur. 1972. "A Half-Sibling Study of Alcoholism." *American Journal of Psychiatry* 128:1132–1136.

Schuckit, M. A., and R. Irwin. 1989. "An Analysis of the Clinical Relevance of Type 1 and Type 2 Alcoholics." *British Journal of Addiction* 84:869–876.

Schuckit, M. A., R. Irwin, and H. I. M. Mahler. 1990. "Tridimensional Personality Questionnaire Scores of Sons of Alcoholic and Nonalcoholic Fathers." *American Journal of Psychiatry* 147:481–487.

Schuckit, M. A., et al. 1969. "Alcoholism, I: Two Types of Alcoholism in Women." *Archives of Environmental Health* 18:301–306.

Schulsinger, F. 1972. "Psychopathy: Heredity and Environment." *International Journal of Mental Health* 1:190–206.

Searles, J. S. 1988. "The Role of Genetics in the Pathogenesis of Alcoholism." *Journal of Abnormal Psychology* 97:153–167.

Seeley, J. 1959. "The W.H.O. Definition of Alcoholism." *Quarterly Journal of Studies on Alcohol* 20:352–356.

Seixas, R. 1978. "Racial Difference in Alcohol Metabolism: Introduction." *Alcoholism: Clinical and Experimental Research* 2:59.

Seligman, M. E. P. 1975. *Helplessness: On Depression, Development, and Death.* San Francisco: W. H. Freeman.

Selzer, M. L. 1971. "The Michigan Alcoholism Screening Test: The Quest for a New Diagnostic Instrument." *American Journal of Psychiatry* 127:1653–1658.

———— 1980. "Alcoholism and Alcoholic Psychoses." In *Comprehensive Textbook of Psychiatry,* ed. H. I. Kaplan, A. M. Freedman, and B. J. Sadock. Baltimore: Williams and Wilkins.

Selzer, M. L., and W. H. Holloway. 1957. "A Follow-up of Alcoholics Committed to a State Hospital." *Quarterly Journal of Studies on Alcohol* 18:98–120.

Shadel, C. A. 1944. "Aversion Treatment of Alcohol Addiction." *Quarterly Journal of Studies on Alcohol* 5:216–228.

Shadwell, A. 1902. *Drink, Temperance and Legislation.* London: Longmans Green.

Shaper, A. G. 1990. "Alcohol and Mortality: A Review of Prospective Studies." *British Journal of Addiction* 85: 854–857.

Shepard, E. A. 1967. "Alcohol and Drug Dependence Division, State of Connecticut." In *The Treatment of Alcoholism: A Study of Programs and Problems,* ed. R. M. Glascote et al. Washington: Joint Information Service.

Sherfey, M. J. 1955. "Psychopathology and Character Structures in Chronic Alcoholism." In *Etiology of Chronic Alcoholism,* ed. O. Diethelm. Springfield, Ill.: C. C. Thomas.

Simmel, E. 1948. "Alcoholism and Addiction." *Psychoanalytic Quarterly* 17:6–31.

Sledge, W. H., J. A. Boydstun, and A. J. Rabe. 1980. "Self Concept Changes Related to War Captivity." *Archives of General Psychiatry* 37:430–433.

Smith, E. M., C. R. Cloninger, and S. Bradford. 1983. "Predictors of Mortality in Alcoholic Women: A Prospective Follow-up Study." *Alcoholism: Clinical and Experimental Research* 7:237–243.

Smith, H. 1955. *The Kidney.* New York: Oxford University Press.

Smith, P. F., et al. 1990. "A Comparison of Alcohol Sales Data with Survey Data on Self-reported Alcohol Use in 21 States." *American Journal of Public Health* 80:309–312.

Smith, R. 1981. "Alcohol and Alcoholism." *British Medical Journal* 283:835–838, 895–899, 972–975.

Smith, S. S., et al. 1992. "Genetic Vulnerability to Drug Abuse." *Archives of General Psychiatry* 49:723–727.

Sobell, L. C., and M. B. Sobell. 1975. "Outpatient Alcoholics Give Valid Self-Reports." *Journal of Nervous and Mental Disease* 16:32–42.

Sobell, M. B., and L. C. Sobell. 1973. "Alcoholics Treated by Individualized Behavior Therapy: One Year Treatment Outcome." *Behavior Research and Therapy* 11:599–618.

———— 1976. "Second Year Treatment Outcome of Alcoholics Treated by Individualized Behavior Therapy: Results." *Behavior Research and Therapy* 14:195–215.

———— 1978a. *Behavioral Treatment of Alcohol Problems.* New York: Plenum Press.

———— 1978b. "Evaluating the External Validity of Ewing and Rouse." *British Journal of Addiction* 73:343–345.

———— 1987. "Stalking White Elephants." *British Journal of Addiction* 82:245–247.

Special Committee of Royal College Psychiatrists. 1979. *Alcohol and Alcoholism.* London: Tavistock.

Spence, J. D., W. J. Sibbard, and R. D. Cape. 1978. "Pseudohypertension in the Elderly." *Clinical Science and Molecular Medicine* 55:3995–4025.

Srole, L., et al. 1962. *Mental Health in the Metropolis: The Midtown Manhattan Study.* New York: McGraw-Hill.

Stall, R., and P. Biernacki. 1986. "Spontaneous Remission from the Problematic Use of Substances: An Inductive Model Derived from a Comparative Analysis of the

Alcohol, Opiate, Tobacco and Food/Obesity Literatures." *International Journal of Addictions* 21:1–23.

Stampfer, J. J., et al. 1988. "A Prospective Study of Moderate Alcohol Consumption and the Risk of Coronary Disease and Stroke in Women." *New England Journal of Medicine* 319:267–273.

Stein, L. I., J. R. Newton, and R. S. Bowman. 1975. "Duration of Hospitalization for Alcoholism." *Archives of General Psychiatry* 32:247–253.

Stinson, D. J., et al. 1979. "Systems of Care and Treatment Outcomes for Alcoholic Patients." *Archives of General Psychiatry* 36:535–539.

Stinson, F. S., and S. F. DeBakey. 1992. "Alcohol-related Mortality in the United States, 1979–1988." *British Journal of Addiction* 87:777–783.

Stivers, R. 1976. *A Hair of the Dog.* University Park: Pennsylvania State University Press.

Stockwell, T. 1986. "Cracking an Old Chestnut: Is Controlled Drinking Possible for the Person Who Has Been Severely Alcohol Dependent?" *British Journal of Addiction* 81:455–456.

Straus, R. 1974. *Escape from Custody.* New York: Harper and Row.

Straus, R., and S. D. Bacon. 1951. "A Study of Occupational Integration of 2023 Male Clinic Patients." *Quarterly Journal of Studies on Alcohol* 12:231–260.

Sugerman, A. A., D. Reilly, and R. S. Albahary. 1965. "Social Competence and the Essential Reactive Distinction in Alcoholism." *Archives of General Psychiatry* 12:552–556.

Sundby, P. 1967. *Alcoholism and Mortality.* Oslo: Universitets Forlaget.

Svanum, S., and W. G. McAdoo. 1991. "Parental Alcoholism: An Examination of Male and Female Alcoholics in Treatment." *Journal of Studies on Alcohol* 52:127–132.

Syme, L. 1957. "Personality Characteristics and the Alcoholic." *Quarterly Journal of Studies on Alcohol* 18:288–301.

Szasz, T. S. 1972. "Bad Habits Are Not Diseases: A Refutation of the Claim that Alcoholism Is a Disease." *Lancet* 2:83–84.

Tabakoff, B., et al. 1988. "Differences in Platelet Enzyme Activity between Alcoholics and Nonalcoholics." *New England Journal of Medicine* 318:134–139.

Tahka, V. 1966. *The Alcoholic Personality.* Helsinki: Finnish Foundation for Alcohol Studies.

Tamerin, J. S., and J. H. Mendelson. 1969. "The Psychodynamics of Chronic Inebriation: Observation of Alcoholics During the Process of Drinking in an Experimental Group Setting." *American Journal of Psychiatry* 125:886–899.

Tamerin, J. S., S. Weiner, and J. H. Mendelson. 1970. "Alcoholics' Expectancies and Recall of Experiences During Intoxication." *American Journal of Psychiatry* 126:1697–1704.

Tarter, R. E. 1981. "Minimal Brain Dysfunction as an Etiological Predisposition to Alcoholism." In *Evaluation of the Alcoholic: Implications for Research, Theory and Treatment,* ed. R. E. Meyer et al. NIAAA Monograph Series. Washington: NIAAA.

Tarter, R. E., et al. 1977. "Differentiation of Alcoholics." *Archives of General Psychiatry* 34:761–768.

Taylor, C., et al. 1985. "Patterns of Outcome: Drinking Histories over Ten Years among a Group of Alcoholics." *British Journal of Addiction* 80:45–50.

Taylor, J. R., J. E. Helzer, and L. N. Robins. 1986. "Moderate Drinking in Ex-alcoholics: Recent Studies." *Journal of Studies on Alcohol* 47:115–121.

Temple, M. T., and E. V. Leino. 1989. "Long-term Outcomes of Drinking: A 20-year Longitudinal Study of Men." *British Journal of Addiction* 84(8):889–899.

Terman, L. M., and M. H. Oden. 1959. *The Gifted Group at Midlife.* Stanford: Stanford University Press.

Terris, M. A. 1967. "Epidemiology of Cirrhosis of the Liver: National Mortality Data." *American Journal of Public Health* 57:2076–2088.

Thomas, C. B., and R. L. Greenstreet. 1973. "Psychobiological Characteristics in Youth as Predictors of Five Disease States: Suicide, Mental Illness, Hypertension, Coronary Heart Disease and Tumor." *Johns Hopkins Medical Journal* 132:16–43.

Thomas, C. B., P. B. Santora, and J. W. Shaffer. 1980. "Health of Physicians in Midlife in Relation to Use of Alcohol: A Prospective Study of a Cohort of Former Medical Students." *Johns Hopkins Medical Journal* 146:1–10.

Thorpe, J. J., and J. T. Perret. 1959. "Problem Drinking: A Follow-up Study." *Archives of Industrial Health* 19:24–32.

Thurstin, A., A. Alfano, and M. Sherer. 1986. "Pretreatment MMPI Profiles of AA Members and Nonmembers." *Journal of Studies on Alcohol* 47:468–471.

Tobin, J., W. Delaney, and W. Doyle. 1993. "The Controlled Drinking Controversy." *Irish Journal of Psychological Medicine* 10:121–123.

Todd, J. E. 1882. *Drunkenness a Vice, Not a Disease.* Hartford, Conn.: Case, Lockwood and Brainard.

Tomosovic, M. 1974. "'Binge' and Continuous Drinkers." *Quarterly Journal of Studies on Alcohol* 35:558–564.

Trice, H. M., and J. R. Wahl. 1958. "A Rank Order Analysis of the Symptoms of Alcoholism." *Quarterly Journal of Studies on Alcohol* 19:636–648.

Trimpey, J. 1989. *Rational Recovery from Alcoholism: The Small Book.* New York, Delacorte.

Trotter, T. 1804. *Drunkenness and Its Effects on the Human Body.* London.

Tuchfeld, B. 1981. "Spontaneous Remission in Alcoholics: Empirical Observations and Theoretical Implications." *Journal of Studies on Alcohol* 42(7):626–641.

Tyndel, M. 1974. "Psychiatric Study of One Thousand Alcoholic Patients." *Canadian Psychiatric Association Journal* 19:21–24.

Ullman, A. D. 1953. "The First Drinking Experience of Addictive and of Normal Drinkers." *Quarterly Journal of Studies on Alcohol* 14:181–191.

Unterberger, H., and L. M. DiCicco. 1973. "Planning Alcoholism Services." *Contemporary Drug Problems* (Winter):697–716.

Utne, H. E., et al. 1977. "Alcohol Elimination Rates in Adoptees With and Without Alcoholic Parents." *Quarterly Journal of Studies on Alcohol* 38:1219–1223.

Vaillant, G. E. 1962. "Tuberculosis: An Historical Analogy of Schizophrenia." *Psychosomatic Medicine* 24:225–233.

——— 1966. "A 12-Year Follow-up of New York Addicts, IV: Some Characteristics and Determinants of Abstinence." *American Journal of Psychiatry* 123:573–584.

——— 1974. "Natural History of Male Psychological Health, II: Some Antecedents of Healthy Adult Adjustment." *Archives of General Psychiatry* 31:15–22.

——— 1977. *Adaptation to Life.* Boston: Little, Brown.

——— 1980a. "Natural History of Male Psychological Health, VIII: Antecedents of Alcoholism and 'Orality.'" *American Journal of Psychiatry* 137:181–186.

——— 1980b. "The Doctor's Dilemma." In *Alcoholism, Treatment and Transition,* ed. G. E. Edwards and M. Grant. London: Croom Helm.

——— 1983. "Natural History of Male Alcoholism, V: Is Alcoholism the Cart or the Horse to Sociopathy?" *British Journal of Addiction* 78:317–326.

——— 1988. "What Can Long-term Follow-up Teach Us about Relapse and Prevention of Relapse in Addiction?" *British Journal of Addiction* 83:1147–1157.

——— 1993. *The Wisdom of the Ego.* Cambridge, Mass: Harvard University Press.

Vaillant, G. E., and E. S. Milofsky. 1980. "Natural History of Male Psychological Health, IX: Empirical Evidence for Erikson's Model of the Life Cycle." *American Journal of Psychiatry* 137:1348–1359.

——— 1982. "Natural History of Male Alcoholism, IV: Paths to Recovery." *Archives of General Psychiatry* 39:127–133.

Vaillant, G. E., and C. O. Vaillant. 1981. "Natural History of Male Psychological Health, X: Work as a Predictor of Positive Mental Health." *American Journal of Psychiatry* 138:1433–1440.

Vaillant, G. E., et al. 1983. "Prospective Study of Alcoholism Treatment: Eight-year Follow-up." *American Journal of Medicine* 75:455–463.

——— 1991. "A Prospective Study of the Effects of Cigarette Smoking and Alcohol Abuse on Mortality." *Journal of General Internal Medicine* 6:299–304.

Vallance, M. 1965. "A Two-Year Follow-up Study of Patients Admitted to the Psychiatric Department of a General Hospital." *British Journal of Psychiatry* 111:348–356.

Vanclay, F. M., and B. Raphael. 1990. "Type 1 and Type 2 Alcoholics: Schuckit and Irwin's Negative Findings." *British Journal of Addiction* 85:683–684.

van Dijk, W. K., and A. van Dijk-Koffeman. 1973. "A Follow-up Study of 211 Treated Male Alcoholic Addicts." *British Journal of Addiction* 68:3–24.

Vesell, E. S., J. F. Page, and G. T. Passananti. 1971. "Genetic and Environmental Factors Affecting Ethanol Metabolism in Man." *Clinical Pharmacology and Therapeutics* 12:192–201.

Viamontes, J. A. 1972. "Review of Drug Effectiveness in the Treatment of Alcoholism." *American Journal of Psychiatry* 128:1570–1571.

Voegtlin, W. L., and W. R. Broz. 1949. "The Conditioned Reflex Treatment of Chronic Alcoholism, X: An Analysis of 3125 Admissions over a Period of Ten and a Half Years." *Annals of Internal Medicine* 30:580–597.

Vogler, R. E., T. A. Weissbach, and J. V. Compton. 1977. "Learning Techniques for Alcohol Abuse." *Behavior Research Therapy* 15:31–38.

Volpicelli, J. R., et al. 1992. "Naltrexone in the Treatment of Alcohol Dependence." *Archives of General Psychiatry* 49: 876–880.

von Knorring, A. L., et al. 1985. "Platelet MAO Activity Is a Biological Marker in Subgroups of Alcoholism." *Acta Psychiatrica Scandinavica* 72:51–58.

———— 1987. "Personality Traits in Subtypes of Alcoholics." *Journal of Studies on Alcohol* 46:388–391.

Wallack, L. 1992. "The Alcohol Industry Is Not Your Friend." *British Journal of Addiction* 87:1109–1111.

Wallerstein, R. S. 1956. "Comparative Study of Treatment Methods for Chronic Alcoholism: The Alcoholism Research Project at Winter V.A. Hospital." *American Journal of Psychiatry* 113:228–233.

Walsh, D. C., et al. 1991. "A Randomized Trial of Treatment Options for Alcohol-abusing Workers." *New England Journal of Medicine* 325:775–782.

Wanberg, K. W., and J. C. Horn. 1970. "Alcoholism Symptom Patterns for Men and Women: A Comparative Study." *Quarterly Journal of Studies on Alcohol* 31:40–61.

Weissman, M. M., et al. 1984. "Psychiatric Disorders in the Relatives of Probands with Affective Disorders." *Archives of General Psychiatry* 41:13–21.

Westermeyer, J., and E. Peake. 1983. "A Ten-year Follow-up of Alcoholic Native Americans in Minnesota." *American Journal of Psychiatry* 140:189–194.

Whitehead, W. E., et al. 1977. "Anxiety and Anger in Hypertension." *Journal of Psychosomatic Research* 21:383–389.

Willems, P. J. A., F. J. J. Letmendia, and F. Arroyave. 1973. "A Two-Year Follow-up Study Comparing Short- with Long-stay In-patient Treatment of Alcoholics." *British Journal of Psychiatry* 122:637–648.

Williams, H. L., and O. H. Rundell. 1981. "Altered Sleep Physiology in Chronic Alcoholics: Reversal with Abstinence." *Alcoholism: Clinical and Experimental Research* 5:318–325.

Wilsnack, R. W., and R. Cheloha. 1987. "Women's Roles and Problem Drinking across the Life Span." *Social Problems* 34:231–248.

Wilsnack, R. W., S. C. Wilsnack, and A. D. Klassen. 1984. "Women's Drinking and Drinking Problems: Patterns from a 1981 National Survey." *American Journal of Public Health* 74:1231–1238.

Wilsnack, S. C. 1979. *The Needs of the Female Drinker: Dependency, Power, or What?* National Institute on Alcohol Abuse and Alcoholism. Washington: U.S. Government Printing Office.

Wilsnack, S. C., and L. J. Beckman, eds. 1989. *Alcohol Problems in Women.* New York, Guilford Press.

Wilsnack, S. C., et al. 1991. "Predicting Onset and Chronicity of Women's Problem Drinking: A Five Year Longitudinal Analysis." *American Journal of Public Health* 81:305–318.

Wilson, G. J., and D. M. Lawson. 1976. "Expectancies, Alcohol, and Sexual Arousal in Male Social Drinkers." *Journal of Abnormal Psychology* 85:587–594.

Winokur, G., D. J. Clayton, and T. Reich. 1969. *Manic Depressive Illness.* St. Louis: C. V. Mosby.

Winokur, G., J. Rimmer, and T. Reich. 1971. "Alcoholism IV: Is There More than One Type of Alcoholism?" *British Journal of Psychiatry* 118:525–531.

Wolff, P. H. 1972. "Ethnic Differences in Alcohol Sensitivity." *Science* 175:449–450.

———— 1973. "Vasomotor Sensitivity to Alcohol in Diverse Mongoloid Populations." *American Journal of Human Genetics* 25:193–199.

Wood, D. R., et al. 1976. "Diagnosis and Treatment of Minimal Brain Dysfunction in Adults." *Archives of General Psychiatry* 33:1453–1460.

Woodruff, R. A., et al. 1973. "Alcoholism and Depression." *Archives of General Psychiatry* 28:97–100.

World Health Organization. In press. *Mental Disorders: Glossary and Guide to Their Classification in Accordance with the Tenth Revision of the International Classification of Diseases.* Geneva: World Health Organization.

Young, M., B. Bernard, and G. Wallis. 1963. "The Mortality of Widowers." *Lancet* 2:454–456.

Zook, C. J., and F. D. Moore. 1980. "High Cost Users of Medical Care." *New England Journal of Medicine* 302:996–1002.

Zucker, R. A., and E. S. L. Gomberg. 1986. "Etiology of Alcoholism Reconsidered." *American Psychology* 41:783–793.

Index

AA. *See* Alcoholics Anonymous

Abstinence: as goal of treatment, 3, 8, 45, 148, 231, 278, 279, 300, 303; spontaneous, 5, 13, 111, 124, 142, 178, 199, 223, 246, 252, 371; and social recovery, 45; and treatment of depression, 85; and health, 134, 141–142, 242, 276–277; and mortality, 139, 152, 204, 208, 209; definitions of, 149, 162, 170, 231, 232; revisited, 233–235, 246–254, 294, 383–384; and relapse, 234-235; and clinic treatment, 235, 236; etiology of, 235–246; and nontreatment factors, 241; and new love relationships, 244, 250; consequences of, 269–277, 382–383; trial, 387

Abuse, alcohol: consequences of, 1, 52; definition of, 4, 26, 27–28, 29, 32, 45, 50, 127, 131, 150, 337; predictors of, 5–8, 67, 101–102, 127, 380–382; cultural factors in, 6, 114, 115, 118, 319; and depression, 13, 77, 80–85, 99; and the heart, 13, 201, 206; and alcohol consumption, 23–24; frequency of, 25, 26, 36; lifetime pattern of, 28, 32, 38, 66, 131–132; as unitary disorder, 36–37, 43, 46, 86, 100, 163, 167, 175; familial, 37, 44, 45, 52–53, 54, 59, 64, 65, 67, 68–69, 73, 75, 85, 86, 96–97, 99, 326–327; symptoms of, 40–45, 282;

cultural factors in, 59–64; familial *vs.* acquired, 69; age of onset of, 70–71, 90, 101, 103, 158, 182, 183–184, 218–219; "secondary," 83, 91–92; and social policy, 112–113; and alcoholism, 120; long-term effect of, 121; gender differences in, 122–124; decline in, 162; and loss of control, 163–164, 176, 223, 279; natural history *vs.* career in, 178; severity of, 283–284; cost of, 389

Accidents, 1, 140, 194, 201, 291; death rates for, 124, 203, 205. *See also* Traffic fatalities

Addiction, alcohol. *See* Dependence, alcohol

Addiction Research Foundation (Toronto), 118, 138, 302–303, 387

Aggression, 48, 77, 214, 225

Al-Anon, 347, 359, 371, 372, 373

Alateen, 373

Alameda County, California, Study, 138

Albany Study, 140

Alcohol: price of, 64, 112, 114, 119, 389n; use of, 109, 113, 150, 158, 160, 183, 193, 236, 378; in Moslem countries, 111; cost of, 200; production of, 200; craving for, 221, 225

Alcoholic, atypical, 184–186, 191, 200, 232, 245

Alcoholics Anonymous (AA): effectiveness of, 3, 13, 254, 255–269, 357, 366, 385,

439